GREEN MEDICINES

Pharmacy of Natural Products for HIV and Five AIDS-related Infections

GREEN MEDICINES

Pharmacy of Natural Products for HIV and Five AIDS–related Infections

KAZHILA C. CHINSEMBU

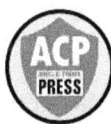

AFRICA IN CANADA PRESS
Kitchener, Ontario
2016

Green Medicines: Pharmacy of Natural Products for HIV and Five AIDS-related Infections

First Printing: 2016

ISBN-13: 978-0-9695307-5-6;   ISBN-10: 0969530757

First Published in Canada by:

AFRICA IN CANADA PRESS
25 Blue Oak Street | Kitchener, Ontario N2R 0K3, CANADA
Tel: 1-647-458-7435 | Fax: 1-416-724-5938
http://www.africaincanadapress.com

Africa in Canada Press is committed to publishing works by authors of African descent in Canada and abroad with excellence.

Ordering Information: Contact the author, Prof. Kazhila C. Chinsembu, email: kchinsembu@gmail.com; kchinsembu@unam.na; P.O. Box 30123, Pioneerspark, Windhoek, Namibia.

Special discounts are available on large quantity purchases by corporations, associations, educators, and others. For more information and orders, please contact the the author at the above listed address.

Book design by: Charles Mwewa
Cover Design: Niranjan Mohammed
                  (http://www.niranjanmohammed.com)

Intellectual, Self-improvement, Health, Medicine, Plants, Natural products
Green Medicines: Medicinal Plants, Natural Products, HIV, AIDS

16.04.01

Dedication

In loving memory of my mother,
Nelly Chikwama Chinsembu,
May Your Soul Rest in Eternal Peace
"I thank my God in all my remembrance of you,"
(Philippians 1:3)

To my wife, Grace and my daughters, Wana and Lusa,
"For with God, nothing shall be impossible,"
(Luke 1:37)

Contents

Chapter 4: Natural Products in the Management of Sexually Transmitted Infections 137

Chapter 5: Natural Products for Oral Health 171

Chapter 6: Natural Products as Anti-Tuberculosis Agents 201

Chapter 7: The World of Malaria: Antimalarial Medicines from Mother Nature 245

Acknowledgements

I thank all the institutions which directly or indirectly helped me with information, data and insights to write this book: University of Namibia, NEPAD/SANBio, CSIR in Pretoria, Ministry of Health in Zambia, Ministry of Health in Namibia, Elsevier Journals and ScienceDirect database, more especially Journal of Ethnopharmacology and all institutions and publications that served as sources of data.

I am very thankful to all the authorities and sources cited in the text and tables, especially: Afolayan et al., 2014; Lall and Kishore, 2014; Mabona and Van Vuuren, 2013; Ochwang'i et al., 2014; Martínez and Barboza, 2010; Ndubani and Höjer, 1999; De Wet and Ngubane, 2014; Naidoo et al., 2013; De Wet et al., 2012; Semenya et al., 2013; Van Vuuren and Naidoo, 2010; Ocheng et al., 2014; Bunalema et al., 2014; Tabuti et al., 2010; McGaw et al., 2008; Tsabang et al., 2012; Traore et al., 2013; Muthaura et al., 2011; Fowler, 2006; Adebayo and Krettli, 2011; Lacroix et al., 2011; and Ngarivhume et al., 2015. Even if I have not yet personally reached out to you, please accept my sincere gratitude.

I thank the following individuals for their help in one way or another: Prof. Aggrey Ambali, Prof. Keto Mshigeni, Dr. Ludwig Sondashi, Dr. John Sivah Kachimba, Prof. Charles Mwewa, Dr. Munyonzwe Hamalengwa, Mr. Zila Kaduma and Dr. Marius Hedimbi. Thank you, Lusa Chinsembu, for editing the references. All individuals who helped me during the research and writing of this book, even those I have failed to mention by name, I thank them most sincerely.

I also thank my awesome family: My wife Grace Mukumbo Chinsembu and daughters Wana Wamweni Chinsembu and Lusa Chinsembu, for all the support during the long hours I was away writing this book. I remain indebted to you. Every fibre of my body says thank you!

Foreword I

There are two fundamental reasons why we should all be excited about this book. Currently, there is no cure for HIV/AIDS. There is also a growing problem of drug resistance to current antiretroviral drugs. These, and many other reasons, point to the need for humanity to look to plants as an alternative, as an abundant, and as an appealing, yet a largely neglected resource from which we can isolate novel biochemicals to develop new and more efficacious drugs. This book is a critical turning-point in this intriguing journey. Indeed, a voyage towards innovation and drug discovery.

As HIV and AIDS wreak havoc in Africa, we need to look more inward to home-grown solutions. Our unique and affluent plant biodiversity, undoubtedly, contains potent molecules that can help us move ahead towards arresting HIV and bypass the AIDS epidemic. The aim of this book is not to create a backlash against antiretroviral therapy. On the contrary, the book speaks about the need for increased usage of medicinal plants and other natural agents as locally-affordable and long-term solutions to HIV/AIDS.

Being a Botanist, I see nothing more rewarding than witnessing the healing power of medicinal plants being brought to light, and the clinical amelioration of HIV infection and AIDS-related diseases, being promoted. For decades now, science has revealed that many plants and other bioresources contain chemicals that block HIV and inhibit pathogens of AIDS-associated diseases, such as tuberculosis, malaria, sexually transmitted infections and skin diseases. But, ironically, for some very strange reasons that continue to defy common sense (maybe common sense is no longer common), these natural anti-HIV and anti-AIDS agents have not been pursued vigorously. This book, *Green Medicines*, sheds new light in that direction, and gives new hope towards changing the current *status quo*, scenario and contradictions.

Through the exposé of empirical and scientific data, *Green Medicines* contains extraordinary and persuasive rhapsodies of acclaim for plants and other natural products that effectively work against HIV. The book is, thus, an important contribution towards building a bridge that may lead us to an AIDS-free future.

I am not new to medicinal plants. I earned my Ph.D in Botanical Sciences at the University of Hawaii (USA) in 1974, and my Bachelor of Science with a major in Botany and Geography at the University of East Africa (Dar-es-Salaam University College campus), in 1969. Subsequently, I became the first Tanzanian full Professor of Botany at the University of Dar-es-Salaam. During the 1980s, I had played a leading role in a collaborative research project on Tanzania's medicinal plants, jointly with eminent scientists from Uppsala University in Sweden. And, indeed, we generated quite a few exciting publications on the subject. In 1990, I worked closely with Tanzania's government, the Ministry of Health and Social Welfare, in organizing a very successful international conference on traditional medicinal plants in Africa. This conference was held in Arusha, Tanzania. Subsequently, I served as editor-in-chief when we published the Conference Proceedings. I am currently Vice-president of the International Medicinal Mushrooms Association.

Given my scientific background and career, I read the substance contained in this new book with great rapture. You will find the wealth of information on nature's pharmacy of natural products for HIV and AIDS-related infections intriguing and wonderful reading. I can say so with confidence, having served as editor-in-chief of the Journal of Discovery and Innovation, a joint peer-reviewed publication of the African Academy of Sciences (AAS), and the World Academy of Sciences (TWAS), for almost two decades.

Recalling my earlier involvements with medicinal plants during my tenure as Vice-chairperson of the Tanzania Commission for Science and Technology, and also formerly as Chair of the Commission's Biotechnology Committee, I am delighted to see that at long last, African academics are stepping up efforts to contribute to the global share of knowledge. Yes, Africa is rising.

Also importantly, as founding Pro-vice Chancellor for Academic Affairs and Research at the University of Namibia (UNAM), and also as an external member of the Council of UNAM, I am very pleased and proud to note that the author of *Green Medicines* is an Associate Professor of UNAM. Professor Kazhila C. Chinsembu has worked on medicinal plants for HIV/AIDS for many years now. He has published many scientific papers on this subject. His latest paper, "Ethnomedicinal plants used by traditional healers in the management of HIV/AIDS opportunistic diseases in Rundu, Kavango East Region, Namibia", published by the South African Journal of Botany, is an enlightening and eye-opening study.

Let me now conclude this Foreword with a word of commendation to Professor Chinsembu for writing this landmark book, *Green Medicines*. I urge you to take time to read the book and to internalize its contents.

Professor Keto E. Mshigeni, PhD

Professor of Botany and Vice Chancellor, Hubert Kairuki Memorial University, Dar es Salaam, Tanzania; Winner of the Association of African Universities (AAU) Higher Education and Research Excellence Award in Africa; Winner of the African Academy of Sciences (AAS)/CIBA Prize for Agricultural Biosciences in Africa; Africa Winner of the Boutros Boutros Ghali Prize; TWAS Medal Recipient in Recognition of Excellence in Scientific Research and Development, World Academy of Sciences (TWAS); TWAS Vice President Representing the Africa Region; and Member of the Pan African University Council.

Foreword II

This study is concerned with the use of natural products to treat HIV and other AIDS related infections. I have known Professor Kazhila C. Chinsembu for some time now. He is a very hardworking scientist who has spent most of his time researching on natural products as a source of treatment, particularly to the HIV pandemic.

As for me, a person who founded the *SF2000*, a natural product which has proved to be a treatment and cure of HIV and AIDS, I can confirm that scientific findings on the *SF2000* have shown that the formula can inhibit HIV and AIDS-related microbes.

In the observational clinical trials which took place in 2006, the studies showed that out of ten patients given to me, six improved their status in viral load and CD4 count. This was a new milestone unknown in the history of herbal remedies.

The fact that herbal remedies can be used to treat this disease has led to further investigations of *SF2000*. A second clinical trial was conducted in Zambia for the sole purpose of ensuring safety for patients. My work as well as this one by Professor Chinsembu, confirm that herbal remedies work.

I, therefore, recommend this treatise by Professor Chinsembu and that leaders would find it revolutionary and a breakthrough.

Dr. Ludwig S. Sondashi, PhD
Inventor of the *Sondashi Formula, SF2000*
Herbal medication for HIV/AIDS
Lusaka, Zambia.

Foreword III

In Africa, herbal medicines are utilized as primary treatment for most ailments, including HIV/AIDS and HIV-related problems. Many patients take advantage of the vast array of natural products that have been in our traditional realm for millennia to treat the primary HIV infection, or when on conventional antiretroviral therapy, to manage HIV-related problems such as dermatological diseases, gastrointestinal complications, general malaise and many other symptoms that arise in patients with HIV/AIDS. Evidence suggests that the use of natural products is widespread, efficacious and will certainly continue among African communities. Many patients seem to draw significant benefits from the use of these products. It is certainly fair to say that some products have therapeutic benefits in this condition. There are significant examples of natural products that, historically, have been effective in antimalarial and anticancer treatments. These are now mainstream conventional therapies. There is no reason why a natural product cannot be the next major treatment for HIV infection.

In writing this remarkable book, *Green Medicines: Pharmacy of Natural Products for HIV and Five AIDS-related infections*, Professor Chinsembu has responded to the fascinating challenge of bringing a complex subject within the understanding of the general public, while appealing to the scientific curiosity of the medical fraternity. Grappling with natural therapies and medicines requires skills in both biomedical sciences and social sciences in a way that lifts the shroud off an intricate and mysterious art of natural treatments (usually traditional), which may hold great potential, but remain poorly researched and documented. This book tackles this challenge heads-on and in a more multifaceted way by providing clinical and laboratory evidence about some treatments that make use of natural products in the treatment of primary HIV/AIDS and AIDS-related infections. It is an interesting, useful and lifestyle changing book in that regard.

The author, a distinguished professor and researcher, presents a detailed treatise with a huge body of evidence to explain the mechanisms of action for natural products, their interactions with conventional antiretroviral treatment and the benefits that mainstream health professionals may take advantage of as they treat their patients. This is a biomedical book which will be a resource to a wide variety of people, from wellness consultants dealing with issues of lifestyle management, to healthcare professionals in clinical practice and yet it is profoundly different as the general reader will find it engaging and educative. The promise is that once you have read this book you will gain a new knowledge of a vast and interesting branch of science with a new vision for the rest of your life, whether you are a healthcare practitioner or a layperson.

After decades of research, major progress has been made in the quest for natural products with potent anti-HIV activity. The number of natural products recognized to date is staggering, and the author proceeds to present the extensive literature that has been documented on these natural products and their beneficial effects toward health and well-being, disease prevention, and disease treatment. What the reader will glean from the opening two chapters is the wide range of potential anti-HIV remedies in nature. It is fascinating that as one reads these opening chapters, one is introduced to the immense benefits that can be gained from relatively mundane habits such as drinking a cup of green tea, taking a portion of ginseng or extracts of a multitude of exotically named plants that occur naturally throughout the Sub-Saharan African region.

The chapters on skin diseases and STIs bring out two distinctly contrasting scenarios with regard to the use of natural products in mainstream medicine. The use of natural skin care products has been widely accepted and aggressively marketed. It is now accepted that for the treatment of skin diseases and the maintenance of skin beauty, nature's products are the best. In stark contrast, the treatment of STIs using natural products is totally frowned upon and any attempt to suggest their use draws negative responses from the medical fraternity. The author presents hundreds of natural products that have proven efficacy in the treatment of STIs, but laments the failure to capitalise on these potential treatments. This is a recurring motif when one reads through this book; natural treatments hold huge potential to be a source of active molecules to treat HIV/AIDS and its related infections. Natural products are not the figments of someone's imagination nor are they myths conjured up by traditional healers, but chemical ingredients that hold practicable and applicable use if investigated and applied scientifically.

The treatment of oral diseases, covered in Chapter 5, highlights a number of key issues that will be of great interest to the reader. Firstly, there is considerable evidence linking poor oral health to chronic conditions, such as HIV/AIDS and diabetes and the incidence of severe oral diseases is increasing. In most Sub-Saharan African countries, the provision of oral health care is virtually non-existent and large populations of dentally disadvantaged individuals exist in our countries. Sadly, these populations are frequently child populations and the poor. The author rightly points out the global need for alternative prevention and treatment options and products for oral diseases that are safe, effective and economical. These alternative treatments, using natural products, will address the rise in oral disease incidence, the opportunistic oral infections in immunocompromised individuals and financial considerations in developing countries that make dental care difficult to provide. The second significant point addressed in this chapter, and is a recurring theme throughout this book, is that there is a long history among rural and traditional societies in Africa of the use of traditional plants and natural products for the treatment of oral diseases. This is evidenced by the lower rates of oral diseases among rural populations that use these natural products to maintain oral hygiene. Many plant-derived medicines used in traditional medicinal systems have been recorded in pharmacopoeias and these are presented in detail. What will be of great interest to the reader is the range of traditional medicinal plant extracts or phytochemicals that have been shown to inhibit the growth of oral pathogens, reduce the development of dental plaque, inhibit the adhesion of bacteria to surfaces and reduce the symptoms of oral diseases. These natural products are presented with the clinical evidence to support their safety and efficacy.

In Chapter 6, Professor Chinsembu explores the role of natural products as a continuing source of novel drugs for tuberculosis. There continues to be tremendous research all over the world in the search for new anti-tuberculosis agents. It is surprising that despite the large number of potential agents in nature, none of the currently used first or second line drugs in the chemotherapy of tuberculosis has been derived from natural products. This chapter presents several reports of anti-tuberculosis activity discovered in many plants belonging to different families and genera. It is interesting to note that the plants with antimycobacterial activities have for centuries been used in traditional societies for the treatment of tuberculosis or related symptoms such as cough and other respiratory diseases. In what is certainly a rallying call to all researchers, especially in the Sub-Saharan region, the author stresses that these natural products are a fertile ground for research in newer drugs and they can also serve as useful templates for the discovery of novel anti-tuberculosis drugs.

The final chapter addresses the role of natural products in the treatment of malaria, a disease that has plagued humankind since early times and a disease whose major treatment has remained quinine – a derivative from a natural product. As a constituent alkaloid derived from the *Cinchona* plants that are well known for their antimalarial properties, quinine exemplifies the immense benefits that can be derived from natural products. This chapter explores numerous natural treatments such as *Artemisia annua* and its active compound, artemisinin, the Chinese traditional treatment of malaria that currently holds considerable promise. With rising resistance to present antimalarial drugs, there is a pressing necessity for the development of new remedies to treat malaria. Research into plants used traditionally for the treatment of malaria by ancient communities is an obvious way to explore the vast experience in the use of medicinal plants and the knowledge in these communities.

After reading through this remarkable book, two salient points are evident. First, it is accepted that the use of traditional medicine and natural products is widespread among those living with HIV infection and not even the hardened sceptic could question the value that patients draw from their use. And second, natural products have been of immense value to the pharmaceutical industry, especially in the areas of infectious diseases and oncology, where numerous natural products and synthetically modified natural product derivatives have been successfully developed for clinical use. The challenge confronting healthcare professionals and researchers in Sub-Saharan Africa, and the world at large, is to learn how best to utilize and apply the vast knowledge of natural products literally lying in our backyard. *Green Medicines: Pharmacy of Natural Products for HIV and Five AIDS-related infections* offers a remarkable look at the immense possibilities for medicine and the benefits that our patients may derive if we were to harness the healing potential of natural products.

Professor Chinsembu has written a powerful, deeply intelligent, thought–provoking and urgently needed book for our present times. My sincere hope is that we take heed of the message of hope and promise that this seminal book has presented and take up the challenge to explore the bounty that nature has to offer in our fight against disease. Natural products may not cure all our illnesses, but investigating them, evaluating their efficacy and opening up their full potential to mainstream healthcare will give society one of its greatest tools in the fight against HIV/AIDS and other diseases. I am certain that this book will stimulate debate, encourage research and ultimately change lives for the better.

Dr. John Sivah Kachimba,
Consultant Urologist, Levy Mwanawasa General Hospital, Lusaka, Zambia; Editor-in-Chief, Medical Journal of Zambia; and Board Member, National Science and Technology Council of Zambia

Preface

All over the world people are now spending more resources - effort, money, time and biomedical products - on increasing their personal health. In this age of increased health awareness, juxtaposed with healthy lifestyles and driven by an insatiable appetite for organic products, natural remedies are the new normal, the mainstay of this new health paradigm.

More than 50,000 flowering plants are used for medicinal purposes across the world. Change towards healthy regimes has rekindled a new anticipation and belief in the power of natural products to prevent and treat human diseases. Understandably, for people living with HIV/AIDS, natural remedies build a protective fortress around the body, a fortress that keeps opportunistic infections at arm's length.

The use of therapeutic natural products continues to take the human body away from the precipice of disease. Ever since antibiotics and antiretroviral drugs began to flounder, public attention has re-shifted to the use of natural products. In the world of drug discovery and HIV/AIDS, natural products now provide a real sense of expectation for something new.

Over the past several years, the use of natural products has shown irrevocable commitment to improving human health. Scientific evidence in this book is unequivocal and explicit that the use of anti-HIV natural products has now crossed the Rubicon. Natural products are now within striking distance of bringing down the curtain on HIV and AIDS-related diseases.

Still, in the management of HIV/AIDS, natural products have been misunderstood by patients, medical doctors and the general public. However, as natural remedies continue to make a dramatic comeback, it is important to know which natural products, specifically, work against HIV/AIDS.

The aim of this book is to demystify the use of natural remedies, to bring to the fore hard scientific data that speak to the antimicrobial and pharmacological efficacy and safety of natural products that inhibit HIV and AIDS-related infections such as skin, sexually transmitted, oral infections, tuberculosis and malaria.

Of course, natural products are not a silver-bullet solution to the HIV/AIDS epidemic. Medicinal plants are not a replacement for antiretroviral therapy, but they do increase the options available to AIDS patients, especially those faced by side-effects due to antiretroviral drugs, HIV resistance and treatment failure. Thus, natural remedies no longer belong to the Dark Ages.

In fact, the use of plants and other natural products presents a brighter spot in the match to knowable therapies for emerging as well as old diseases. Phytotherapy, especially the application of African medicinal plants, may soon cause a quantum leap in the discovery of novel medications that will rein in stubborn and drug-resistant microbial infections such as HIV/AIDS.

There is now a new yearning to mainstream the use of natural products in the management of HIV and AIDS-related infections. HIV/AIDS policy, especially in resource-limited settings, will become more caring and effective by shifting towards the integration of natural remedies.

As therapeutic plant products continue to cut loose the impacts and shackles of HIV, the anti-AIDS benefits of natural products become more and more visible and invaluable. In the fight against AIDS, natural products are, in all honesty, a game-changer - the new frontier where we can all dream about the novel medicines of tomorrow.

In this book, over 1,500 studies do submit with gusto a corpus of overwhelming empirical evidence in support of natural products - plants, fungi and algae - that purge HIV infection and AIDS-related diseases. The case for natural products as anti-HIV/AIDS agents is now beyond conjecture.

The data for anti-HIV and anti-AIDS natural products are no longer anecdotal and circumspect. Suffice to state that the experimental data in this book do point to one epic biomedical reality, that is, the hope of using natural products - our priceless heritage - to combat HIV/AIDS is clearly tenable.

For those who think natural products are dangerous and should be banned, this book has bad news for them because it offers experimental evidence that will compel a rethink of their positions. There is need to deconstruct the role of medicinal plants. This book represents what is best about plants: The power to heal the nations. The point really is that the burden of proof is no longer on the antimicrobial efficacy and safety of natural products. Consistent with experimental data, the key idea in this book is that natural products urgently deserve a proportionate inclusion into the arsenal of pharmaceutical and biomedical interventions against HIV/AIDS.

The example of Chinese medicine which embraces natural remedies and provides a distinct window of dispensary, is instructive of the new reality that anti-HIV natural products are a critical building block in the battle against AIDS. We have enough time to reconsider the importance of medicinal plants and get them on board of customized and generic interventions for HIV/AIDS.

Even in their raw form, natural products are not only essential in preventing and managing HIV/AIDS, they are also a *sine quo non* in the bioprospecting and discovery of novel drugs for HIV infection and AIDS-related diseases. This is not medical utopia; this is not a quest for relevance of plant remedies.

Going forward, the unequivocal anti-HIV and anti-AIDS evidence presented in this book will provide a fresh quest to look at the critics of natural products in the eye, telling them that the world has an incorrect view about the efficacy and safety of natural products. In the fight against HIV and AIDS-related infections, this work emphasizes the need to turn to the healing power of natural products.

Like Rachel Carson's *Silent Spring*, this book inspires not a special interest but a popular lens and culture through which to view and utilize plants and other natural materials as agents for managing HIV and AIDS opportunistic infections. Through scientific evidence and rationalization of the use of plant preparations in the management of these diseases, the book goes beyond marketplace knowledge and understanding of herbal products.

Stated differently, this book is invaluable in that it brings an utterly new perspective to help change the misplaced view that undermines the use of natural remedies in the management of HIV/AIDS. Looking ahead, antimicrobial evidence in this book will provide a vantage point for natural products to gain traction in medicine. Thus, hopefully, natural products will become the new window of dispensary in the management of HIV and AIDS-related infections.

Pause and think for a moment. We are living in unprecedented times. Each year, there are millions and millions of drug resistant microbial infections. In the USA alone, 2 million bacterial infections are resistant to drugs each year. These resistant infections are caused by drug-resistant super bugs; methicillin-resistant *Staphylococcus aureus* (MRSA) is one such hard-to-treat infection.

We are running out of options. One way to stay ahead of drug resistant microbes is to return to Mother Nature, to 'pharm' and use natural products that possess chemical ingredients that the microbes have never seen before. Bioprospecting for new natural products will reveal potential novel antimicrobial molecules with different mechanisms of action. This will help bring new drugs that may even overcome drug-resistant super bugs.

Here is one critical question to consider: Are herbal medicines really useful in the management of HIV/AIDS? Yes and no. Mostly "yes" because much of the available evidence demonstrates that plants contain plenty of useful anti-HIV and antimicrobial agents that inhibit AIDS-related infections like skin, sexually transmitted, oral infections, tuberculosis and malaria. But "no" in the sense that plants may also possess poisonous substances, chemical compounds that may be cytotoxic to the body, and active chemical ingredients that may be anti-synergistic with mainstream HIV/AIDS medications.

Undoubtedly, there are good and bad natural products. In the management of HIV/AIDS, use of the good products should be credited and encouraged, and that of bad products should be shunned and frowned upon. But separating the bad from the good natural products is not easy because there has been no in-depth discernment of the pharmacological and toxicological properties of plants and other natural products.

We, therefore, need an honest assessment of all natural products, on a case-by-case basis, because every natural remedy has its own unique pharmacological and toxicological properties. While care and caution should be taken in the selection and use of natural products; in this book, there are inescapable and amazing scientific data of natural agents that steel and fortify the body against HIV/AIDS, especially before one embarks on antiretroviral therapy.

With respect to the management of HIV, this book firms up the due credit we should give to the use of the many good natural products that are very efficacious and non-toxic. Just as we must never throw away the baby with the bath water, we should also not throw away the effective and non-toxic natural products together with those that are ineffective and toxic.

We are fortunate that the tools of modern science now more than ever before do help us to discern and separate the good natural products from the bad ones. But, as others have warned before, we should remember that Mother Nature has had three billion years to refine her chemistry, yet we are only now scratching the surface in exploring Nature's molecular diversity.

All in all, this book is an empirical advocacy for and about the good natural products that possess repertoires of chemical compounds for fighting HIV infection and AIDS-related diseases. Use of this pharmacy of natural products puts HIV infection on the back foot. It de-escalates progression to AIDS. The bottom line is that this book is all about staying the course.

The trove of antimicrobial data in this treatise epitomizes a unique vantage point, a long-range lens through which to view the power of natural products to alleviate HIV/AIDS-related conditions. Therefore, this study is a significant push to the tipping point in the use of natural products to manage HIV and AIDS conditions.

It is argued that with respect to HIV infection and AIDS-related conditions, medicinal natural products, much like synthetic antiretroviral drugs, can bolster and augment patient management and, in the not-so-distant future, may become a co-equal narrative of healthcare.

This book offers a competent basis and platform for a re-evaluation of our notions about natural medicines for the management of HIV/AIDS. Especially now that HIV infection is a chronic ailment, much like high blood pressure, bonding with and increasing the use of effective natural products will promote a pro-healthy orientation towards living with the virus.

Studies in this book show consistent support that leveraging the use of medicinal plants during HIV infection improves the body's health status by circumventing attack from malaria, TB, oral diseases, skin diseases and STIs. The more the use of natural products, the less vulnerable to opportunistic infections, and the slower will be the progression to AIDS. Natural products fence off the body from opportunistic diseases.

Here is the best case example. A man was diagnosed with HIV infection in Lusaka, Zambia. His CD4 count dwindled to 190. His viral load climbed to 90,000. Despite that, he never had flu, cough, TB, and serious opportunistic diseases characteristic of AIDS. He was not yet on antiretroviral therapy. What was his secret weapon to keeping health? He drank green tea every day. Drinking green tea has multiple benefits which kept him healthy.

Impressively, our use of natural products is determined to meme itself into a signature footprint that will characterize humanity's evolutionary path to more innovative organic medicines and a healthier future.

Since time immemorial, medicinal natural products have given animal and human bodies the steely ability and indomitable capacity to overcome disease. The chemistry of human physical wellbeing has co-evolved with the chemistry of medicinal plants. In both animals and plants, Darwinian evolution has selected for chemical ingredients that are useful in body defences against natural enemies such as predators and disease-causing pathogens.

This book cannot be appreciated in isolation. It is part of our humanity's medical history to use plants to fend off disease. Knowledge of medicinal natural products is our priceless endowment. It is part of our cultural and genetic blueprints for healthier selves. It is part of our DNA.

Use of medicinal plants embodies the very basic instinct of human survival. In the provision of broader, safer, cheaper and more effective healthcare, the use of medicinal plants still shakes up the *status quo*. It expands the imaginations, options and boundaries of healthcare provision.

Humans and other animals depend on oxygen produced by plants through photosynthesis. Without this oxygen from green plants, there would be no human and animal life on earth. In the same way, human and animal health depends on natural medications from green plants. Our health is dependent on green medicines, healing chemicals found in green plants. We depend on the power of green medicines from green plants to cure many diseases. Without plants, we can wake up dead!

Introduction

We cannot ignore the achievements of the pharmaceutical drug manufacturing industry and the advances of modern-day medicine. However, the proliferation of drug-resistant microbes makes patients appreciate the power of natural products. Thus, over 55% of synthetic drugs are derived from natural products.

It is a hyperbole, a mistake, to expect that all plants and natural products of all hues are safe to use as medicines even if they are advertised by persuasive marketers. In fact, some plant products are very dangerous and can kill better and faster than synthetic poisons.

In today's world of pharmaceutical drugs, humanity has a complicated relationship with natural products. For HIV/AIDS, the human-herbal relationship is even more complicated now in this era of antiretroviral therapy than at any other time. As flattering as these natural products may seem, their medicinal efficacies are incredible and credible enough to pull humankind out of the mire of HIV/AIDS. The best is yet to come.

This is not the first work on natural products. However, this book will draw the curiosity of the global community to Mother Nature's little-known anti-HIV and anti-AIDS medicinal agents. Putting it succinctly, the natural medicinal agents in this book will become the staple for those that live with HIV infection and those that suffer from AIDS complications.

The use of natural products is not a journey to return humankind to the Dark Ages. It is not *juju*. The shift to natural products is a global recognition of humanity's age-old medicobotanical knowledge, most of this knowledge is now disappearing due to menacing environmental degradation, pollution and mortality of older folks - the adept storytellers and repositories of this tacit know-how.

A West African adage says: "When an old person dies, a library of knowledge burns to the ground."
Despite its huge potentials, modern-day humans have not yet grasped and revered the universality and the curative powers of medicinal agents from Mother Nature. This book helps change that perception as it brings to the fore scientific data about medicinal properties of natural products.

Human ignorance and inertia can no longer defer the promise of green medicines and other natural products to combat HIV and AIDS-related infections. At the minimum, evolution designed and built green medicines and natural products for combating HIV and AIDS-related infections. In its tactical plan, the balance of Mother Nature has this intrinsic ability to put down, disinfect, and clean up the human body of stubborn infectious agents like HIV and its attendant opportunistic microbial infections.

In the longer term, natural products that possess medicinal functions would ensure the human body can successfully compete and remarkably survive in a world full of deadly germs. Natural products are the original frontier for containing human infections.

By continuously taking in medicinal natural agents, the body systemically becomes hardwired to disinfect itself and thwart HIV and AIDS-related infections. Over a much longer evolutionary time course, anti-infective chemical agents in nature's pharmacy may completely attenuate the lethality of HIV.

Use of natural remedies, therefore, comes with real perks for HIV/AIDS. Unfortunately, in this thriving era of antiretroviral therapy - never mind its myriad challenges - administration of natural products for managing HIV/AIDS is an awfully endangered practice, often downplayed and overly criticized as dumb or mediocre.

On 25 March 2015, Bill Gates said, "The world needs to arm itself for a different war - a war against germs." We cannot win this war, especially the war against drug-resistant microbes, or the fight against HIV/AIDS, without sustainably utilizing the wealth of chemical ingredients imbued in plants and other natural products.

As an African, a Zambian, I feel inclined to urge our African governments and entrepreneurs to invest resources in the discovery of better drugs from our priceless heritage of medicinal plants, to defeat HIV and AIDS-related diseases.

Health economists tell us that diseases hamper our productivity. Preventing and treating diseases increase crop yields and household incomes. Stated differently, the use of medicinal plants is a great economic stimulus. It can conquer diseases and increase food security and boost revenues.

Medicinal plants can also be converted into pharmaceutical drugs, creating high earning jobs in manufacturing, innovation and industrialization. This is the way to go, the way of the knowledge economy, the green economy, and green health sustained by green medicines.

Granted, screening of plants for pharmacological activity and characterization of their anti-HIV active chemical compounds is expensive. But the risk is worth the reward. African institutions such as the African Development Bank and the Common Market for Eastern and Southern Africa (COMESA) should lead the pack of other investors including banks to promote start-ups and value-addition of green medicines from plants and other natural products. Even Aliko Dangote and Tony Elumelu should invest in the production of novel drugs, especially for HIV/AIDS, from Africa's wealth of medicinal plants.

Green medicines and medicinal natural products are low hanging fruits already ripe for harvest and yawning to be harnessed into Africa's new money spinner– biotechnology and phytotrade.

The African continent should move from bioprospecting to R&D and quickly bring novel anti-HIV phytochemical products to the market. Western countries cannot invest in this kind of work because it threatens the market niche of synthetic pharmaceutical drugs manufactured by their multinational companies.

As Kenyan President, Uhuru Kenyatta, said, "Africa should get its own solutions to keep its people healthy." Evidently, many of these 'own' solutions and domestic resources include our abundant green medicines to treat HIV and AIDS-related infections.

On 23 September 2014, writing on his Facebook page, President Uhuru Kenyatta said: "I attended the Africa Rising Forum at the Africa Centre in New York where I was the chief guest and a panelist. I called on the people of Africa to liberate their thinking to harness the enormous resources on the continent." Kenyatta would not have been more apt, because, if Africans liberate their thinking, they would harness the abundant wealth of anti-HIV natural products into novel antiretroviral drugs for HIV/AIDS.

Again, I concur with the Kenyan President who, at a high-level meeting on Health Financing, United Nations Headquarters, New York, on 22 September 2014, said that: "Africa is rising economically but the fruits of this transformation will only be sweet if proper investments are channelled towards health. Africa should get its own solutions to keep its people healthy. We have always depended on external help for health services but we have to mobilise domestic resources to find our own solutions instead of moving from one crisis to another."

Unfortunately, through biopiracy, Africa is fast losing her heritage of anti-HIV plants and other natural products to other continents. This is shocking, to say the least. Hopefully, data provided in this book will help unlock Africa's potential to harness her repertoire of anti-HIV natural products.

In retrospect, the presence of this wealth of anti-HIV molecules in natural products perhaps points to a recurring theme in the evolution of parasites, that is, the evolution of HIV would not have been designed to completely wipe out all the human hosts. Mother Nature ubiquitously provides correctives to HIV in most of the natural products around us - in the plant foods we eat, in the drinks, in organisms at the bottom of the oceans, in rivers and on land. Indeed, nature knows no bottom.

The current generation of humans is too greedy, too complacent, or too incompetent to harness the available pharmacy of natural products - our common heritage - to clamber out of this biomedical and social quagmire called AIDS. It is shocking that this generation of humans is so busy with cellphones that it continues to neglect this natural pharmacy of products that holds the answer to the question of HIV/AIDS. We often forget that we shall

3

never use cell-phones once we are dead. Anti-HIV natural products represent the future of antiretroviral therapy.

Plants and other natural products are the reason we should all be optimistic about finding better and safer treatments for HIV/AIDS in the future. After reading this book, you will find nine important reasons why this book is special, for it helps to:

1. Unlock new opportunities for entrepreneurship, innovation, local pharmaceutical manufacturing and income generation;
2. Improve alternatives and options for healthcare, even usher in diverse and novel molecules to conquer drug-resistant super-bugs;
3. Signify the importance of conserving forests and natural resources so as to continue harvesting products that improve health and incomes;
4. Reduce poverty and diseases;
5. Encourage more research, bioprospecting and scientific validation of natural products;
6. Spur the introduction of new curricula, courses and training in medicinal natural products including indigenous knowledge systems;
7. Provide local content and reading material in the form of a book showcasing local and global natural products with medicinal properties;
8. Inspire a new hope to look to our immediate surroundings (Mother Nature's own pharmacy), not just foreign synthetic drugs, to combat diseases; and
9. Show that while ARVs are incredibly important in our fight of HIV/AIDS, the power to defeat HIV infection and AIDS is not far away, it is intrinsically linked to nature and its sustainable stewardship at personal and community levels.

This book also fits into the Science, Technology and Innovation Strategy for Africa (STISA) - a policy document adopted in June 2014 by the African Union (AU) - to address the critical socioeconomical priority areas of disease prevention and control.

The following is the summary of each chapter in this book:

Chapter 1: HIV/AIDS, Antiretroviral Therapy and Natural Products

Antiretroviral therapy has greatly improved the health of people living with HIV infection. There is no denying this fact. There is no replacement for synthetic antiretroviral drugs, because they're immensely important.
In spite of that fact, the challenges to antiretroviral therapy will always remain. In many resource-limited settings, these drugs are not always present. Stigma still prevents people from accessing medicines from the hospitals. Many HIV-infected persons are also unaware of their seropositive status, and cannot, therefore, access antiretroviral drugs. Testing for HIV is not widespread, and even if it was widely accessible, HIV testing is not mandatory by law, in many settings.

Physiological challenges also remain, including the immune reconstitution syndrome, resistance to antiretroviral therapy and adverse reactions in certain individuals. In Africa, resistance to antiretroviral therapy is growing, well over 6%. This means that antiretroviral therapy is ineffective in persons where the virus is now resistant. So, such individuals must find alternative therapy, usually green medicines from nature's pharmacy.

Long distances to hospitals, long queues, long waiting hours, unhelpful public health workers with 'rotten' attitudes and drug shortages all force patients to abandon antiretroviral therapy, or reduce adherence to medications.

In short, some patients begin to see plants and other natural products as a viable window of dispensary. They use green medicines to reduce HIV viral loads and manage opportunistic infections like malaria, TB, oral diseases, STIs and skin diseases.

Given the strong belief in the use of plants to heal diseases, especially in rural areas, many people can never do away with green medicines.

But this book is not an excuse for the use of plants. This book is about why plants are sometimes equal and even more powerful than synthetic drugs in preventing and managing HIV and AIDS-related infections. Plants are blessed with chemical agents, green medicines that cure infections.

Of course, administration of green medicines is not well regulated. Charlatan traditional healers are plenty, cheating desperate patients. Poisonous plants also exist - they kill - and some plant products reduce the efficacy of antiretroviral drugs.

Still, the good side of plants cannot be overemphasized, as many synthetic drugs are made from or designed after plant chemicals. Consider the birds of the air. Whenever they are ill, they do not fly to hospitals to get treatment. Their health depends on natural remedies. Even before the 1928 discovery of penicillin, the first true antibiotic, by Alexander Fleming, Profes-

5

sor of Bacteriology at St. Mary's Hospital in London, humans were already using curative green medicines.

For thousands of years, human survival has been and will still be inextricably linked to the green side of plants. Now that HIV infection is a chronic condition, the use of plants to boost immunity, to lower viral loads and keep the body from progressing to AIDS will continue to become very important.

The data presented in this book make for a compelling case to debunk the myths associated with the healing abilities of plant remedies. Any Doubting Thomas of medicinal agents of plants, green medicines, should surely read this book. It is written for them!

Many medical doctors, pharmacists and nurses at public and private hospitals have been the hardest critics of the medicinal powers of plants. They pour scorn on and scoff at natural remedies. This attitude is wrong, it is unreasonable, and lacks the merits of experimental evidence as most plant products clearly have very beneficial ingredients to heal the body.

Yes, there are challenges with traditional medicines and medicinal plant products, as in many systems of Western conventional medicines. In this regard, we need to quickly understand the correct dosages, the routes of administration, the bioavailability, and the cytotoxicity of green medicines in the body. But cases of over-dosing and under-dosing are not only restricted to the use of medicinal plants. Even the use of pharmaceutical drugs finds itself with the same dilemma.

Scientists should, therefore, conduct more research in the field of posology, in order to better understand the correct dosages for safely administering medicinal plant remedies. Cellular safety, bioavailability, pharmacokinetics, cytotoxic effects, genotoxicity and mutagenicity of green medicines should also be checked in lab assays and in *vivo*.

Chapter 2: Anti-HIV Natural Products

This chapter details plants and other natural products that inhibit HIV replication. What this means is that green medicines lower HIV viral loads. Chemical agents in green tea, red wine, marijuana, ginseng, mangroves, pine cones and *Daphne* species, contain various chemical compounds that stop HIV replication. This chapter presents experimental data of plants in many countries and many habitats that contain anti-HIV chemical agents.

Again, products in this chapter are not a replacement for ARVs. Moreover, these products do safeguard the health of people who are not yet on antiretroviral therapy. A normal habit of drinking green tea can lower the load of HIV and delay the deterioration of the immune system. ARVs are being given when CD4 counts ebb to 500. Taking green agents enumerated in this chapter can keep the CD4 levels well above 500 for a much longer time.

Anti-HIV natural medicines in Botswana, China, Thailand, Indonesia, Malaysia, Ethiopia, South Africa and Namibia are detailed in this chapter. Also, many natural agents in this chapter inhibit HIV entry, reverse transcriptase, protease, integrase, syncytium formation and the killing of human body cells by HIV.

Although some natural medicinal agents reduce HIV by 20-30%, their cumulative protective effects cannot be overemphasized. In many cases, medicinal products of green plants are the reasons why most people are still looking very healthy, even if they are infected with HIV.

Humans have a lot to learn from their close relatives, the monkeys, which despite being infected with simian immunodeficiency virus (SIV) never develop AIDS. The secret is closely guarded in what monkeys eat, medicinal plants found in Mother Nature.

Chapter 3: Pharmacopoeia of Natural Remedies for Skin Diseases

The health of the outer skin is a reflection of the health of the inner self, especially the gut. Microbial interactions in the gastrointestinal tract do influence the health of the outer skin. It follows, therefore, that many plant products that stop microbial infections in the gut enhance the good health of the skin.

During HIV infection, skin diseases proliferate. They get worse as immunity deteriorates and their management becomes difficult as the body moves to AIDS. Microbial skin diseases overtly and visibly signal a person's progression to AIDS; they are very difficult to conceal. Even zits can invite AIDS stigma.

Green medicines for skin infections work by inhibiting microbial infections. Others reduce skin oxidation by removing free radicals. And some natural products act as anti-inflammatory agents, blocking body chemicals that cause rashes and swellings of the skin. Natural products, therefore, work by counteracting skin oxidation, inflammation and microbial infections.

But to say that the products detailed in this chapter are only useful for persons with HIV would be erroneous. Maladies of the skin do occur in everybody, they are ubiquitous, with oxidation occurring more frequently in persons exposed to the sun, inflammation and infections also becoming prevalent in conditions thriving with germs. This is the reason why many faiths like Christianity and Islam have attached significance to skin diseases.

Skin diseases are also linked to loss of beauty. It is against this backdrop that many skin care products contain natural products. Skin care is a booming commercial industry, much more responsive to the functions of beauty than disease.

Most women already use skin care products containing aloe, tea, avocado, jojoba, marula, cocoa, and etc. Through this chapter, they will discover the medicinal values of these natural products. Plant species that heal microbial infections ranging from eczema to herpes zoster and other skin conditions like cancer are described.

What is clear in this chapter is this: There is overwhelming experimental evidence that natural products improve skin health because they are powerful antimicrobial agents, strong antioxidants and potent chemical messengers against inflammation. Common natural products that improve skin care and health are described, and the chapter explains exactly what ingredients they contain that make them function the way they do, on the skin. Natural products for the skin in several countries are presented as well.

African skin health products in Botswana, Ethiopia, Kenya, Namibia, South Africa, Rwanda and Zambia are detailed in this chapter. From Asia - Indian, Pakistani, Filipino and Chinese natural products that restore skin health - are covered in this chapter. And so are natural products from Russia. The fact that skin diseases are the biggest problem during a person's active life, including during HIV infection, is surely reflected in the sheer size of this chapter; it is massive.

Chapter 4: Natural Products in the Management of Sexually Transmitted Infections

Since 1996, the author has been working in the field of STIs, starting at Clinic 3 at the University Teaching Hospital (UTH) in Lusaka, Zambia where he worked with the late Dr. Patrick Matondo, a consultant dermatologist. In their book, *Sexually Transmitted Diseases: Text and Atlas*, they clearly illustrate, with photographs, how common STIs become very aggressive in persons with HIV/AIDS.

In this chapter, the author feels much more at home as synergies between HIV infection and classical STIs are really beyond speculation. During HIV infection, frequency and severity of STIs increase. Gonorrhoea, chancroid and syphilis, as well as genital warts, genital herpes, candidiasis and trichomoniasis all become very common opportunistic infections in persons with HIV/AIDS. Conventional STIs are, undoubtedly, linked to HIV infection.

Over the years, treatment of STIs at hospitals has been stonewalled by increasing resistance of pathogens to drugs. STIs also attract a lot of AIDS-related stigma, making patients shy away from seeking care at public health facilities. For such patients in hiding, their only hope is the use of green medicines from traditional healers whom they consult in the darkness of the night.

At the beginning, the chapter provides 52 medicinal plants for treating STIs in Sesheke, Western Province, Zambia. This new case study is accompanied by an earlier study of 19 ethnomedicinal plants for treating STIs in Chia-wa, south-east of Lusaka, Zambia. Even stubborn STIs like *bola-bola* are treated using plant remedies.

Elsewhere, many plants used to manage STIs have been documented. Plants in Bangladesh, Botswana, Cameroon, Kenya, Madagascar, Namibia, Nigeria, South Africa, Uganda and Zimbabwe are described in this chapter. In tantalising detail, the chapter describes plant remedies for gonorrhoea, syphilis, genital warts, genital herpes, and chancroid and candida infections. The chapter also describes plant remedies for *Trichomonas vaginalis* and *Gardnerella vaginalis*. Even more exciting is the fact that STIs resistant to synthetic drugs at hospitals are now amenable to green medicines from plants. Commercialization of these medicinal plant products is urgently needed.

Chapter 5: Natural Products for Oral Health

As a small boy growing up in Chileng'a village of Zambezi, a small town in north-western Zambia, the author was well used to a plant, *Mchenja*, often used to whiten teeth and disinfect the mouth, producing a pleasant smell. The scientific name of *Mchenja* is *Diospyros mespiliformis*, now known to contain anti-bacterial chemical substances. So the use of *Mchenja* as a chewing stick in our age old traditions in Zambia and neighbouring countries is not in vain; it is founded on sound antimicrobial imperatives for oral health.

The taste of *Mchenja* is unmistakable. And even 30 years after leaving the village, Chinsembu would in November 2014 still warm up to the taste of *Mchenja*, now as an ingredient of a herbal mouthwash and toothache formulation produced by an amateur entrepreneur in Kabwe, Zambia. The production and use of Toothache Master in Kabwe, formerly Broken Hill town, is in sharp contrast to Broken Hill man, whose fossils indicate this early man suffered from severe periodontal disease because he did not use toothpicks.

In many poor societies, plant products are the only means of oral care and hygiene, often ensuring the health of all the people including those living with HIV/AIDS.

Oral infections are very common in persons progressing to AIDS. Mouth sores and gum diseases characterize dental caries and periodontal diseases in persons with HIV infection. In such patients, even chewing solid foods is difficult as the gums are inflamed and painful.

Oral thrush, produced by yeast infection, is common in HIV disease. Foul smell is even difficult to hide. In the course of HIV infection, the mouth becomes a fertile ground for the growth of viruses, fungi, protozoa and bacteria. Thus, toothache and loss of teeth are warning bells for AIDS. HIV-infected persons also develop more aggressive forms of gingivitis and periodontitis. Even the tongue gives in to bacterial infection, developing whitish stuff with terrible smell. Oral microbes are also developing resistance to common synthetic antimicrobials. This, and other reasons, make bioprospecting for natural products all the more urgent.

Therefore, many plant species and other natural products are being studied for use in oral care formulations. This chapter notes that natural agents for improved oral health are present in chewing sticks like miswak and *Mchenja*, algae, pomegranate, chamomile, essential oils, probiotics, milk, coffee, green tea, honey, mushrooms, grapes, rhein, raisins, red wine and peppermint among other common natural products for oral hygiene. Some of these products are now ingredients of commercial toothpastes like Colgate and mouthrinses.

Medicinal plants and other natural products being studied for oral care in various pharmacopoeias in Africa, Australia, Asia Middle East, Europe and South America are also reviewed. Selected active chemical compounds that confer their antimicrobial functions are also mentioned. This is the smallest chapter of this book. Yet, it is dedicated to green products for a part of the human body that harbours the highest number of bacterial species (>500). Many of these are innocuous when immunity is fully functional, but cause opportunistic oral infections in persons progressing to AIDS, when CD4 counts dip below 200.

Chapter 6: Natural Products as Anti-tuberculosis Agents

A conservative estimate is that global TB deaths in 2015 stand at 1.1 million people. Before that, TB was believed to kill 2-3 million people every year. This is literally like yearly wiping out the entire 2.1 million population of Namibia. Projections suggest over the next 15 years leading up to 2030, about 10 million people will be saved from dying of TB. But this will only happen if additional resources - not just money - are thrown at the disease.

Investing more resources into diagnosis, care and treatment of drug-sensitive and drug-resistant *Mycobacterium tuberculosis* will greatly aid the global campaign against TB and save close to 10 million people from TB deaths. With additional resources, the forecast is that global TB deaths may dwindle to 247,800 in the year 2030.

With respect to the treatment of drug-resistant TB - which is killing many people, plants and other natural products - will obviously play a much bigger role in saving these 10 million lives, especially to provide novel chemical compounds for creating new anti-TB drugs that inhibit these stubborn super-bugs. Experimental evidence in this chapter shows many natural products already possess powerful chemical ingredients active against drug-resistant *M. tuberculosis*.

Drug-resistant TB is very common in people infected with HIV. In fact, TB was amenable to drugs until HIV infection made TB pathogenesis and therapy go haywire. Luckily, nature knows no limit. We now have potent green medicines from plants and other natural products capable of bringing down HIV/TB co-epidemics. We can use pharmacognosy as a vehicle to discover powerful drugs to combat drug-resistant TB.

This chapter explores anti-TB agents from endophytes, common natural products like St. John's Wort, green tea, curry, miswak, marijuana, honey/propolis, and *Vernonia* species. Pharmacopoeias of anti-TB plants used in many different parts of the world are considered.

Chapter 7: The World of Malaria: Antimalarial Medicines from Mother Nature

Given the progress in the elimination of malaria that has taken place in many parts of the world now free of this mosquito-borne disease, I am optimistic that malaria is going the way of smallpox, to be totally wiped off the face of the earth. But to achieve this, malaria must get additional resources, and more importantly, global attention, which it has ceded over the past three decades to HIV/AIDS.

Big pharmaceutical companies should take fresh interest in malaria, to make innovative antimalarial drugs from plants and other natural products, instead of labelling malaria a low-profit disease. The discovery of artemisinin and quinine are, to most people, the most telling reminders of the biomedical significance of green medicines. Plant products work.

The control and treatment of the global burden of malaria is at the tipping point, the point where small changes will soon become significant enough to cause a significant and more important leap 'over the hill' to the other side of a malaria-free world. We should now employ all the weapons at our disposal.

In this final chapter, the die is cast. Use of antimalarial plants has crossed the Rubicon. Malaria's world is shrinking, and shrinking very fast. The war against malaria is now irreversible. It will soon be won.

1

HIV/AIDS,
ANTIRETROVIRAL THERAPY
AND NATURAL PRODUCTS

Introduction

What is the current status of antiretroviral therapy (ART)? What challenges do governments that provide ART and people taking antiretroviral drugs (ARVs) face? Why is there a renewed interest in natural products and anti-HIV medications from Mother Nature? This chapter seeks to provide the reader with pertinent information that should help answer these questions. Five major themes are discussed in relation to HIV/AIDS:

- Status of public sector antiretroviral therapy in Africa
- Challenges of antiretroviral therapy
- The notion of the best of both worlds - using both antiretroviral therapy and natural products
- Mainstreaming and institutionalization of natural products, and
- The renewed search to recruit natural products to the frontline of efforts to fight the epidemic.

HIV and AIDS

Human immunodeficiency virus (HIV) is the causative agent of AIDS - acquired immunodeficiency syndrome, a manifestation of diseases that has claimed millions of lives since its discovery in 1983. HIV is a retrovirus belonging to the genus of lentiviruses (lente-, Latin for "slow"), viruses with a long incubation period. Retroviruses have the ability to use their ribonucleic acid (RNA) and host deoxyribonucleic (DNA) to make viral DNA. Like other retroviruses, HIV infects the body, has a long incubation period (clinical latency), and ultimately causes the signs and symptoms of AIDS. HIV causes severe damage to the immune system and eventually destroys it.

Experts agree that there are two types of HIV, namely HIV-1 and HIV-2. Both types are transmitted through sexual intercourse, through blood, and from mother to child, and they appear to cause clinically identical forms of AIDS. However, it seems that HIV-2 is less easily transmitted, and the incubation period, that is the time between initial infection and illness, is longer in the case of HIV-2. Globally, the leading virus is HIV-1, and generally when people refer to HIV without specifying the type of virus they will be referring to HIV-1. HIV-2, initially endemic to West Africa, is spreading worldwide.

HIV-2 demonstrates a closer genetic relationship and geographic distribution to the simian immunodeficiency virus (SIV), long endemic to Central Africa, than to HIV-1. Sequencing studies of early HIV-2 isolates showed a 75% nucleic acid homology with SIV but only a 40-50% homology with HIV-1. Thus, it is hypothesized that HIV-2 may be the prototype virus that was originally transmitted from monkeys to man.

The World Health Organization (WHO) estimated that about 36.9 million people were living with HIV/AIDS in 2014. Globally, there were over 2 million annual deaths due to AIDS in 2009, and 1.5 million people died of AIDS-related illnesses worldwide in 2013. At the end of 2014, about 14.9 million people, out of a total of 28 million people eligible for treatment, were on ART. Sub-Saharan Africa still bears an inordinate share of the global HIV burden. Although the rate of new HIV infections has decreased, the total number of people living with HIV continues to rise. In 2012, that number reached 25 million, accounting for 71% of the global epidemic. AIDS, however, is not uniformly expressed in all individuals. A small proportion of persons infected with the virus develop AIDS and die within months following primary infection, while approximately 5% of HIV-infected individuals exhibit no signs of disease progression even after 12 or more years.

Anti-HIV Agents Target Steps in HIV Life Cycle

The life cycle of HIV consists of ten steps that act as targets for chemotherapeutical interventions. Most of the anti-HIV chemical substances, whether synthetic pharmaceutical ART drugs or natural products, work by interfering with one of these steps in the HIV life cycle. There are specific steps in the lifecycle of HIV (Kostova, Raleva, Genova, & Argirova, 2006): (1) viral adsorption to the cell membrane; (2) fusion between the viral envelope and the cell membrane; (3) uncoating of the viral nucleocapsid; (4) reverse transcription of the viral RNA to pro-viral DNA; (5) integration of the proviral DNA into the cellular genome; (6) DNA replication; (7) transcription of the proviral DNA to RNA; (8) translation of the viral precursor messenger RNA to mature messenger RNA; (9) maturation of the viral precursor proteins by proteolysis, myristoylation and glycosylation; and (10) budding, virion assembly and release. Note that step 4, involving HIV reverse transcriptase, is the main target for ART; it is different from the replicative cycle of other viruses. Another target for therapeutic intervention is step 9, particularly the proteolysis of precursor proteins by HIV protease. Many chemotherapeutic strategies focus on the development of enzyme inhibitors that target one or more steps in the lifecycle of HIV.

Status of Antiretroviral Therapy

The discovery of antiretroviral drugs, the most prominent of which was zidovudine (also called azidothymidine, AZT), showed that treating HIV infection was a possible biomedical achievement (Broder, 2010). Although zidovudine is no longer used in most countries, this earliest antiretroviral drug breached a critical technological barrier and illuminated the path to the discovery of other drugs.

There are four types of antiretroviral drugs:

1. Nucleoside reverse transcriptase inhibitors (NRTIs) such as AZT interfere with HIV-1 replication by inhibiting viral reverse transcriptase.
2. Non-nucleoside reverse transcriptase inhibitors (NNRTIs) cause conformational changes at the active site of reverse transcriptase thereby inhibiting its activity.
3. Protease inhibitors such as indinavir, ritonavir and nelfinavir prevent the cutting of the precursor polypeptide that is processed into smaller core proteins, and
4. Entry inhibitors: These drugs prevent the passage of HIV into host cells.

ART is the treatment of people infected with HIV using anti-HIV drugs. The standard treatment consists of a combination of at least three drugs which significantly reduces the viral load. This standard treatment protocol is known as triple combination therapy or highly active antiretroviral therapy (HAART). There are now triple-in-one pills which combine all the three standard drugs. The cost of HAART has reduced due to the manufacturing of generic drugs. Monotherapy is limited due to the rapid development of resistant HIV strains. The use of standardized and affordable first-line combinations of antiretroviral drugs, including two NRTIs and one NNRTI, has also been crucial in allowing the scale-up of ART (Hamers, Wallis, Kityo, Siwale, Mandaliya, & Conradie, 2011).

Indeed, ART has changed the face of AIDS, not least from emaciated bodies to plump ones. No doubt, ART has brought about a substantial decrease in mortality and morbidity due to HIV-1 infections, changing AIDS from a rapidly lethal condition into a chronic and manageable disease, compatible with very long survival (Broder, 2010); even more than 25 years after infection. So, globally, antiretroviral drugs have dramatically slashed deaths due to HIV/AIDS. Since the advent of public sector ART, Africa is leading the world in expanding access to antiretroviral treatment, with 7.6 million people across the continent receiving ART by December 2012, including 7.5 million people in Sub-Saharan Africa (World Health Organization, 2013).

According to WHO, Eastern and Southern Africa doubled the number of people on treatment between 2006 and 2012. At least ten countries (Botswana, Cape Verde, Eritrea, Kenya, Namibia, Rwanda, South Africa, Swaziland, Zambia and Zimbabwe) reported reaching 80% or more of adults eligible for antiretroviral therapy, under the 2010 WHO guidelines. However, new WHO guidelines on HIV treatment in 2013 have since made many more people eligible for treatment.

The good news for HIV-infected persons came in 2013 when WHO directed all member countries that ART should be initiated for all adult patients with a CD4 count equal or less than 500 cells per mm^3. Symptomatic patients with WHO clinical stage 3 (advanced) and 4 (severe) disease, and symptomatic individuals with a CD4 count equal or less than 350 cells per mm^3, should be treated as a priority. According to the WHO, ART should be initiated as soon as it is tolerated in all HIV positive adults with active TB irrespective of CD4 count. Patients should not wait until TB treatment is completed to initiate ART.

Moreover, ART should be given to HIV positive adult patients with active hepatitis B co-infection with evidence of severe liver disease, irrespective of CD4 cell count or WHO clinical stage. Liver disease is emerging as a leading cause of death in HIV-hepatitis B co-infected patients and some antiretroviral drugs used on HIV treatment also are active against hepatitis B virus (HBV), emphasizing the benefit of treatment of dual infection. WHO stated that ART should be initiated for all HIV-infected pregnant and breastfeeding women irrespective of CD4 cell count or WHO clinical stage. It brings benefits to mothers' health, prevents the exposed child from becoming infected, and may offer additional benefits for prevention of the sexual transmission of HIV.

In addition, WHO has advised that ART should be offered to all HIV-infected partners in a serodiscordant relationship irrespective of CD4 cell count. Results of HPTN052 trials and other observational studies strongly support the use of ART to prevent HIV transmission among serodiscordant couples. Under the WHO 2013 guidelines, about 20.2 to 22.7 million people are eligible for ART in Africa. The average number of Africans eligible for ART was 21.2 million in 2013 under the 2013 WHO guidelines. Of the 21.2 million people in Africa eligible for ART, only 7.6 million were receiving anti-HIV medication as of December 2012. Considerable work and resources are needed to reach all people eligible for HIV treatment, with ART reaching only about one in three eligible, according to the WHO 2013 guidelines.

The trend towards increased ART coverage across Africa masks significant national gaps. In at least 14 countries in Africa, 80% or more of people who were estimated to be eligible for treatment under the 2013 WHO guidelines were not on ART as of December 2012. Some of those on ART do not stay on treatment long enough to maximize benefits. According to WHO, nine out of every ten people have an unmet need for ART in Sub-Saharan African countries such as Angola, Cameroon, Central African Republic, Chad, Cote d'Ivoire, Democratic Republic of the Congo, Ethiopia, Ghana, Kenya, Lesotho, Malawi, Mozambique, Nigeria, South Africa, South Sudan, Togo, Uganda, United Republic of Tanzania, Zambia and Zimbabwe.

These countries face a plethora of acceptability, feasibility and operational challenges in rolling-out ART to those in need. In addition, key questions remain to be answered on the best use of ART, adverse drug reactions, how patients should be maintained on treatment and how to institutionalize support structures for improved monitoring of treatment failure. ART for children is also a topical issue that has not received much attention. In 2007, less than 10% of all HIV-infected children in need ART in Sub-Saharan Africa were actually receiving therapy (Eley & Nuttall, 2007). Today, this situation has not significantly changed. Many constraints prevent children from gaining access to appropriate treatment and care, including the magnitude of the paediatric epidemic, competing interests of adult care, health system inadequacies, technical challenges and patient-related factors.

Challenges to ART

While many countries have made remarkable progress in the provision of ART to those in need, ART is still limited by its cost, the requirement of life long adherence, side effects and the presently unknown effects of long-term treatment (Richman, Margolis, Delaney, Greene, Hazuda, & Pomerantz, 2009). Therapeutic choices for HIV/AIDS treatment are even more compromised in developing countries due to a persistent lack of access to antiretroviral drugs, limited healthcare capacities, and other factors that counteract the benefits of ART, for example malnutrition and poverty (Leteane, Ngwenya, Muzila, Namushe, Mwinga, & Musonda et al., 2012).

Moreover, intensified use of antiretroviral drugs gives way to the emergence of drug-resistant strains which dramatically increase the genetic and immunological variability of HIV (Montagnier, 2010). This makes it difficult to rely on the use of few standard antiretroviral drugs. Mutations in the HIV genome that confer drug resistance, acquired during ART failure, limit the response to subsequent lines of treatment (Hamers et al., 2011). The threat of increased onward transmission of drug-resistant HIV strains to newly infected people, what is called primary drug resistance, has the potential to compromising the effectiveness of first-line ART regimens. In Europe and the United States of America, about 9–15% of antiretroviral-naive individuals harbour HIV strains with at least one drug-resistance mutation, and, therefore, pre-treatment resistance testing is done before starting therapy (Hamers et al., 2011).

Data show that in Africa- Kenya, Nigeria, South Africa, Uganda, Zambia, and Zimbabwe- the overall prevalence of HIV resistance is 5.6%, which includes 3.3% associated with NNRTIs, 2.5% resistance to NRTIs, and 1.3% to protease inhibitors (Hamers et al., 2011). The prevalence of primary drug resistance varies substantially between cities and countries, ranging from 1.1% in Pretoria, South Africa, to 12.3% in Kampala, Uganda. The prevalence of primary HIV resistance in Zambia is about 5%. Prevalence of primary drug resistance in antiretroviral-naïve persons is substantially higher in Uganda where ART was first introduced, compared with other African countries. Resistance is mostly confined to a single drug-class, most commonly NNRTIs. HIV resistance leads to ART failure and complications, causing patients to seek other options, including herbs, for treatment.

ART is also associated with the development of lipodystrophy, a condition characterized by peripheral fat loss (lipoatrophy) and central fat accumulation which may result in thin facial pads, thin arms and legs, pot-bellies, or 'buffalo humps', leaving patients stigmatized (Lindegaard, Keller, Bruunsgaard, & Pedersen, 2004). In other cases, chronic ART can bring about cardiac and metabolic side-effects, including dyslipidemias, insulin resistance, abnormal body fat re-distribution, and related disorders, which can in turn increase the risk of developing heart disease and type 2 diabetes (Broder, 2010). Other scientists argue that there is probably a higher risk of coronary artery disease in patients who receive protease inhibitors. Thus, several challenges remain in the current paradigm of ART, with special impact in the developing world.

Thus, while acknowledging that current antiretroviral drugs are vitally important in improving the quality and prolonging the life of HIV/AIDS patients, the drugs still have many shortcomings including drug resistance, drug failure, complications, side-effects, toxicity, limited availability, high cost and lack of any curative effect (Vermani & Garg, 2002). Ramana, Anand, Sethuraman, and Krishnan (2014) also lamented that antiretroviral drugs have challenges such as resistance, lack of compliance to long-term therapy, adverse drug-drug interactions, poor bioavailability and lack of access to tissues and reservoirs which amass and hide away HIV particles.

In malaria-endemic areas, co-administration of antimalarial and antiretroviral drugs increases the risk of toxicity. Let us examine the case of ART-induced liver toxicity. Severe liver toxicity affects 8-23% of HIV-infected patients receiving ART (Lemoine & Ingiliz, 2012). There are various patterns of acute or progressive ART-induced hepatotoxicity: Immune reconstitution syndrome, hypersensitivity reactions, mitochondrial toxicity, direct cell stress, liver steatosis and nodular regenerative hyperplasia. In Africa, clinical management of ART-induced liver damage is very difficult. Consequently, as affected patients blame ART for damaging their livers, they encourage others to shun the same.

Hamzah and Post (2009), note that ART is associated with the poisoning of kidneys (nephrotoxicity). Citing several studies, these two authors write that impaired kidney function and nephrotoxicity have been observed with several antiretrovirals, although most often with indinavir and tenofovir. Indinavir, a protease inhibitor, may crystallize in the urinary tract and cause acute obstruction or sub-acute decline in renal function. Tenofovir may cause acute renal failure, progressive decline in glomerular filtration rate, tubular dysfunction as manifested by Fanconi syndrome, hypophosphataemia with urinary phosphate wasting, glycosuria, renal tubular acidosis or nephrogenic diabetes insipidus. Tenofovir-induced tubular injury may result in severe osteomalacia-soft bones, resembling rickets in children. The risk of kidney complications is increased when tenofovir is co-administered with protease inhibitors.

Another antiretroviral drug that has caused many side-effects is stavudine. Like many other antiretroviral drugs, stavudine selling under the trade names d4T and Zerit, is associated with a number of side-effects. Inflammation of the pancreas (pancreatitis) occurs in some patients taking stavudine. Symptoms of pancreatitis include a tender or swollen abdomen, nausea, vomiting, fever, rapid heart rate and rapid breathing. Stavudine also leads to lactic acidosis. In simple language, this means a lot more lactic acid accumulates in the blood. Wester, Okezie, Thomas, Bussmann, Moyo, and Muzenda et al. (2007), working in Botswana, found a high incidence of lactic acidosis in patients taking stavudine. The incidence of lactic acidosis was significantly higher than that found in industrialized countries.

These investigators observed that the development of lactic acidosis was higher in women, especially if they were overweight, or aged over 40 years. About 65% of lactic acid is converted to carbon dioxide and water, 20% into glycogen, 10% into protein and 5% into glucose. The breakdown of glucose or glycogen produces lactic acid and hydrogen ions. The presence of hydrogen ions, not lactic acid, makes the muscles acidic and this eventually halts muscle function.

As hydrogen ion concentration increases, the blood and muscles become acidic. This acidic environment slows down enzyme activity, reduces the breakdown of glucose and prevents energy production. Acidic muscles also aggravate associated nerve endings, causing pain and irritation of the central nervous system. Hence patients taking stavudine become nauseous. Typical symptoms of increased lactic acid accumulation include feeling weak or tired, muscle pain, breathing problems, abdominal pain, feeling cold, dizziness, persistent nausea, vomiting, shortness of breath, enlarged liver and weight loss.

The normal lactic acid circulating in the blood is 1-2 milli moles per litre of blood. Increased lactic acid concentration above 10 millimoles per litre of blood has been associated with an 80% mortality rate in patients. Due to these side-effects, WHO has recommended that stavudine should not be given as part of first-line therapy. However, noting that stavudine was cheaper than alternative drugs, it was the most accessible option for people in resource-limited settings. Stavudine was donated and distributed in large quantities in Africa. Too bad, the damage done by stavudine is still visible today. As they say, beggars cannot be choosers.

Taken together, all these shortcomings of conventional ART continue to open new vistas in the use of ethnomedicinal plants and other natural products for the management of HIV/AIDS. Besides these clinical challenges, Chinsembu (2009) bemoaned that many public sector ART programmes in southern Africa, the epicentre of the HIV/AIDS epidemic, are a candle in the wind as they battle to glimmer against the inevitable possibility of dying from another form of AIDS - 'Acquired Income Deficiency Syndrome'. There are concerns that free public sector ART programmes are not sustainable due to their heavy reliance on donor funding. Unfortunately, access to treatment still has many rivers to cross, including: lack of confidentiality, lack of bed space, lack of transport to hospitals, shortages of qualified health workers, long queues and serious side-effects now causing new forms of stigma.

To further put the challenges of ART into perspective, let us look at a few examples. In 2006, the United Nations High-Level Meeting on HIV/AIDS in New York hailed Namibia's AIDS treatment programme as the best in southern Africa (Government of the Republic of Namibia, 2009). At the end of August 2009, there were approximately 70,000 Namibians on ART (Chinsembu, 2009), but this number rose to 122,300 by 2014. During the 2008/09 financial year, the total cost of ART in Namibia was approximately US$ 21 million. Of this amount, 68% was financed through donations by the Global Fund and the United States Centres for Disease Control. The Namibian government subsidy was 23%, the Clinton Foundation paid for 8%, and Supply Chain Management Systems contributed the remaining 1% (Government of the Republic of Namibia, 2009).

Clearly, these figures show that Namibia's free public sector ART programme is not sustainable due to its heavy reliance on donor funds. Moreover, access to ART in Namibia is still challenged by low levels of human and infrastructural resources required to roll-out services particularly in the pre-ART and ART clinics (Government of the Republic of Namibia, 2009). Specifically, more trained professionals are needed, not only for pharmaceutical services but also for doctors, clinical officers, and nurses in hospitals, health centres, and clinics.

The staffing situation for the Namibian public health sector is currently inadequate. Estimates suggest that the vacancy rates for public sector doctors, nurses and pharmacists are 40%, 25%, and 58%, respectively (Chinsembu & Mutirua, 2008). Health facilities that provide ART services also need to be renovated in order to adequately accommodate patients. Further, since Namibia is the second most sparsely populated country in the world, providing full ART services to the rural population requires a fully decentralized and community-based model with strong policies and leadership from the central level.

However, insufficient numbers of skilled technical personnel and limited managerial capacity at all levels have impaired the challenges of decentralization, and access to services remains a Herculean obstacle for those living in sparsely populated areas. As a country with one of the highest *Gini* coefficients and levels of income disparity in the world, Namibia's household poverty and nutrition scenarios also pose major questions to ART access, treatment adherence and success (Chinsembu & Mutirua, 2008). It is not an overestimation to suggest that the challenges of ART in Namibia mirror those in most developing African countries.

In Zambia, Chinsembu and Hedimbi (2009) observed that access to treatment is challenged by inadequacy of the healthcare system, which suffers from high patient numbers, lack of physical space and infrastructure and attrition of health workers. Notably, there is a critical shortage of doctors. In 2006, there were only about 646 doctors working in Zambia; this was under a third of the doctor-patient ratio recommended by WHO, which also deemed 26 other countries in Sub-Saharan Africa as 'crisis countries' because of having densities of physicians, nurses and midwives lower than the WHO minimum recommendation of 2.3 per 1,000 population.

Characteristics of the HIV epidemic and the human resources shortages in African countries have been reviewed by Zuber, McCarthy, Verani, Msidi and Johnson (2014). The figures reveal critical shortages of medical doctors, especially in Ethiopia, Malawi, Rwanda, South Sudan, Tanzania, Zambia and Zimbabwe. The ratio of nurses, general ART coverage, prevention-of-mother-to-child-transmission and ART for children is still very poor in these African countries. Due to severe shortages of public health workers, provision of ART in these countries is severely constrained. Thus, overall, the average number of people on ART in Africa is 63.5%. Suffice to state that several limitations of current ART programmes continue to push patients towards the use of plants and other natural products to manage HIV/AIDS.

ART and Natural Products: The Best of Both Worlds

While acknowledging that current antiretroviral drugs are vitally important in improving the quality and prolonging the life of HIV/AIDS patients, the drugs still have many disadvantages including resistance, toxicity, limited availability, high cost and lack of any curative effect (Chinsembu, 2009). These shortcomings of conventional ART continue to open new vistas in the use of ethnomedicinal plants and other natural products for the management of HIV/AIDS. In many countries, the inclusion of ethnomedicines and other natural products in official HIV/AIDS policy is an extremely sensitive and contentious issue.

It is sensitive because anti-HIV ethnomedicines and other natural products can easily become a scapegoat for denial and inertia to roll-out ART. This is what may have happened in South Africa during Thabo Mbeki's presidency when the government was blamed for apparently failing to initiate and operationalize large-scale antiretroviral treatment to those in need, urging instead the patients to use beetroots.

It is also contentious because in various resource-poor settings, government-sponsored ART programmes discourage the use of traditional medicines, fearing that the efficacy of antiretroviral drugs may be inhibited by such natural products, or that their pharmacological interactions could lead to toxicity (Hardon, Desclaux, Egrot, Simon, Micollier, & Kyakuwa, 2008). Reliance on anti-HIV plants and other natural products can also lead to poor adherence to ART. Thus, Chinsembu (2009) observed that many governments still have contradictory attitudes towards the use of traditional medicines and natural products in the management of HIV/AIDS, discouraging them within ART programmes, and supporting them within other initiatives of public health and primary healthcare.

In essence, many HIV-infected persons have access to antiretroviral drugs, but some still use ethnomedicinal plants and other natural products to treat opportunistic infections and offset side-effects from antiretroviral medication. Medicinal plants and other natural products such as mushrooms are used as primary treatment for HIV-related problems such as skin disorders, nausea, depression, insomnia and body weakness (Babb, Pemba, Seatlanyane, Charalambous, Churchyard, & Grant, 2004). In the case of rural communities, formal biomedical services are also hardly accessible.

Therefore, whilst the majority of HIV/AIDS patients rely on ART, some still have faith in the use of traditional medicines from plants and mushrooms. Genuine traditional healers deserve respect because they have dispensed ethnomedications to treat opportunistic infections associated with HIV even before the massive roll-out of cheaper generic ARVs. Understandably, HIV/AIDS patients are vulnerable in their choice of treatments, such that some of them do vacillate from conventional ART programmes to traditional medicines and vice versa; they want to have the best of both worlds (Hardon et al., 2008). However, caution should be taken when using natural products because, unlike conventional ARVs, correct dosages for natural remedies are difficult to determine; they are not always available and standardized. Some natural products are also poorly packaged. Their shelf-lives may be unknown, and some are cytotoxic, or contaminated by metals.

According to Calixto (2000), some traditional medicines strengthen the immune systems of gravely ill individuals and improve their appetite for food. This is important for the management of HIV-related opportunistic infections. Certain natural products including foods contain minerals that improve immunity to HIV/AIDS. Symptoms of AIDS can be reversed by correct nutritional supplementation even in patients close to death. Supplementation of the diet with mushrooms and other organic foods rich in L-selenomethione, L-glutamine, hydroxytryptophan, and N-acetyl cysteine can reverse the symptoms of AIDS and prevent HIV-infected patients from rapidly progressing to AIDS. To fight opportunistic infections, good nutrition is a key component in the care and support for people living with HIV and AIDS. One good example is the plant *Solanum nigrum* which contains nutrients and micronutrients that are important for AIDS patients (Kamatenesi, 2010).

Mainstreaming and Institutionalization of Natural Products

As early as 1989, WHO had already voiced the need to evaluate ethnomedicines and other natural products for the management of HIV/AIDS. A memorandum of the WHO (1989: p. 613) stated as follows: "In this context, there is need to evaluate those elements of traditional medicine, particularly medicinal plants and other natural products, that might yield effective and affordable therapeutic agents. This will require a systematic approach."

Later, African governments expressed the need for a concerted, systematic and sustained effort at both local and regional levels to support and biochemically validate African traditional medicines. To popularize this commitment, the Organization of African Unity (later renamed the African Union) Heads of State and Government declared the period 2000-2010 as the Decade of African Traditional Medicine. In addition, the Director General of WHO, declared 31st August of every year as the African Traditional Medicine Day. All these initiatives demonstrate the need to mainstream and institutionalize natural products into the formal healthcare system.

The importance of investing in the high growth sectors of biotechnology and phytomedicine is also articulated in the founding document of the New Partnership for Africa's Development (NEPAD), and adopted by the African Biosciences Initiative (NEPAD, 2001; African Biosciences Initiative,

2005). Due to the renewed public interest in phytomedicines, NEPAD's Southern Africa Network for Biosciences (SANBio) has a flagship project on validation of ethnomedicines for effective and affordable treatment of HIV/AIDS. Scientific validation of ethnomedicinal plants is done at the Council for Scientific and Industrial Research (CSIR) in Pretoria, South Africa.

Why do plants and other natural products hold this renewed promise to clinically-safer and financially-cheaper drugs? Well, medicines from natural products provide rational means for the treatment of many diseases that are stubborn and incurable in western systems of medicine. Phytomedicines are particularly regaining patient acceptance because they have fewer side effects, are relatively less expensive, are easy to use, and have a long history of use (Vermani & Garg, 2002). Medicinal effects of plants also tend to normalize physiological function and correct the underlying cause of the disorder. Furthermore, medicinal plants are renewable in nature unlike synthetic drugs that are obtained from non-renewable sources of basic raw materials such as fossil sources and petrochemicals. Cultivation, gathering and selling of medicinal plants can also be a source of income for poor families (Reihling, 2008); thus killing two birds- disease and poverty- with one stone.

Despite the appeal presented by natural products, Chinsembu and Hedimbi (2010) bemoaned that only a handful of workers in Africa such as Abere and Agoreyo (2006), Bessong, Obi, Andréola, Rojas, Pouységu and Igumbor et al. (2005), Boyd, Hallock, Cardellina, Manfredi, Blunt, McMahon, Buckheit, Bringmann and Schaeffer (1994), Igbinosa, Igbinosa and Aiyegoro, (2009), and Klos, van de Venter, Milne, Traore, Meyer and Oosthuizen (2009) have screened medicinal plants for anti-HIV activity, especially prior to the NEPAD/SANBio initiative. There are a few exceptions, however, such as in South Africa, where CSIR has a bioprospecting programme which screens plants for medicinal properties. In 2007, Namibia embarked on similar bioprospecting initiatives, albeit, very late, and on a very small scale. In order to scientifically validate traditional medicines for HIV/AIDS, Chinsembu (2009) described a model and experiences of initiating collaboration between biomedical scientists and Namibian traditional healers. Many traditional healers are willing to subject their traditional medicines to scientific tests.

Collaboration was institutionalized at a one-day workshop on the use of traditional medicines to treat HIV/AIDS, held at Windhoek's Safari Hotel on 20th November 2007. The one-day workshop was sponsored by the Namibian government's Ministry of Education as part of an initiative to form a National Biosciences Forum. The workshop was also part of the NEPAD initiative to scientifically validate traditional medicines to treat HIV/AIDS and related opportunistic infections.

Officially opening the workshop, University of Namibia (UNAM) Pro-Vice-Chancellor for Academic Affairs and Research Professor Osmund

Mwandemele reaffirmed NEPAD's commitment to developing the continent through the use of science and technological innovations. Mwandemele is also chairman of NEPAD's steering committee for the Southern African Network for Biosciences (SANBio). Speaking at the workshop, SANBio Director Professor Luke Mumba stressed that because Southern Africa is the epicentre of the HIV/AIDS pandemic, SANBio is interested in finding affordable and effective traditional medicines for treating HIV/AIDS.

Mumba informed workshop participants that SANBio was facilitating the scientific validation of *SF2000*, a traditional medicine from Dr. Ludwig Sondashi, a healer from Zambia. Matshidiso Moroka, a scientist from South Africa's Council for Scientific and Industrial Research (CSIR), where *SF2000* was being tested, confirmed that some of the herbs had shown interesting laboratory results. She could not elaborate further due to intellectual property and patent constraints. *SF2000* is believed to contain HIV integrase inhibitors.

Meanwhile, UNAM's Faculty of Science was designated as the focal point for the SANBio flagship project on scientific validation of traditional medicines for HIV/AIDS in Namibia. This meant that UNAM, together with other stakeholders in Namibia, was to spearhead research on traditional medicines for HIV/AIDS. A national steering committee on scientific validation of traditional medicines in Namibia was formed. The steering committee is still chaired by Prof. Kazhila C. Chinsembu.

In Namibia, as in many other African countries, traditional medicines are still not well-researched and Africans' knowledge of natural products used to remedy HIV/AIDS opportunistic infections is not scientifically validated. For this reason, bioprospecting for anti-HIV plants can surely unlock the promise to manufacture our own antiretroviral drugs. In a way, this is exactly what former Nigerian President Goodluck Jonathan meant when he urged other African leaders to de-emphasize reliance on external funding and importation of essential medicines for the treatment of HIV/AIDS, TB and malaria. President Jonathan was speaking on Monday, 15th July 2013 at the opening of the Abuja+12 Special Summit of the African Union on HIV/AIDS, TB and malaria.

The New Search for Natural Products

There is an urgent need to increase the search for newer and more affordable anti-HIV medications. One of these search strategies takes us back to Mother Nature. There, scientists scour forests for plants and other natural products that provide leads or can be directly converted into anti-HIV drugs. The search for natural products has received renewed attention in recent years due to their general structural diversity and uniqueness. Natural products also present new modes of action, have the ability to offset side effects produced by synthetic antiretroviral drugs, and can block multiple steps and enzymes in HIV. Because of these characteristics, many scientists believe that natural products are promising candidates in the fight against HIV resistance to current antiretroviral drugs (Hupfeld & Efferth, 2009).

Sub-Saharan Africa has rich plant biodiversity and a long tradition of medicinal use of plants with over 3,000 species of plants used as medicines (Van Wyk & Gericke, 2000). Several of these plants may contain novel anti-HIV compounds. Corollary, there has been a sustained bioprospective effort to isolate the active leads from plants and other natural products for preventing transmission of HIV and the management of AIDS. Screening of plants and other natural products based on ethnopharmacological data increases the potential of finding novel anti-HIV compounds.

Indigenous knowledge of medicinal plant use also provides leads towards therapeutic concept thereby accelerating drug discovery. This is now being called reverse pharmacology (Chinsembu, 2009). Thus, it is important to search for novel antiretroviral agents which can be added to or which can replace the current arsenal of drugs against HIV. Despite the rich African repertoire from which to select medicinal plants, traditional herbal medicines are still not well-researched and African knowledge of herbal remedies used to manage HIV/AIDS is scanty, impressionistic and not well documented (Kayombo, Uiso, Mbwambo, Mahunnah, Moshi, & Mgonda, 2007). Africa is also awash with fake AIDS cures (Amon, 2008), one of these is Tetrasil from Zambia.

However, there is a new reality in which natural products have now found a renewed promise to surmount current shortcomings associated with ART. About 21 drugs sold in 2007 to treat HIV-1 infection were all obtained by chemical synthesis, and none from natural products. Yet, natural products provide a rich and diverse source of bioactive compounds with practical value as anti-HIV therapy. In PubMed alone, a search for "anti-HIV plants" produced 800 search results on 24th August 2014. Natural products can be selected for biological screening based on ethnomedicinal usage, random collection and a chemotaxonomic approach, that is, screening of species of the same botanical family for similar compounds. However, the follow-up and selection of plants based on leads from the literature would seem to be the most cost-effective way of identifying plants with anti-HIV activity (World Health Organization, 1989).

Medicinal plants now present a whole new dynamic and paradigm in the search for leads to novel antiretroviral drugs. Since Africa is the birthplace of humankind, Africans are historically endowed with indigenous knowledge of phytomedicines. Singh, Singh and Goel (2011) noted that many plant anti-HIV chemical compounds are widely distributed in nature. By 2006, more than 50 chemical compounds with varying levels of anti-HIV activity had been isolated from plants. It goes without saying that evaluation of medicinal plants provides an opportunity for the discovery of novel anti-HIV-1 medications with lower or no cytotoxicity at all. But, evidence about anti-HIV natural products is anecdotal.

In retrospect, Mother Nature has given us an arsenal of plants and other natural products with which to fight HIV/AIDS. The missing link is the lack of political and scientific initiatives to bring these resources to the cutting-edge of our efforts to combat AIDS. As a consequence, while AIDS is largely an African problem, the hotbeds of research for new treatments of HIV/AIDS are still outside Africa. To win the fight against AIDS, we can only do better if we look deeper into the past. Our human past is inextricably linked to Mother Nature. Let us go back to our 'roots'.

Finally, throughout this book, the recurring motif is that HIV and AIDS-related infections in Africa and other parts of the developing world are inextricably linked to poverty. Poor individuals and communities predominantly use medicinal plants and other natural products. Since many poor folks cannot afford to buy pharmaceutical drugs, they resort to the use of medicinal plants to manage HIV and AIDS-related ailments. Good food and good nutrition ring-fence the body from infection, any infection, including HIV and AIDS-related diseases. Sadly, poverty-stricken individuals hardly afford nutritious foods - their bodies are open to infection; and because of their weakened immune systems, they are very susceptible to HIV and AIDS-related infections. In my informed opinion, the successful management of HIV and AIDS-related diseases should go hand in hand with the fight against poverty.

Conclusion

Despite considerable progress in the provision of ART, many people who are eligible for ART under WHO's new guidelines are not yet enrolled onto treatment. Several challenges continue to plaque and slow down the roll-out of ART in most African countries. Key among these are clinical issues that subtract from the acceptability and cellular safety of antiretroviral drugs, infrastructural and human resources shortages that impede expansion, and funding constraints that threaten the sustainable supply of ART. At a personal level, many of these challenges make people needing treatment to seek out the use of anti-HIV natural products including ethnomedicinal plants and mushrooms that compliment, rather than substitute, the efficacy of ART. To formalize the use of natural products, public health policy is embracing scientific validation of natural products, in order to ascertain their anti-HIV properties and cytotoxicity. Going forward, bioprospecting and evaluation of natural products may also lead to the discovery of novel antiretroviral drugs that are less toxic and more efficacious.

Essential Points

- The demand for ART services exceeds the supply. Many people are not yet receiving treatment.
- Patients that encounter ART failure because of resistant HIV strains usually seek the use of putative anti-HIV natural products.
- Individuals that suffer liver, kidney and pancreas damage due to ART likely switch to anti-AIDS natural products.
- Persons that experience symptoms of lactic acidosis, for example, nausea and vomiting, prefer natural products to ART.
- In most African countries, laboratory facilities are too inadequate to determine the extent of ART-induced liver, kidney and pancreas impairment.
- The insufficient number of skilled workers at public health ART clinics leads to long patient queues. This exasperates patients seeking ART services. Consequently, when push comes to shove, patients give up and find solace in the use of natural products.

References

Abere, T.A., & Agoreyo, F.O. (2006). Antimicrobial and toxicological evaluation of the leaves of *Baissea axillaries* Hua used in the management of HIV/AIDS patients. *BMC Complementary and Alternative Medicine, 6*:22.

African Biosciences Initiative (2005). *Business Plan 2005-2010.* Pretoria: NEPAD Office of Science and Technology.

Amon, J.J. (2008). Dangerous medicines: unproven AIDS cures and counterfeit antiretroviral drugs. *Globalization and Health, 4,* 5.

Babb, D.A., Pemba, L., Seatlanyane, P., Charalambous, S., Churchyard, G.J., & Grant, A.D. (2004). Use of traditional medicine in the era of antiretroviral therapy: experience from South Africa. Int Conf AIDS, Bangkok, Thailand, 11-16 July 2004.

Bessong, P.O., Obi, C.L., Andreola, M.L., Rojas, L.B., Pouysegu, L., Igumbor, E., Meyer, J.J., Quideau, S., & Litvak, S. (2005). Evaluation of selected South African medicinal plants for inhibitory properties against human immunodeficiency virus type 1 reverse transcriptase and integrase. *Journal of Ethnopharmacology, 99*(1), 83-91.

Boyd, M.R., Hallock, Y.F., Cardellina II, J.H., Manfredi, K.P., Blunt, J.W., McMahon, J.B., Buckheit Jr, R.W., Bringmann, G., & Schaeffer, M. (1994). Anti-HIV michellamines from *Ancistrocladus korupensis. J Med. Chem., 37*(12), 1740-1745.

Broder, S. (2010). The development of antiretroviral therapy and its impact on the HIV-1/AIDS pandemic. *Antiviral Research, 85*(1), 1-18.

Calixto, B.J. (2000). Efficacy, safety, quality control, marketing and regulatory guidelines for herbal medicines (phytotherapeutic agents). *Braz J Med Biol Research, 33,* 2.

Chinsembu, K.C. (2009). Model and experiences of initiating collaboration with traditional healers in validation of ethnomedicines for HIV/AIDS in Namibia. *Journal of Ethnobiology and Ethnomedicine, 5*:30.

Chinsembu, K.C., & Hedimbi, M (2009). A survey of plants with anti-HIV active compounds and their modes of action. *Medical Journal of Zambia, 36* (4), 178-186.

Chinsembu, K.C., & Hedimbi, M. (2010). Ethnomedicinal plants and other natural products with anti-HIV compounds and their putative modes of action. *International Journal for Biotechnology and Molecular Biology Research, 1*(6), 74-91.

Chinsembu, K.C., & Mutirua, T. (2008). Validation of traditional medicines for HIV/AIDS treatment in Namibia. A report of the study visit to Zambia and South Africa. Windhoek, Namibia: University of Namibia.

Eley, B., & Nuttall, J. (2007). Antiretroviral therapy for children: challenges and opportunities. *Annals of Tropical Paediatrics: International Child Health*, *27*(1), 1-10.

Government of the Republic of Namibia. (2009). United Nations General Assembly Special Session (UNGASS) country report, reporting period 2008-2009. Windhoek: Ministry of Health and Social Services.

Hamers, R.L., Wallis, C.L., Kityo, C., Siwale, M., Mandaliya, K., Conradie, F., ... & de Wit, T.F.R. (2011). HIV-1 drug resistance in antiretroviral-naive individuals in Sub-Saharan Africa after rollout of antiretroviral therapy: a multi-centre observational study. *The Lancet Infectious Diseases*, *11*(10), 750-759.

Hamzah, L., & Post, F.A. (2009). HIV and kidney disease. *Medicine*, *37*(7), 365-367.

Hardon, A., Desclaux, A., Egrot, M., Simon, E., Micollier, E., & Kyakuwa, M. (2008). Alternative medicines for AIDS in resource-poor settings: insights from exploratory anthropological studies in Asia and Africa. *Journal of Ethnobiology and Ethnomedicine*, *4*:16.

Hupfeld, J., & Efferth, T. (2009). Drug resistance of human immunodeficiency virus and overcoming it by natural products. *In vivo*, *23*(1), 1-6.

Igbinosa, O.O., Igbinosa, E.O., & Aiyegoro, O.A. (2009). Antimicrobial activity and phytochemical screening of stem bark extracts from *Jatropha curcas* L. *African Journal of Pharmacy and Pharmacology*, *3*(2), 058-062.

Kamatenesi, M.M. (2010). 1053 Nutri-medicinal plants usage in the management of immuno-compromised ailments in Uganda. *Pediatric Research*, *68*, 523-523.

Kayombo, E.J., Uiso, F.C., Mbwambo, Z.H., Mahunnah, R.L., Moshi, M. J., & Mgonda, Y.H. (2007). Experience of initiating collaboration of traditional healers in managing HIV and AIDS in Tanzania. *Journal of Ethnobiology and Ethnomedicine*, *3*(1), 6.

Klos, M., van de Venter, M., Milne, P.J., Traore, H.N., Meyer, D., & Oosthuizen, V. (2009). *In vitro* anti-HIV activity of five selected South African medicinal plant extracts. *Journal of Ethnopharmacology*, *124*, 182-188.

Kostova, I., Raleva, S., Genova, P., & Argirova, R. (2006). Structure-activity relationships of synthetic coumarins as HIV-1 inhibitors. *Bioinorganic Chemistry and Applications*, *2006*.

Lemoine, M., & Ingiliz, P. (2012). Liver injury in HIV monoinfected patients: Should we turn a blind eye to it? *Clinics and Research in Hepatology and Gastroenterology*, *36*(5), 441-447.

Leteane, M.M., Ngwenya, B.N., Muzila, M., Namushe, A., Mwinga, J., Musonda, R., ... & Andrae-Marobela, K. (2012). Old plants newly discovered: *Cassia sieberiana* DC and *Cassia abbreviata* Oliv. Oliv. root extracts inhibit *in vitro* HIV-1c replication in peripheral blood mononuclear cells (PBMCs) by different modes of action. *Journal of Ethnopharmacology*, *141*(1), 48-56.

Lindegaard, B., Keller, P., Bruunsgaard, G., & Pedersen, B.K (2004). Low plasma level of adiponectin is associated with stavudine treatment and lipodystrophy in HIV-infected patients. *Clin. Exp. Immunology*, *135*(2), 273-279.

Montagnier, L. (2010). 25 years after HIV discovery: prospects for cure and vaccine. *Virology*, *397*(2), 248-254.

NEPAD. (2001). The New Partnership for Africa's Development Founding Document. Abuja: Nigeria.

Ramana, L.N., Anand, A.R., Sethuraman, S., & Krishnan, U.M. (2014). Targeting strategies for delivery of anti-HIV drugs. *Journal of Controlled Release*, *92*, 271-283.

Reihling, H.C.W. (2008). Bioprospecting the African renaissance: the new value of muthi in South Africa. *Journal of Ethnobiology and Ethnomedicine*, 4:9.

Richman, D.D., Margolis, D.M., Delaney, M., Greene, W.C., Hazuda, D., & Pomerantz, R.J. (2009). The challenge of finding a cure for HIV infection. *Science*, *323*(5919), 1304-1307.

Singh, D., Singh, B., & Goel, R.K. (2011). Traditional uses, phytochemistry and pharmacology of *Ficus religiosa*: A review. *Journal of Ethnopharmacology*, *134*(3), 565-583.

Van Wyk, B.E., & Gericke, N. (2000). *People's plants: A guide to useful plants of Southern Africa*. Briza Publications.

Vermani, K., & Garg, S. (2002). Herbal medicines for sexually transmitted diseases and AIDS. *Journal of Ethnopharmacology 80*, 49-66.

Wester, C.W., Okezie, O.A., Thomas, A.M., Bussmann, H., Moyo, S., Muzenda, T., ... & Marlink, R.G. (2007). Higher-than-expected rates of lactic acidosis among highly active antiretroviral therapy-treated women in Botswana: preliminary results from a large randomized clinical trial. *Journal of Acquired Immune Deficiency Syndrome*, *46*(3), 318-322.

World Health Organisation. (1989). *In vitro* screening of traditional medicines for anti-HIV activity:memorandum from a WHO meeting. Bulletin of the World Health Organization 87: 613–618.

World Health Organization (2013). Consolidated guidelines on the use of antiretroviral drugs for treating and preventing HIV infection: Recommendations for a public health approach. WHO: Geneva.

Zuber, A., McCarthy, C.F., Verani, A.R., Msidi, E., & Johnson, C. (2014). A survey of nurse-initiated and-managed antiretroviral therapy (NIMART) in practice, education, policy, and regulation in East, Central, and Southern Africa. *Journal of the Association of Nurses in AIDS Care* (*in press*).

2 Anti–HIV Natural Products

Introduction

Do plants and other natural products have a role to play in protecting the human body from HIV/AIDS? Absolutely! In the battle against HIV, plants and other natural products are not just the rear-guard; they are at the frontline. In the fight against AIDS, natural products can deliver a better future. Natural products are not a distant prospect in the treatment of HIV infection and management of AIDS. They are the new reality, a biomedical and health imperative. Human health and natural products are inseparable. Natural products provide intelligent molecules to combat HIV.

For centuries, natural products have been used to treat various diseases. The significance of plants, mushrooms, microorganisms, marine organisms, and animal products in the management of human ailments cannot be overstated. Therefore, this chapter describes and analyses the storeroom of natural products that possess anti-HIV properties. But then again, some of the anti-HIV natural products are fascinating as they elicit one or two questions:

- Surely, can drinking tea help slow the spread of HIV in infected individuals?
- Should African governments allow the use of marijuana as an anti-HIV agent?

The aim of this chapter is threefold, and this will provide the answers to the two questions above: to showcase the pharmacy of natural products - plants, fungi, algae, marine organisms, and etc. - with anti-HIV activities; to describe the active ingredients present in the natural products and to determine the mechanisms or modes of action by which the active compounds inhibit strategic and specific steps in the HIV life cycle.

Empirically, many scientists including Yu, Morris-Natschke and Lee (2007) acknowledge that natural products contain anti-HIV active ingredients such as terpenoids, coumarins, alkaloids, polyphenols, tannins and flavonoids. Gambari and Lampronti (2006) also affirm that several plant compounds have inhibitory effects against different steps of the HIV life cycle, including virus–cell fusion and virus absorption, reverse transcription, integration and proteolytic cleavage. Plants and other natural products present multiple barricades to HIV infection. No doubt, medicinal plants are an excellent source of clinically relevant anti-HIV molecules. Let's start with a nice cup of tea. Drinking tea, lots of tea, can help alleviate HIV/AIDS.

Tea

Many parts of the plant *Camellia sinensis* including leaves, leaf buds and internodes are processed by various techniques into raw products for making tea. Tea is an aromatic beverage mainly prepared by pouring hot or boiling water over cured leaves of the tea plant. After water, tea is probably the most widely consumed beverage in the world. Since time immemorial, tea is a beverage that has been imbibed for social and health reasons. Depending on the geographical origins, processing methods and the degree of fermentation, a couple of different teas can be distinguished: Green tea, white tea, yellow tea, oolong tea, black tea and Pu-erh tea.

Hajiaghaalipour, Kanthimathi, Sanusi and Rajarajeswaran (2014) opine that white tea is an unfermented tea made from young tea leaves or unopened buds covered with tiny, silvery hairs, and the leaves are harvested once a year in the early spring. The leaves are then steamed rapidly and dried with a minimum amount of processing to prevent oxidation. On the other hand, green, oolong and black teas are processed to a greater extent compared to white tea, though green tea is also unfermented. Huang, Yang, Li, Zheng, Wang, Yang, and Zheng (2012) say Pu-erh tea is produced through microbial fermentation of leaves harvested from a large-leaf variety of *C. sinensis*.

Since the 1980s, the health benefits of tea have become a subject of scientific interest. Huang and others assert that Pu-erh tea has various health benefits including slowing or preventing of carcinogenesis, alleviating heart disease, easing symptoms of rheumatoid arthritis and repairing the immune system. In Paris, a study of 131,401 people aged 18 to 95 years showed that drinking tea cuts the risk of dying early by a quarter. Antioxidant ingredients in tea are good for the heart. Teas contain naturally occurring chemical compounds called catechins. Catechin derivates have a wide spectrum of biological actions, including (Hajiaghaalipour et al., 2014): antioxidant, antiviral, anticancer, antibacterial, antifungal, antitoxoplasmal, antitrypanosomal, anticoccidial, antinematodial and antihelminthic.

Many of the health benefits of tea are due to the role of catechins in scavenging for reactive oxygen species, modification of signal transduction at cell cycle checkpoints and during apoptosis and the regulation of various enzymes that interfere with drug metabolism. Indeed, the results of

Hajiaghaalipour et al. (2014) are unequivocal that white tea protects normal human cells from DNA damage, and has antioxidant and antiproliferative outcomes against malignant cells. Serafini, Del Rio, Yao, Bettuzzi and Peluso (2011) also agree that the health benefits associated with drinking tea are due to the antioxidant and free radical scavenging activities of flavonoids, including catechins and other polyphenols.

It goes without saying that regular intake of tea can help preserve good health and guard the body against disease. Do teas work against HIV? Well, they actually do. In fact, you need to drink more and more tea because tea provides many health benefits.

Laboratory experiments show that catechins in green tea stop HIV from binding to host cells (Huang et al., 2012). Besides blocking HIV's post-adsorption entry into host cells, catechins also inhibit HIV reverse transcriptase. Catechins from black tea also disrupt the molecular architecture of the HIV-1 gp41 envelope protein, resulting in the failure of HIV to fuse to the host cell membrane. Other tests have shown that extracts from Pu-erh tea have low cytotoxicity and do inhibit HIV-induced cytopathic effects (Huang et al., 2012). Pu-erh tea also acts in synergy with antiretroviral drugs such as AZT.

A study by Nance, Siwak and Shearer (2009) showed that catechins are present in green and black teas. Catechins are an important group of polyphenols which make up approximately 13-30% of the dry weight of green tea leaves. The four main catechin derivatives include the isomers epicatechin, (-)-epicatechin gallate, (-)-epigallocatechin, and (-)-epigallocatechin gallate (EGCG). EGCG is the most ubiquitous and active catechin derivate of green tea because of the pyrogallol and galloyl moieties with physiological concentrations ranging from 0.1 to 10 mmol per litre. Zhao, Jiang, Liu, Chen, and Yi (2012) found that catechins with a galloyl moiety, isolated from tea, inhibit HIV-1 integrase, the enzyme that inserts the HIV cDNA into the genome of infected human cells.

Seven cups of green tea (containing 118 mg EGCG each) would result in a mean peak plasma level within the physiologically relevant range of 1.0 mmol per litre. Among the biomodulative properties of EGCG are the anti-inflammatory and antiallergic effects such as inhibition of type IV allergic responses and histamine release, as well as antioxidative, antitumour and antiviral activities. Nance et al. (2009) resolved that epigallocatechin gallate inhibits HIV-1 replication by targeting several steps in the HIV-1 life cycle, such as interfering with the reverse transcriptase and protease activities, blocking gp120-CD4 interaction by binding to CD4 cells, and inactivating HIV particles, though almost all of these results are at high non-physiological dosages greater than 10 mmol per litre of EGCG.

In terms of binding, EGCG mimics gp120 and binds in the same molecular pocket on CD4 as HIV-1 gp120. EGCG, at 0.170 mmol per litre, a concentration equivalent to that obtained by the consumption of two cups of green tea, reduces the attachment of gp120 to CD4 by a factor of between 10- and 20-folds (Nance et al., 2009). In this way, blocking of HIV-1 gp120 binding to the CD4 receptor by the green tea catechin EGCG is specifically responsible for the inhibition of HIV-1 infectivity at physiologic concentrations. Likewise, the EGCG-induced inhibition is effective in a broad range of HIV-1 subtypes without compromising the survival of lymphocytes.

The work of Nance and fellow workers is fascinating because epigallocatechin gallate inhibits HIV-1 infectivity of human CD4 cells and macrophages in a dose-dependent fashion. At a physiologic concentration of 6 mmol per litre, EGCG drastically halts HIV-1 p24 antigen production in several HIV-1 clinical isolates and subtypes. By preventing the attachment of HIV gp120 to the CD4 molecule, EGCG inhibits HIV-1 infectivity. Since this inhibition is achieved at human body concentrations, the anti-HIV agent EGCG, present in black and green teas, is an excellent natural ingredient for HIV therapy.

Liu, Lu, Zhao, He, Niu and Debnath et al. (2005) maintain that theaflavins and catechins are the major polyphenols in black tea and green tea, respectively. Several tea polyphenols, especially those with galloyl moiety, inhibit HIV-1 replication with multiple mechanisms of action. Liu and others illustrated that theaflavin derivatives have more compelling anti-HIV-1 activity than catechin products. Theaflavin and its derivatives, commonly known as theaflavins, are antioxidant polyphenols formed from the condensation of flavan-3-ols in tea leaves.

Tea polyphenols prohibit HIV-1 entry into target cells by blocking HIV-1 envelope glycoprotein-mediated membrane fusion. Their results signify that tea, especially black tea - with high levels of theaflavins, is a magnificent source of anti-HIV agents. Theaflavin derivatives are being studied as lead compounds for developing HIV-1 entry inhibitors targeting gp41. All in all, teas are a welcome resource that should become part of the therapeutic arsenal of anti-HIV natural products.

The next anti-HIV natural product, marijuana, quite contentious as it may be, decreases HIV's devastation and spread.

Marijuana

In many parts of the world, the use of the herb *Cannabis sativa*, commonly called marijuana, engenders strong feelings on either side of the issue. Politics and morality override science and the medical benefits of marijuana and patients needing the medicinal uses of the plant are caught in the middle of the fight. But many voices are now calling for the decriminalization of cannabis. It is not a secret that marijuana is more widespread than any other street drug, with more than 227 million users worldwide (2012 estimate).

Therefore, marijuana is among the most widely used illicit drugs. The main active substance in marijuana is tetrahydrocannabinol, THC, which affects cannabinoid receptor 1 in the brain and cannabinoid receptor 2 in the periphery, producing psychoactive effects that make people feel high. *C. sativa* is not a uniform plant or product, varying considerably in genotype, cultivation tech niques and methods of processing. The resulting phenotypes have remarkable temporal and spatial variations in potency.

Seventy-six per cent of medical doctors in the United States of America say they would approve the use of marijuana to help ease a woman's pain from breast cancer. Use of marijuana in the United States of America is not new. According to Dr. Sanjay Gupta, chief medical correspondent for Cable News Network (CNN), marijuana was until 1943 part of the United States of America drug pharmacopoeia. One of the conditions for which it was prescribed was neuropathic pain. Dr. Gupta writes that between 1840 and 1930, several papers describe the use of medical marijuana to treat neuralgia, convulsive disorders and emaciation, among other things. The last condition, emaciation, is where marijuana may really be used to manage wasting due to HIV/AIDS.

In the United States of America, the approved cases for which cannabis may be doctor-recommended vary at the state level, but most States allow medical use of cannabis for certain medical disorders and problems such as cancer, severe and chronic pain and HIV/AIDS. In 2008, it was shown that *C. sativa* has anti-HIV-1 activity. A study found that *C. sativa* contains denbinobin, a natural 1,4-phenanthrenequinone that prevents HIV-1 reactivation (Sánchez-Duffhues, Calzado, de Vinuesa, Caballero, Ech-Chahad, & Appendino et al., 2008). Denbinobin does not inhibit HIV reverse transcription and integration. However, other than stopping HIV reactivation, denbinobin also works as an antioxidant and an anti-inflammatory agent.

There is growing recognition that individuals with HIV report greater cannabis use than the general population. Occasional cannabis use is associated with increased adherence to ART and general relief of HIV symptoms (Bonn-Miller, Oser, Bucossi, & Trafton, 2014). People living with HIV/AIDS, including those on ART, use marijuana to prevent nausea and stimulate appetite (Mukhtar, Arshad, Ahmad, Pomerantz, Wigdahl, & Parveen, 2008). Whereas the scientific evidence regarding the use of marijuana in HIV/AIDS may be overwhelming, harmonisation of the medical and moral questions over the use of marijuana perhaps still requires wet towels on our heads.

Marijuana is a good medicinal drug for HIV-infected persons. People living with HIV use marijuana to offset side effects ensuing from ART medications. A 2014 study shows that taking marijuana - a daily dose of THC -

decreases HIV's destruction of immune cells in addition to reducing the spread of HIV infection. Scientists in the United of States of America have uncovered a novel inhibitory function of THC during HIV-1 infection of macrophages. A study by Williams, Appelberg, Goldberger, Klein, Sleasman and Goodenow (2014) says administration of THC during macrophage differentiation renders the cells less susceptible to HIV-1 infection.

The researchers reveal that THC treatment of monocytes during differentiation into macrophages results in decreased HIV-1 receptor levels. Their results raise the possibility that extended marijuana use might decrease macrophage susceptibility to HIV-1 infection. How does the THC in marijuana decrease macrophage destruction by HIV? Williams and co-workers opine that the mechanism of THC suppression of HIV-1 infection is due to a reduction in the expression of cell surface HIV receptors CD4, CCR5 and CXCR4. Reduction of these receptors diminishes the efficiency of HIV to enter and destroy human immune cells.

According to the United Nations 2014 Drug Report, cannabis use in West and Central Africa is estimated at 12.4%, significantly higher than the global average of 3.8%. This scenario may partly be explained by the plethora of medical uses of cannabis - especially its benefits for HIV/AIDS patients - in traditional African societies, including Southern Africa, where cannabis is known by the name *Mbanje*. The United Nations report says the main exporter in Africa is South Africa, followed by Zambia, Nigeria, Egypt and Kenya. Best estimates for prevalence of cannabis use are 14.3% (Nigeria), 9.5% (Zambia), and 3.6% (South Africa).

Ginseng

As early as the 1st century, *Panax ginseng*, family Araliaceae, was already famous as one of the most important Chinese and Korean herbal medicines for the promotion of body power and resistance to infections. Many studies describe the diverse physiological functions of ginseng in diseases such as cancer, neurodegenerative disorders, insulin resistance and hypertension. Ginseng maintains homeostasis of the immune system and increases the body's resistance to sickness and microbial infections.

By the year 2005, more than 40 ginsenosides had been isolated from ginseng. Among these, some triterpene saponins have anti-HIV protease activity. Similarly, triterpene aglycones from ginseng have potent anti-HIV protease activity. Scientists from China and Japan have also shown that triterpenoids and oleanolic acid from ginseng hinder the function of HIV protease (Wei, Ma, & Hattori, 2009).

Mangroves

The plant genus *Excoecaria,* family Euphorbiaceae, is a part of the mangroves of Southeast Asia. In Thailand, extracts from this plant genus induce contractions of the uterus, thus they contain uterotonic chemical agents. One of the species is *Excoecaria acerifolia,* widely distributed in the dry hot valleys of Yunnan and Sichuan provinces of Southwest China, where it is used as an ethnodrug (Gua-jing-ban) with antidote, anti-malaria and antiviral properties (Huang, Zhang, Ma, Zheng, Xu, & Peng et al., 2013). These authors have now traced the anti-HIV purposes of the mangrove *E. acerifolia* to phenols, triterpe noids, and diterpenoids. These compounds decrease HIV replication. Yu, Morris-Natschke and Lee (2007) stated that diterpenoid lactones, phenolic diterpenes and phorbol diterpenes have anti-HIV activities.

iKhataso and Other anti-HIV Plants in Southern Africa

In South Africa, rhizomes and roots of *Alepidea amatymbica* are used as herbal medicine for the treatment of colds, chest complaints, asthma, flu, diarrhoea, abdominal cramps, sore throat and rheumatism (Louvel, Moodley, Seibert, Steenkamp, Nthambeleni, & Vidal et al., 2013). Known under the Zulu name iKhataso, the plant *A. amatymbica* contains several diterpenoid kaurene derivatives and phenolic acids. Louvel and colleagues discovered that *A. amatymbica* has moderate anti-HIV activity. However, coupled with poor bioavailability, its direct use to treat HIV/AIDS is quite limited.

Hurinanthan (2013) screened South African medicinal plants for anti-HIV activity. She found that *Cleome monophylla, Leonotis leonurus* and *Dichrostachys cinerea* aqueous leaf extracts had anti-HIV-1 reverse transcriptase activities. *Dichrostachys cinerea,* which inhibits 82% of reverse transcriptase action, is also known by the names *Museledele* in siLozi (Namibia and Zambia), and *Mwege* (*Mweghe*) in the Kavango languages of Namibia. In Namibia and Zambia, *Muselesele* is used to manage oral candidiasis and venereal diseases. *Mwege* is also applied against stomach ache, dysentery and malaria. Clearly, *D. cinerea* is a multi-use ethnomedicinal plant species whose functions are well suited to manage the myriad of disorders associated with AIDS in Southern Africa. The predominant polyphenol 3,4,5 tri-O-galloylquinic acid in the Namibian and South African resurrection plant species *Myrothamnus flabellifolia* inhibits HIV-1 reverse transcriptase.

In her laboratory assays, Hurinanthan (2013) demonstrated that water extracts of *D. cinerea* have the best anti-HIV action with a selectivity index of 43.5. Also, the plant *D. cinerea* has high antioxidant activity and considerable inhibitory activity against HIV-1 reverse transcriptase. In HIV positive persons, oxidative stress and free radicals increase the rate at which HIV infection progresses to AIDS. Corollary, use of *D. cinerea*, with its high antioxidant content, slows progression to AIDS. Biochemical analyses suggest that the anti-HIV actions of *D. cinerea* are due to the presence of catechins, the plant's active principle, as well as the rich content of tannins, saponins, flavonoids and alkaloids.

Hurinanthan (2013), quoting several authors, lists several plants with anti-HIV activities: *Adansonia digitata, Aspilia pluriseta, Aleurites moluccana, Calotropis gigantean, Cuscuta sandwichiana, Eugenia malaccensis, Justicia reptans, Neurolaena lobata, Pipturus albidus, Pluchea indica, Pouteria viridis, Psychotria hawaiiensis, Rumex bequaertii* and *Scaevola sericea*. The common baobab tree, *A. digitata*, known as *Mubuyu* in the siLozi language of Namibia and Zambia, or *Euyu* in Rukwangali tribe of Namibia, is also a well-known remedy for AIDS-related opportunistic infections such as coughs, sexually transmitted infections, malaria, dysentery and diarrhoea. Extracts from the following plants also have anti-HIV reverse transcriptase activities: *Jatropha curcas, Acalypha macrostrachya, Combretum molle, Hyptis lantanifolia, Momordica balsamina, Terminalia sericea, Tuberaria lignosa* and *Phyllanthus myrtifolius*.

Daphne and *Trigonostemon*

Huang, Zhang, Li, Kong, Jiang, Ma and co-workers (2012) say that the plant *Daphne acutiloba* grows in the wet valleys of South-western China at 2,000 metres above sea level. It is a member of the family Thymelaeaceae, which also includes the plant *Daphne genkwa*, a well-known species whose fragrant flowers are commonly used in folk Chinese medicine for anticancer functions. Huang and associates have shown that plant species in the genus *Daphne* contain various compounds including coumarins, lignans, and daphnane-type diterpene esters with anti-HIV activities. Zhang, Huang, Gu, Yang, Chen, and Zheng et al.. (2014), working in China, isolated wikstroelide M, a daphnane diterpene from *Daphne acutiloba* (family Thymelaeaceae) with potent HIV-1 and HIV-2 inhibitory activities whose mechanisms of action include inhibition of reverse transcriptase.

The first daphnane diterpenoid was isolated from the plant *Trigonostemon reidioides*. Some members of the genus *Trigonostemon* (family Euphorbiaceae), widely distributed in China, for example, *Trigonostemon chinensis, T. lii, T. thyrsoideum, T. filipes, T. howii, T. heterophyllus* and *T. xyphophylloides*, contain diverse compounds including diterpenoids, alkaloids and phenanthrenes (Cheng, Chen, He, Zhang, Li, & Tang et al., 2013). These constituents have a variety of biological properties such as anti-flu and anti-mosquito larval activities, inhibition of HIV-1-induced cytopathic effects, and antimicrobial activities.

Studies show that daphnane-type and tigliane-type diterpenoids exhibit antiviral activities. Cheng et al. (2013) corroborate that five daphnane diterpenoid compounds, isolated from the methanol extract of the twigs and leaves of *Trigonostemon thyrsoideum*, have potent anti-HIV-1 activity, with effective concentration values of 0.015–0.001 nM and therapeutic index values of 1,618–17,619. *Trigonostemon lii* has moderate anti-HIV activity (Li, Zhang, Huang, Zheng, Di, & Li et al., 2013). Their mode of action is mainly through inhibition of the cytopathic effects of HIV on CD4 cells. The hallmark of AIDS is depletion of CD4 cells, which is partly due to the direct cytopathic effect of the virus.

Artemisia annua, *Callophyllum inophyllum* and *Bersama engleriana*

The Chinese medicinal herb *Artemisia annua*, family Asteraceae, is mainly used to treat malaria. The most important active ingredient of this plant is artemisinin. Although *A. annua* is native to Asia, it now being introduced to other parts of the world, primarily because of its antimalarial efficacy. Interestingly, Lubbe, Seibert, Klimkait and Van der Kooy (2012) observed that local people use *A. annua* to treat HIV/AIDS in Cameroon, Kenya and Uganda. *Artemisia* also inhibits hepatitis B and HIV replication. The compounds responsible for inhibiting HIV replication are two flavonoids, arcapillin and isorhamnetin, and a coumarin called aesculetin. Therefore, in many regions of Africa where malaria is endemic and widespread, *Artemisia* presents a potential malaria-HIV/AIDS combination therapy.

Callophyllum inophyllum, the most abundant species of this genus, is an evergreen tree in the tropical lands of Africa, America and Asia. In French Polynesia, the plant is locally called as *Tamanu* where it is used in traditional medicine. Laure, Raharivelomanana, Butaud, Bianchini, and Gaydou (2008) affirm that dipyranocoumarins extracted from members of the *Calophyllum* genus generally exhibit anti-HIV-1 properties. Specifically, (+)-calanolide A, a 4-propyl-dipyranocoumarin, inhibits HIV-1 reverse transcriptase.

In Cameroon, West Africa; Mbaveng, Kuete, Mapunya, Beng, Nkengfack, Meyer and Lall (2011) found that the plant *Bersama engleriana* from Bafou in the western region has anticancer properties. Besides, Mbaveng and collaborators revealed that *B. engleriana* has anti-HIV properties.

Anti-HIV Plants in Botswana

Several plants are used to manage HIV and AIDS-related opportunistic infections in Botswana. These plants include: *Dichrostachys cinerea (Moselesele)*, *Maerua angolensis (Moretete/Moreketi)*, *Mimusops zeyheri (Mmupudu)*, *Albizia anthelmintica (Monoga)*, *Plumbago zeylanica (Masigomabe)*, *Combretum imberbe (Motswiri)*, *Indigofera flavicans (Tshikadithata)*, *Clerodendrum ternatum (Legonyana)*, *Solanum panduriforme (Thulathulane)*, *Capparis tomentosa (Motawana)*, *Terminalia sericea (Mogonono)* and *Maytenus senegalensis (Mothono)*. Many Tswana traditional healers use the plant *Cassia abbreviata*, family Caesalpiniaceae, to manage backache, abdominal pains, diarrhoea, constipation, toothache, fever, sexually transmitted infections and ulcers. Others use *Cassia sieberiana* as an ethnomedication for bilharzia, leprosy, dysentery, diarrhoea, haemorrhoids, sexually transmitted infections, malaria and eczema.

Experiments have elucidated that *C. sieberiana* root and bark extracts block HIV replication (Leteane, Ngwenya, Muzila, Namushe, Mwinga, & Musonda et al., 2012). Also, *C. abbreviata* inhibits HIV entry into human cells. But caution should be exercised when dealing with plant extracts containing lots of tannins because tannins cause non-specific interference with HIV replication. While crude plant extracts can show non-specific anti-HIV properties due to the presence of tannins, the Botswana experiments involving *C. sieberiana* and *C. abbreviata* extracts inhibited HIV even after the removal of the tannins.

Phut-nam-but or *Rak-na* in Thailand

Certain ethnomedicines possess anti-HIV properties but are also cytotoxic, which makes them of less therapeutic value. This is the case with *Gardenia carinata*, a member of the Rubiaceae family. According to Kongkum, Tuchinda, Pohmakotr, Reutrakul, Piyachaturawat and Jariyawat et al. (2012), the genus *Gardenia* consists of more than 80 species, widely distributed in the tropical forests of the world. In Thailand, *G. carinata*, also known as *Phut-nam-but* or *Rak-na*, is rich in flavonoids which possess anti-HIV and, unfortunately, cytotoxic properties too.

Peltophorum africanun

Mazimba (2014), at the University of Botswana, has reviewed the pharmacology and phytochemistry of *Peltophorum africanum*, a plant widely used in African traditional medicine. The root and bark decoctions are used to treat eye infections, joints and back pains, toothache, abdominal disorders, diarrhoea, dysentery, infertility, skin rashes, blisters, sexually transmitted infections, depression, parasites, coughs and sore throat. Other medicinal roles involve the use of the bark as a cure for fever besides inducing vomiting and cleansing the liver.

In Zimbabwe, Mazimba, quoting other workers, writes that *P. africanun* root decoctions and infusions detoxify blood, treat infertility, heal wounds and relieve toothache. The plant also has ethnoveterinary applications and is used against major human diseases including tuberculosis and HIV/AIDS. It is known as *Muzeze* in the Nhema communal area of Zimbabwe. Known as *Muparara* in the Rukwangali tribe of Namibia, *P. africanum* is traditionally used to manage HIV/AIDS-related diseases such as tuberculosis, diarrhoea, dysentery, gonorrhoea, syphilis, coughs and sore throat.

In Zambia, the stem bark and roots of the tree *P. africanum*, known as *Munyele* among the Lozi people of Western Province, is used to heal sexually transmitted infections. South Africans use *P. africanum*, called *Mosehla* by the Bapedi people, to treat HIV/AIDS (Semenya, Potgieter, & Erasmus, 2013). In terms of ethnomedicinal remedies, *P. africanum* is, no doubt, a multi-use plant.

A study by Theo, Masebe, Suzuki, Kikuchi, Wada and Obi et al. (2009) revealed that *P. africanum* contains an anti-HIV agent known as betulinic acid. Although betulinic acid may have some toxic properties (Killinger, Shah, & Moszczynska, 2014), several betulinic acid derivatives are potent and highly selective inhibitors of HIV-1. Betulinic acid works by inhibiting HIV fusion as well as interfering with one of the steps in HIV maturation.

Phyllanthus

The genus *Phyllanthus*, family Euphorbiaceae, is widely distributed throughout most of tropical and subtropical countries. Kalidas and Mohan (2009) posit that several *Phyllanthus* species have become a topical issue because of their therapeutic uses in folk medicine, mainly due to their diverse secondary metabolites. In Indonesia, a decoction of *Phyllanthus amarus* is used for kidney and liver ailments. In Nigeria, sexually transmitted infections, chest pains and smallpox are treated using *P. amarus*.

Eldeen, Seow, Abdullah and Sulaiman (2011) assert that in many parts of Asia, Southern Africa and South America, symptoms of cough, jaundice, gonorrhoea, dysentery, diabetes, skin ulcers, headache, stomach-ache, sore throat, dysentery and wounds are alleviated by the use of *Phyllanthus acidus, Phyllanthus debilis, Phyllanthus pulcher, Phyllanthus reticulatus, Phyllanthus urinaria* and *Phyllanthus myrtifolius*. Some of these conditions are associated with AIDS-related microbial infections and oxidative stress.

Eldeen et al. (2011) detected strong inhibition of HIV reverse transcriptase in extracts of Malaysian *P. pulcher, P. urinaria* and *P. myrtifolius*. In the mid-1990s, Chang, Lin, Lee, Liu, Hsu and Lin (1995) illustrated that two lignans, phyllamycin B and retrojusticidin B, isolated from the Chinese plant *P. myrtifolius*, have a strong inhibitory effect on HIV-1 reverse transcriptase activity.

Pine Cones

In traditional Chinese medicine, pine cones are used in the treatment of bronchitis, cough, asthma and other diseases. Cone extracts from some species of *Pinus* in the Pinaceae family possess antiviral, antitumour and immunomodulatory properties. Now, Chinese scientists Zhang, Yang, Liu, Liu, Zheng, Lv, Li and Zheng (2012) have shown that pine cone extract from *Pinus yunnanensis* has anti-HIV action.

Pine cone extracts block HIV entry into cells, inhibit HIV reverse transcriptase, stop HIV-induced breakdown of cells and impede fusion of HIV-infected cells with uninfected cells. Most importantly, pine cone extracts are active against HIV-resistant strains. Five active compounds are found in *P. yunnanensis*: dihydrokaempferol, 7,15-dihydroxydehydroabietic acid, protocatechuic acid, vanillic acid and n-dodecane.

Combretaceae

In Ethiopia, extracts from the plant *C. molle* inhibited HIV reverse transcriptase (Asres & Bucar, 2005). Similar results were obtained in South Africa where the methanol extract of the roots of *C. molle* had the highest inhibitory effect on the ribonuclease H activity of HIV-1 (Bessong, Obi, Andréola, Rojas, Pouységu, & Igumbor et al., 2005). The Ethiopian study indicated that an acetone fraction has the highest selective inhibition of HIV-1 replication.

Phytochemical investigations of this fraction revealed that the HIV inhibitory properties could be mediated by two tannins and two oleanane-type pentacyclic triterpene glycosides. A natural agent, gallotannin, isolated from *C. molle*, inhibits RNA-dependant-DNA polymerase activity of HIV-1 reverse transcriptase. Another member of the Combretaceae, *Terminalia chebula*, contains gallic acid and galloyl glucose which hamper the activity of HIV enzymes reverse transcriptase and integrase (Narayan, Rai, & Tewtrakul, 2013).

Terminalia sericea is used to treat many AIDS-related bacterial infections such as diarrhoea and sexually transmitted diseases. Known as *Muhonono* in the Lozi dialects of Namibia and Zambia and *Mugoro* in the Kavango and *Omwoolo* in the Owambo tribes of Namibia, *T. sericea* has many applications in the management of HIV/AIDS-related diseases (Chinsembu & Hedimbi, 2010). Studies conducted by one of Chinsembu's doctoral research students, Marius Hedimbi, at the CSIR in South Africa, have shown that extracts from stem barks, roots and leaves of *Omwoolo* from northern parts of Namibia inhibit HIV reverse transcriptase at very low concentrations. *Omwoolo*, too, has very low cytotoxicity, meaning it is safe for use as an anti-HIV ethnodrug in humans. Similar anti-HIV and cytotoxicity data were obtained for *Terminalia pruniodes*, known as *Omunghama* in Ovamboland.

Tshikalange, Meyer, Lall, Munoz, Sancho, Van de Venter and Oosthuizen (2008) found that *T. sericea* extract (IC_{50} = 92 mg/ml) has greater alpha-glucosidase inhibitory activity than that of acarbose (IC_{50} = 131 mg/ml). In their reverse transcriptase assay, *T. sericea* also displayed far much higher inhibitory activity (IC_{50} = 43 mg/ml) than that of the reference drug adriamycin IC_{50}

= 100 mg/ml). But, some workers sound caution over the human safety of *T. sericea*, saying the plant is toxic. *T. sericea* contains a bioactive compound called anolignan B, which has anti-inflammatory action and broad-spectrum activity against bacteria; 3.8 μg/ml against *Bacillus subtilis* (gram-positive bacteria) to 31 μg/ml against *Escherichia coli* (gram-negative bacteria) (Eldeen, Elgorashi, Mulholland, & van Staden, 2006).

Although *T. sericea* demonstrates very strong activity against the HIV-1 RNA-dependent DNA polymerase and HIV-1 RNase enzymes with 98% and 99% inhibition, respectively (Bessong, Obi, Igumbor, Andreola, & Litvak, 2004), the same plant may contain high levels of toxic tannins (Ndhlala, Ncube, Okem, Mulaudzi, & van Staden, 2013; Wink & Van Wyk, 2008). In experiments performed in Tanzania, Moshi and Mbwambo (2005) concluded that, with the exception of the dichloromethane and petroleum ether extracts, all the intermediate and polar extracts of *T. sericea* were toxic to brine shrimps giving lethal concentration values ranging from 5.4 to 17.4 mg per ml, while that of cyclophosphamide, a standard anticancer drug, was 16.3 mg per ml.

While differences in the reported toxicities of *T. sericea* may be confounding, it is plausible that extracts of *T. sericea* from Namibia are less cytotoxic because the plants are different biotypes, growing under different climatic and soil conditions, which may confer them with altered profiles of secondary metabolites. Plus, depending on the methods and solvents for extraction, the resultant substances may have different levels of cytotoxicity. As a result, in Moshi and Mbwambo's analysis, dichloromethane and petroleum ether extracts of *T. sericea* were not significantly toxic.

Rhus chinensis

The etthnomedicinal plant *Rhus chinensis* is part of the indigenous flora of China and Japan. It has been used for the management of flu, fever, cough and malaria. Wang, Gu, Wang, Zhang, Yang and Zhou et al. (2008) have worked on the medicinal plant R. *chinensis*. Wang and co-workers showed that stem extracts of R. *chinensis* repress HIV-1 activity by targeting late stages of the life cycle.

During laboratory assays, compounds from the plant subjugated syncytium formation. A benzofuranone-type compound, believed to be a novel anti-HIV-1 agent, curbs late steps of the HIV-1 life cycle. Compound 13, which inhibits HIV-1 replication, also blocks the integration of HIV into the human genome. Wang, Gu, Yang, Chen, Li and Zheng (2006) found that R. *chinensis* also interrupts syncytium formation and blocks the HIV-1 p24 antigen.

Marine Organisms

Oceans and seas contain ernomous biological diversity and concurrent chemical diversity. The first census of marine life (2000–2010) inventorized high levels of marine biodiversity and increased known marine species from approximately 230,000 to nearly 250,000 (Zhou, Liu, Yang, Lin, Yang, & Liu, 2013). With tens or even hundreds of millions of microbial species, Graig Venter's metagenomics expeditions have identified more than 1.2 million new genes.

In a review of 132 anti-HIV natural products from marine sources obtained during the period 2002–2011, Mehbub, Lei, Franco and Zhang (2014) state that sponges contribute more than half of all anti-HIV natural products from marine organisms. These include alkaloids and cyclic depsipeptides such as cortistatin A, a recently discovered natural steroidal alkaloid isolated from the marine sponge *Corticium simplex.* Cortistatin A potently suppresses Tat-dependent HIV transcription. Cyclodepsipeptides from marine sponges also inhibit HIV entry.

Brown algae, which have a high concentration of phlorotannins, possess anti-HIV activity. An active chemical compound called 6,6'-bieckol, one of the main phloroglucinol derivatives naturally occurring in the brown alga *Ecklonia cava*, potently inhibits HIV-1 induced syncytia formation, lytic effects, and viral p24 antigen production (Artan, Li, Karadeniz, Lee, Kim, & Kim, 2008).

Vo and Kim (2010) have reviewed anti-HIV agents from marine biological resources. They mention marine-derived anti-HIV agents such as phlorotannins, sulfated chitooligosaccharides, sulfated polysaccharides, lectins and bioactive peptides. According to these authors, lectins or carbohydrate-binding proteins are found in a variety of different species, ranging from prokaryotes to corals, algae, fungi, plants, invertebrates and vertebrates. Vo and Kim (2010) posit that lectins have the potential to block the binding of HIV to target cells, preventing HIV infection and dissemination.

The bad news is that although marine organisms are excellent sources for anti-HIV agents, development of marine natural prodrugs into pharmaceuitical drugs still faces several challenges such as toxic side effects, problems of large-scale production and cultivation and drug resistance. However, biochemical techniques hope to remove or modify toxic groups in order to produce new chemical derivatives with safer and more superior potencies than the original compounds. Thus, going forward, marine organisms will still prove very useful in the discovery of novel drugs for HIV/AIDS.

Homalanthus nutans

Narayan et al. (2013) describe *Homalanthus nutans* as a plant with remarkably potent anti-HIV activities. Its active ingredient is a 12-deoxyphorbol molecule called prostratin, a powerful activator of HIV replication and expression in latently infected T-cells. Therefore, as part of ART, prostratin from *H. nutans* is used to bring 'out of hiding' latent HIV particles from reservoirs such as lymph nodes.

Prostratin may be likened to the loud sounds of a *vuvuzela*, the long horn blown by football fans in South Africa. The action of prostratin produces a big shout out to HIV, calling the latent HIV particles out of hiding from lymph nodes and other cellular sanctuaries and reservoirs, so that the virus is exposed to lethal concentrations of the antiretroviral drugs.

Search for Anti-HIV Agents - Part 1

Chinsembu and Hedimbi (2010) reviewed ethnomedicinal plants and other natural products with anti-HIV active compounds and their putative modes of action. In October-December 2009, they searched for the key words "plants with anti-HIV activity" in PubMed Central, the United States of America National Library of Medicine's digital archive of biomedical and life sciences journal literature. PubMed is a free database comprising more than 24 million citations for biomedical literature from MEDLINE, life science journals and online books. Citations include links to full-text content from PubMed Central and publisher websites. During the literature search, up to 250 journal publications were reviewed.

The search documented 40 plant families containing 65 plant species, two fungal families containing four mushroom species (*Ganoderma lucidum*, *Grifola frondosa*, *Ganoderma pfeifferi* and *Inonotus obliquus*), and one blue-green algae (*Nostoc ellipsosporum*), respectively, with known anti-HIV active compounds. It was fascinating that some of the pharmacological data that were downloaded, dating as far back as 1989, had not been included in previous reviews. The species of plants and other natural products with known anti-HIV activity and their modes of action are described in Table 2.1. After that, Table 2.2 shows natural products whose active compounds and mechanisms of action are not clearly known.

Inhibitors of General Replication

Citing several studies, Chinsembu and Hedimbi (2010) confirm that many active compounds inhibit general HIV replication (Table 2.1). Among these are diterpene lactones from *Andrographis paniculata* and *Tripterygium wilfordii*, triterpene lactone and lancilactone from *Kadsura lancilimba*, biflavonoids from *Rhus succedanea*, and lanostane-type triterpenes from *Polyalthia suberosa*. Others are suksdorfin from *Lomatium suksdorfii*, wedelolactone (a coumarin) and orobol (an isoflavone derivative) from *Arctium lappa*, caffeic acid tetramers from *Arnebia euchroma*, and celasdin from *Celestrus hindsii*.

Rhus succedanea, a plant in the family Anacardiaceae, secretes two biflavonoids, robustaflavone and hinokiflavone, that stop HIV replication. The fruit extracts of two Leguminosae plants, *Gleditsia japonia* and *Gymnocladus chinensis*, produce two triterpenoid saponins which block replication of HIV in human white blood cells. Suksdorfin, a coumarin from *Lomatium suksdorfii*, also has anti-HIV activity. It suppresses HIV replication in lymphocytes.

Since their isolation from *Calophyllum lanigerum* in 1992, the calanolides have been reported to be active against early stage reproduction of HIV-1. The alkaloid, papaverine, produced by the plant *Papaver sominiferum* inhibits HIV replication and suppresses the production of HIV proteins (Yadav, Jaiswal, Singh, Mishra, & Jain, 2009). Then there is nuciferine, an aporphine alkaloid from *Argemone mexicana*, which inhibits HIV in human lymphocytes. Another triterpene, suberosol, extracted from *Polyalthia suberosa*, inhibits HIV replication activity in lymphocytes.

Entry Inhibitors

Table 2.1 illustrates that most of the entry inhibitors were lectins such as agglutinins from *Galanthus nivalis* and *Hippeastrum* hybrids which stop the spread of HIV among cells. BanLec, a jacalin-related lectin that binds to glycosylated viral envelopes, blocks HIV-1 entry into cells. Cyanovirin, an 11 kilo Dalton protein isolated from *Nostoc ellipsosporum*, targets gp120 proteins and blocks fusion of HIV-1 to lymphocyte membranes. Glycoprotein complexes from *Ganoderma* mushrooms inhibit HIV-1 gp120 binding to CD4 cells. A code-named compound, PJ-S21, from *Punica granatum* inhibits the binding of gp120 to cells expressing CXCR4 receptors.

Reverse Transcriptase Inhibitors

Many different chemical compounds are active against HIV reverse transcriptase (Table 2.1). Some HIV reverse transcriptase inhibitors include michellamines, triterpenes, triterpene lactone, coumarins, isoflavone derivatives, caffeic acid tetramers, calanolide A, hypericin, 3-hydroxy lauric acid, gallotannin, flavonone-xanthone glucoside, linearol, catechins, cepharanthine, galloylquinic acids, velutin, nitidine, oleanolic acid, nigranoic acid, sulfated polysaccharides and harmine.

Integrase Inhibitors

Table 2.1 reveals that some known active compounds are HIV integrase inhibitors: Flavonoid gallate ester from *Acer okamotaanum* of the Aceraceae family, dicaffeoylquinic acids from *Achyrocline satureioides* of the Asteraceae family, gallic acid and galloyl glucose from *Termainalia chebula* of the Combreataceae family and curcumin from *Curcuma* species in the Zingiberaceae family. In Zambia, for example, the Sondashi formula *SF2000*, developed by Dr. Ludwig Sondashi, consists of extracts from four plants that are believed to synergistically decrease viral load by blocking HIV integrase.

Protease Inhibitors

Other active compounds are HIV protease inhibitors. These include ganoderiol, ganodermanontriol and ganoderic acid B (a triterpene) from *Gonoderma* mushrooms; lignins from *Gonoderma* and *Inonotus obliquus*, commonly known as chaga mushroom; uvaol and ursolic acid from *Crataegus pinatifida*, and maslinic acid (a triterpene acid) from the plant *Geum japonicum*; limonoids, including limonin and nomilin and secondary metabolites from citrus fruit species belonging to the Rutaceae family (Table 2.1).

Inhibitors of Syncytium Formation and Cytopathic Effect

Various active compounds inhibit syncytium formation, a property of HIV that makes infected and healthy CD4 cells to fuse and form one giant cell with as many as 500 nuclei. Syncytia-inhibiting compounds include: diterpene lactones, michellamines A and B, and limonoids. Other natural compounds prevent HIV-induced cytopathic effects: sulfated lentinan, sulfonated polysaccharides, xanthohumol, cordatolides, laxofloranone, ganoderiol, ganodermamontriol, ganoderic acid, sulfated (1-3)-β-D-glucan with (1-6)-β-D-glucosyl branches and palicourein which inhibits cytopathic effects of HIV. The alkaloid castanospermine from the Australian tree *Castanospermum australe* blocks the glycosylation stage of HIV replication - it stops glycoprotein processing via inhibition of glucosidase I located in the endoplasmic reticulum.

Inhibitors of Multiple and Unknown Targets

Coumarins and naturally occurring benzopyrene derivatives from several plant species possess antioxidant, anti-inflammatory, antithrombotic, antiviral, anticarcinogenic, antiallergic, hepatoprotective and anti-HIV properties (Kostova, Raleva, Genova, & Argirova, 2006). Furthermore, fifty different compounds - including tannins, terpenoids, flavonoids, flavones, alkaloids, coumarins, lignans, lignin-polysaccharide complexes and lectins - found in many different plant species, inhibit adsorption, viral fusion, HIV reverse transcriptase, HIV integrase, HIV protease and snyctium formation.

According to Yadav et al. (2009), the mushroom *G. lucidum* produces terpenes that constrain HIV-1 induced cell death in addition to inhibiting HIV-1 protease activity. Glycyrrhizin, from renowned Chinese folk medicine licorice root (*Glycyrrhiza* spp.), is another anti-HIV terpenoid. Glycyrrhizin partially stops the adsorption of HIV-1 particles to CD4 cells.

Chinsembu and Hedimbi (2010) reviewed that L-canavanine from *Sutherlandia frutescens* has activity against HIV but interacts with the efflux of nevirapine. D-pinitol, also from *S. frutescens*, has been suggested as a treatment for wasting in cancer and AIDS patients. Recent evidence shows that D-Pinitol, chemically known as 3-O-methyl-D-chiro-inositol, is an active ingredient of *Diospyros mespliformis* leaves, whose crude extracts inhibit HIV. D-Pinitol is also known to possess anti-diabetic activity. Chinsembu and Hedimbi (2010) showed that catechin (a flavonoid), bergenin (a C-galloyl-glycoside) and betulinic acid have been isolated from *Peltophorum africanum*, an important Southern African ethnomedicinal plant for diarrhoea, dysentery, sore throat, HIV/AIDS and other sexually transmitted infections.

Diterpene lactones isolated from the ethanol extract of *Tripterygium wilfordii* (Celastraceae) exhibit potent anti-HIV activity in lymphocytes. *Actaea racemosa*, formerly called *Cimicifuga racemosa*, is a species of flowering plants in the family Ranunculaceae. The rhizome of this plant, commonly known as black cohosh, produces a terpenoid saponin called actein which has an anti-HIV principle. Cucurbitacins isolated from the leaves of *Cowania mexicana* (Rosaceae) also show anti-HIV properties. Acacetin-7-O-beta-D-galactopyranoside, a natural flavonoid isolated from the methanol extract of the flower heads of *Chrysanthemum morifolium*, has also shown strong anti-HIV action.

Search for Anti-HIV Agents - Part 2

In August-September 2014, a search for the words "plants for HIV/AIDS" was conducted in ScienceDirect.com, a leading pay-to-view full-text scientific database offering journal articles and book chapters from nearly 2,500 journals and 26,000 books. It is a website operated by the Anglo-Dutch publisher Elsevier. The search produced 416 results which were analyzed for the presence of anti-HIV agents.

Inhibitors of General Replication

Several inhibitors of HIV replication exist in natural products. The climb-er plant *Momordica balsamina*, also known as *Lombwalombwa* in the siLozi language of Zambia, is used by traditional healers in Nigeria to manage HIV/AIDS. Bot, Mgbojikwe, Nwosu, Abimiku, Dadik and Damshak (2007) confirmed that *M. balsamina* fruit pulp is a potent inhibitor of HIV replication. In Zambia, *Lombwalombwa* is used to treat gonorrhoea, syphilis, and AIDS-related opportunistic infections.

Scientists in the United States of America have discovered that altertoxins, isolated from endophytic fungi *Alternaria tenuissima* inhabiting the stem tissue of the plant *Quercus emoryi*, totally inhibits replication of HIV-1 (Bashyal, Wellen-siek, Ramakrishnan, Faeth, Ahmad, & Gunatilaka, 2014). According to these authors, plant-associated microorganisms, especially endophytic fungi, are rich sources of novel and bioactive secondary metabolites. *A. tenuissima* is a sapro-phytic fungal pathogen inhabiting various plant species. Many *Alternaria* sp. contain perylene oxides and alterperylenols which possess antibacterial, anti-fungal, mutagenic and phytotoxic activities.

Perera, Berna, Scott, Lemaitre-Guillier and Bernier (2008) describe a DING protein, isolated from St John's Wort (*Hypericum perforatum*), which in hibits HIV replication. Proteins belonging to the so-called DING family of proteins, named for their conserved N-terminus which starts with DINGGG, are still poorly studied although they are ubiquitous in animals. In the one letter code for amino acids, DING represents Asp (D)-Ile (I)-Asn (N)-Gly (G). The DING proteins are also present in a few prokaryotes and plants.

Chemical compounds from the root bark of the plant *Zanthoxylum ailan-thoides* significantly inhibit HIV replication in H9 lymphocyte cells (Cheng, Lee, Tsai, & Chen, 2005). Then there is *Daphne odora*, a species of flowering plants in the family Thymelaeaceae, native to China, Japan and Korea. Three flavans, daphnodorins A, B and C isolated from *D. odora*, wield their anti-HIV-1 action through inhibition of the early stages of replication and attachment of the viri-ons to subsequent cells (Yusa, Oh-hara, Tsukahara, Baba, Taniguchi, & Kozawa et al., 1994).

A study by Zhang, Wang, Chen, Zhang, Tam and Zheng (2005) says the chemical compound scutellarin, purified from the plant *Erigeron breviscapus*, in-hibits several processes in HIV-1 replication. *E. breviscapus* is an important herbal drug for the treatment of glaucoma, blood pressure, cardiovascular and cerebral vessel diseases. It grows in the high plateaus of south-west China. Ta-ble 2.3 presents several natural products that inhibit the general HIV replicative cycle.

Inhibitors of HIV Entry and Spread

Bedoya, Abad, Sánchez-Palomino, Alcami and Bermejo (2010), while screening plants from the Iberian Peninsula for anti-HIV activity, explain that an ellagitannin-enriched fraction (EFF) of *Tuberaria lignosa* exhibits antiviral activity against HIV in infected cells, with an IC_{50} value of 2.33 µg/ml (selectivity index greater than 21). Inhibition of HIV infection by this EEF appears to be mediated by CD4 down-regulation, the main receptor for HIV entry.

Earlier, Bedoya, Sanchez-Palomino, Abad, Bermejo and Alcami (2001) evaluated ethanolic and aqueous extracts of 15 medicinal plants widely used in the folk medicine of the Iberian Peninsula. They pointed out that the extracts of *T. lignosa* and *Sanguisorba minor* subsp. *magnolii* exhibit *in vitro* anti-HIV activities. Both plant extracts show no significant cytotoxicity to human cells, meaning active ingredients from these two plants may be developed into antiretroviral drugs.

In Guatemala, Bedoya, Álvarez, Bermejo, González, Beltrán and Sánchez-Palomino et al. (2008) found that extracts from three plants *Justicia reptans*, *Neurolaena lobata* and *Pouteria viridis* inhibit transfer of HIV from dendritic cells to lymphocytes; this is the major route that HIV uses to spread in the body. Table 2.4 presents other natural products that block HIV fusion, entry and spread.

Inhibitors of Reverse Transcriptase

Woradulayapinij, Soonthornchareonnon and Wiwat (2005) studied the *in vitro* HIV-1 reverse transcriptase inhibitory activities of Thai medicinal plants. They tested water and 80% ethanol extracts of 20 Thai medicinal plants used to treat AIDS for their HIV-1 reverse transcriptase inhibitory activity. The water extracts of *Ipomoea carnea* subsp. *fistulosa* (aerial parts), *Vitex glabrata* (branch), *Vitex trifolia* (aerial part), *Vitex negundo* (aerial part), *Canna indica* (rhizome), and *Justicia gendarussa* (aerial part) showed HIV-1 reverse transcriptase inhibition ratio higher than 90% at a 200 µg/ml concentration.

In South Africa, Bessong, Obi, Andréola, Rojas, Pouységu and Igumbor et al. (2005) screened seventeen aqueous and methanol extracts of nine South African medicinal plants. The plants were ethnobotanically selected and evaluated for inhibitory properties against HIV-1 reverse transcriptase. Inhibitory action was seen with the stem-bark of *P. africanum* (Fabaceae) (IC_{50} 3.5 µg/ml) and the roots of *C. molle* (Combretaceae) (IC_{50} 9.7 µg/ml). Extracts of the leaves of Sudanese *Combretum hartmannianum* totally inhibits HIV-1 reverse transcriptase at a concentration of 66 µg/ml (Ali, König, Khalid, Wright, & Kaminsky, 2002).

The known compounds bergenin and catechin and a red coloured gallotannin composed of meta-depside chains of gallic and protocatechuic acids esterified to a 1-O-isobutyroly-β-D-glucopyranose core, were isolated from the methanol extract of the roots and stem-bark of *P. africanum* (Bessong et al., 2005). Gallotannin inhibits HIV reverse transcriptase but catechin and bergenin have no effect on the same enzyme.

Other experiments by Chukwujekwu, Ndhlala, De Kock, Smith and van Staden (2014) attest that *Centratherum punctatum* leaves have HIV-1 reverse transcriptase inhibitory activity (IC_{50} = 52.4 µg/ml). The plant *C. punctatum*, family Asteraceae, is commonly known as the Brazilian bachelor button, a refreshing pineapple-scented bushy perennial plant. In Brazilian traditional medicine, it is used as a treatment for heart ailments. Its leaves have antimicrobial, antioxidant and antiproliferative properties.

Scores of oceanic natural products, too, have pharmacological activities against HIV. In Brazil, Cirne-Santos, Souza, Teixeira, Fontes, Rebello and Castello-Branco et al. (2008) discovered that a dollabelane diterpene (8,10,18-trihydroxy-2,6-dolabelladiene), now called dolabelladienetriol, isolated from the marine brown alga *Dictyota pfaffii*, inhibits HIV-1 reverse transcriptase (EC_{50} = 16.5 µM) and HIV-1 infection of macrophages and peripheral blood mononuclear cells, EC_{50} of 1.7 and 8.4 µM, respectively. These authors established that dolabelladienetriol provides an additive effect when applied together with the nucleoside reverse transcriptase inhibitor AZT, and a synergistic effect with the protease inhibitor atazanavir sulphate.

Using a large panel of HIV-1 isolates harbouring NNRTI resistance mutations, there was no cross-resistance between dolabelladienetriol and available NNRTIs. Therefore, dolabelladienetriol has potent activity against HIV-1 isolates carrying common NNRTI resistance mutations. Dolabelladienetriol, which also inhibits *Leishmania donovani*, is a potentially new agent for HIV-1 therapy, especially drug-resistant strains. Table 2.5 presents other natural products that inhibit HIV reverse transcriptase.

Inhibitors of Integrase

Water soluble extracts of the herbal plant *Salvia miltiorrhiza* have potent effects against HIV-1 integrase activity *in vitro* (Abd-Elazem, Chen, Bates, & Huang, 2002). Methyl gallate, a compound from the edible mushroom *Pholiota adiposa*, inhibits HIV-1 integrase with an IC_{50} value of 228.5 µM (Wang, Zhou, Ng, Wong, Qiao, & Liu, 2014). The plant *Morinda citrifolia*, which has many ethnomedicinal applications in India, especially for the treatment of HIV/AIDS, is rich in flavonoids, anthroquinone and alkaloids. Its different extracts are known to inhibit HIV integrase (Selvam, Maddali, Marchand, & Pommier, 2010). Another Indian plant, *Wrightia tinctoria*, widely used to manage HIV/AIDS, contains indirubin and indigotin which interfere with HIV integrase and cytopathic effects (Selvam, Maddali, & Pommier, 2010). Some more inhibitors of HIV integrase are shown in Table 2.6.

Inhibitors of HIV Protease

Dioscorea membranacea shows appreciable activity (IC_{50} = 48 µg/ml) against HIV-1 protease (Tewtrakul, Itharat, & Rattanasuwan, 2006). A study by Klos, Van de Venter, Milne, Traore, Meyer and Oosthuizen (2009), done in South Africa, shows that ethanol extracts of *Bulbine alooides* and *Leonotis leonurus* inhibit HIV-1 protease. Other natural products that inhibit HIV protease are given in Table 2.7.

Blocking HIV-induced Cytopathic Effects

N-acetylglucosamine-specific lectin isolated from the sea worm *Serpula vermicularis* mitigates the cytopathic effects induced by HIV-1 (Molchanova, Chikalovets, Chernikov, Belogortseva, Li, & Wang et al., 2007). Extracts from another marine worm *Chaetopterus variopedatus* inhibit HIV cytopathic effects (Wang, Kong, Li, Molchanova, Chikalovets, & Belogortseva et al., 2006).

According to El-Mekkawy, Meselhy, Nakamura, Hattori, Kawahata and Otake (2000), five phorbol diesters isolated from the seeds of *Croton tiglium* block HIV-induced cytopathic consequences. While analysing several plants from Panama, Matsuse, Lim, Hattori, Correa and Gupta (1998) also observed that the water extracts from the branches of *Jatropha curcas* (Euphorbiaceae) strongly inhibit HIV-induced cytopathic effects with low cytotoxicity to humans. Other inhibitors of HIV cytopathic effects are presented in Table 2.8. Natural products with other modes of action are presented in Table 2.9.

Search for Anti-HIV Agents - Part 3

The last search was conducted in PubMed using the search terms "anti-HIV plants". It was limited to the years 2008-2014. While many of the search results are presented in Table 2.10, some of the results are discussed below.

A study by Kuo, Qian, Morris-Natschke and Lee (2009) found that moronic acid isolated from Brazilian propolis has remarkable anti-HIV activity. These authors also discovered that betulinic acid has inhibitory effects against HIV-1 replication, with an EC_{50} value of 1.4 µM. Betulinic acid is now a preeminent molecular scaffold in the development of triterpene analogues as anti-HIV drugs. One of the chemicals modified from betulinic acid, bevirimat, is potent against HIV-1 isolates resistant to current reverse transcriptase and protease drugs.

After researchers from Panacos Pharmaceuticals Inc. and the National Institutes of Health zoomed into the action of bevirimat, they illustrated that bevirimat inhibits the processing of the HIV capsid precursor p25 to mature capsid p24. According to these workers, the impaired cleavage of p25 to p24 leads to the production of morphologically defective, non-infectious, and immature HIV particles. Essentially, bevirimat works as an amaturation inhibitor; this is a new class in the antiretroviral family. In 2009, bevirimat was in Phase IIb clinical trials.

Xue, Di, Luo, Cheng, Wei and Shi (2014) have also studied resveratrol (3,4',5-trihydroxystilbene), first isolated from the roots of white hellebore, *Veratrum grandiflorum*. This compound is found in at least 72 plant species, 31 genera and 12 families including Vitaceae, Leguminosae, Gnetaceae, Dipterocarpaceae, and Cyperaceae. It is also widely available in edible foods and beverages such as mulberries, peanuts, grapes and red wines. Resveratrol is classified either as a polyphenol or stilbene and is produced by plants to protect themselves against damage or infection in response to stresses such as heat, insects, bacteria and fungus.

Since 2004, resveratrol has attracted attention due to its potential to treat contemporary human diseases such as cancer, neurodegenerative disease, vascular disease, cardiovascular diseases and aging. Resveratrol oligomers exhibit a plethora of biological actions such as antibacterial, antifungal, anticancer, anti-HIV and antioxidant activities. One of the resveratrol oligomers is hopeaphenol, a tetramer isolated from *Shorea ovalis* and red wines from North Africa.

Studies show that hopeaphenol suppresses the growth of human cancer cells in addition to its antimicrobial and anti-HIV properties. Due to poor bioavailability and cellular uptake, resveratrol only reduces HIV replication by 20-30%, but the potential to use resveratrol in the treatment and prevention of HIV/AIDS has been eloquently discussed by Singh and Pai (2014).

Even the Bible, 1 Timothy 5:23, says: "Stop drinking only water, and use a little wine because of your stomach and your frequent illnesses." There you have it.

Another anti-HIV agent from natural products is genistein, a tyrosine kinase inhibitor present in a couple of plants such as soybeans. Genistein (4', 5, 7-trihydroxyisoflavone) is an isoflavone compound with potential applications in cancer therapy. It is undergoing tests for treatment of diseases such as leukemia and prostate cancer. According to Guo, Xu, Rasheed, Yoder, Yu and Liang et al. (2013), genistein inhibits stromal cell-derived factor 1 mediated chemotaxis of CD4 T cells. These authors have now shown that genistein also inhibits HIV infection of resting CD4 T cells and macrophages by mainly interfering with actin dynamics and HIV post-entry DNA synthesis and, to a lesser extent, HIV DNA nuclear migration in resting T cells. Besides demonstrating that genistein blocks HIV infection, their results raise the possibility of harnessing novel therapeutic strategies that disrupt HIV-mediated signal transduction of actin dynamics.

In a discussion of antiviral natural products and herbal medicines, Lin, Hsu and Lin (2014) say a tricyclic coumarin derived from the stem bark of *Calophyllum brasiliense* inhibits HIV replication by suppressing nuclear factor-kappa B activation. They also cite a novel anti-HIV agent called melittin, which is the active component of bee venom. A nanoformulated melittin product has robust efficiency in capturing and inactivating HIV particles by disrupting the viral lipid envelope. They suggest that there is great potential for natural antivirals against HIV to yield novel therapeutics that may play an important role in overcoming the current pressure to discover safer and more efficacious anti-HIV therapies.

Table 2.10 shows more natural products with anti-HIV properties. These natural products include mushrooms, sea weeds and traditional medicines used in China, India, South Africa and Tanzania.

A Final Look at Anti-HIV Natural Products

Bioprospecting for natural products - including their secondary metabolites - that can be harnessed into anti-infective agents and novel therapeutic drugs promises a more robust revolution than the current age of Information and Communication Technologies. In the face of HIV/AIDS, given the many challenges that subtract from effective ART, and because, in any case, ART is not curative, we need not look further than Mother Nature. Natural products with anti-HIV functions are beckoning right in front of our eyes.

It is amazing that nature knows no bottom. Metaphorically, as long as nature holds up its hands, the human body wins the fight against HIV/AIDS. But, whenever nature lowers its hands - or when nature stands akimbo, HIV delivers a devastating blow and wins. When the balance of nature falls apart, HIV becomes more and more transmutable. It becomes more virulent and resistant to drugs. Yet, for many people living with HIV/AIDS, access to natural products with anti-HIV activities means the difference between life and death.

Think for a second. Primates naturally infected with SIV, including SIV-infected chimpanzees, do not seem to develop immunodeficiency or AIDS. A similar retrovirus to HIV, SIV does not cause AIDS in monkeys and chimpanzees. Ever wondered why? The answer may be firmly anchored in nature. Perhaps, monkeys and chimpanzees, through eating wild organic medicinal natural products, utilize and maximise the benefits of Mother Nature's provisions of anti-AIDS agents. Arguably, a breakdown in the anti-HIV balance of nature may have contributed to SIV from chimpanzees (*Pan troglodytes*) and SIV from sooty mangabeys (*Cercocebus atys*) to become transmutable and even cross the species barrier to generate HIV-1 and HIV-2. The evolution of HIV may be closely linked to human destruction of the balance and equilibrium of nature that may have kept HIV in check.

In this chapter, hundreds of species representing plants, fungi, algae, bacteria and other natural products contain anti-HIV chemical compounds. When one digests the data on anti-HIV natural products, several things come to light. The first common thread in this chapter is the remarkable knowledge that a number of natural products with anti-HIV actions are actually common plants and products such as green tea, marijuana, ginseng, mushrooms, mangroves, sea weeds, pine cones, *Jatropha*, mulberries, peanuts, grapes, red wines, soybeans, bee sting, propolis, microbes and several abundant plant species belonging to the genera *Artemisia*, *Cassia*, *Peltophorum*, and *Terminalia*.

The second theme that emerges from this chapter is that a lot of efforts are being directed at elucidating the anti-HIV agents in natural products. These anti-HIV agents target and block specific steps in the HIV replicative life cycle. Indeed, the chapter unravels agents that inhibit entry and general HIV replication as well as HIV enzymes such as reverse transcriptase, protease and integrase.

Albeit, a modest attempt, this chapter pinpoints scientifically proven anti-HIV natural products. Plants and other natural products are an excellent source of clinically relevant anti-HIV molecules that are in fact an epitome of novel anti-HIV chemotherapeutic leads that should be brought to bear on AIDS. Undoubtedly, extracts from many medicinal plants and other natural products have anti-HIV properties not only *in vitro* but also *in vivo*. This means that consumption of these anti-HIV natural products in sufficient amounts may help to alleviate HIV infection.

Be that as it may, a closer look at anti-HIV natural products reveals a very sad reality about Africa. As a continent, Africa has failed to do with its abundant anti-HIV medicinal plants what China has done. Africa is not doing enough to harness its treasure of anti-HIV natural products. The problem in Africa is Africa itself: Africa has not invested much in Research and Development (R&D) and value-addition of anti-HIV natural products. In other words, Africa has not harnessed the full benefits of its anti-HIV natural products chiefly because the continent lacks the research capacity to isolate, characterize and commercialize anti-HIV agents from natural products.

Even when one looks at the research publications on anti-HIV natural products cited in this chapter, about 4 out of 10 are authored by the Chinese. While the Chinese represent about 41% of all research efforts and publications on anti-HIV natural products, the African share of research on anti-HIV natural products is a paltry 16%. This tells us that the next big discovery of novel natural products to treat HIV/AIDS will be from China, from Chinese medicine. China is the world leader in R&D for innovative anti-HIV agents from natural products.

Hence, although Sub-Saharan Africa accounts for about 70% of all HIV infections, it is ironic that the search for novel anti-HIV treatments and the hotbeds of R&D for anti-HIV natural products are in China, where HIV prevalence rate is less than 0.1% among adults. Africa is not investing enough of her resources in the search for new anti-HIV natural products. This means that Africa will continue to look to the outside world for novel drugs to manage AIDS. Africa has failed to sow the seed of self-reliance in terms of searching for new natural remedies to combat HIV/AIDS. This is disheartening considering that Africa is endowed with abundant anti-HIV natural products.

Elucidating the chemical structures of various anti-HIV natural products is an essential step in the R&D of possible lead compounds into drugs. When the chemical structure of the anti-HIV compound is elucidated, and when the interactions of the compound with cellular receptors are known, the drug molecule can be improved by analysing for structure activity relationships before artificial synthesis, pharmaceutical manufacturing and clinical trials. One can also say that to artificially synthesize the anti-HIV active compound is important in order to avoid the risk of depleting plant bioresources because continuous harvesting of anti-HIV plants can lead to extinction of over-used species.

This chapter is part of a fresh corpus of scholarly works which draws on new empirical evidence to deconstruct the medicinal efficacy of plants and other natural products against HIV infection. The data in this chapter overthrow the long-standing notion held by the medical and pharmaceutical fraternities that crude extracts of medicinal plants, even as used by traditional healers, are ineffective against HIV. In persons with HIV infection, use of anti-HIV plants can make the odds to live healthier and longer lives change dramatically for the better as the ferocious intensity of infection begins to fade and wane steadily. With some hindsight and reflection, this chapter reminds us that plants and HIV are so readily and naturally at war with each other. The co-evolution of medicinal plants and HIV infection has been an antagonistic process, nothing near an amicable coexistence. For ages, plants have devoted their chemical ingredients to the fight against infectious agents and diseases, including HIV/AIDS.

So, let us get this straight: HIV carries distinctive molecular signatures that are naturally thwarted by many chemical anti-HIV agents in medicinal plants. Over the most recent evolutionary past, the anti-HIV capabilities of medicinal plants have increased dramatically. If there is a long-term remedy for HIV/AIDS, it must lie in nature's abundant endowment to humans: Potent antimicrobial plants and other natural products. We should not leave the use medicinal plants to chance or during difficult times, when pharmaceutical drugs have failed- for example, when resistant strains of HIV develop. To maintain healthy bodies, the use of medicinal plants should become etched in our daily lives; it is a goodness of fit that completes the balance of nature.

In closing, five issues need highlighting:

1. Nature is the stronghold of anti-HIV agents. Natural products provide our bodies with the natural defences to fight off HIV and AIDS.
2. But, while we destroy nature's anti-HIV strongholds, when we pollute nature's anti-HIV agents, we open up the human body to HIV, its attendant opportunistic infections and AIDS.
3. Progressing to AIDS is the price we pay for neglecting Mother Nature's provisions of organic antidotes to HIV. As the balance and unity of nature falls apart, HIV becomes more transmutable, more virulent and more resistant to drugs.
4. To this day, man's destruction of the natural environments such as forests and pollution of soils and oceans, is depleting the reservoirs of natural products meant to naturally protect us from HIV.
5. At a personal level, a continuous decline and break down in the consumption of adequate protective anti-HIV natural products, including products with antioxidant activity, quickens progression to AIDS.
6. When not matched by sound empirical data, the use of anti-HIV natural products may easily go awry.

Conclusion

In this chapter, I serve as a guide through the journey of scientific insights into natural products useful in defeating HIV infection. This voyage is aimed at bringing greater understanding to some of the most perplexing anti-HIV properties of plants and other natural products in the world around us.

Many natural products inhibit enzymatic steps during HIV replication and can, therefore, be developed into drugs for treating HIV/AIDS. There are many natural anti-HIV agents that block HIV entry and spread, reverse transcriptase, integrase, protease, syntium formation and cytopathic effects. Some of the natural products actually work much better than current synthetic pharmaceutical antiretroviral drugs. Whereas synthetic pharmaceutical drugs block one enzymatic or replicative step, some natural agents inhibit more than one enzyme and more than one replicative step of HIV. There are some natural products with multi-inhibitory functions.

Primary data of known active compounds and mechanisms of action are mostly available from studies done outside Africa. Most of the studies done in Africa are inconclusive about either the active compounds or mechanisms of action, or both. Although Africa has a wealth of anti-HIV plants and other natural products, the search for anti-HIV agents and isolation of active compounds are carried out elsewhere in Asia, Europe and the Americas. A lack of long-term funding and inadequate infrastructure has conspired to exacerbate Africa's dependency on overseas laboratories for screening for active compounds. Africa's capacity to conduct *in vitro* and *in vivo* tests of natural products against HIV is also poor. This apathy is a perfect recipe for biopiracy.

At the international level, there is an urgent need to fast-track HIV/AIDS clinical trials of candidate drugs developed from novel compounds isolated from plants and other natural sources. This will ensure that the millions of people who require HIV/AIDS treatment will have access to newer, more effective and less toxic antiretroviral drugs. By ignoring many anti-HIV natural products, AIDS interventions fail. Natural products ought to be at the centre of interventions against HIV/AIDS. We cannot overlook the importance of anti-HIV natural products that can help the millions of people already suffering from toxicity and failure of current ART regimes.

Finally, there is an army of natural products that can break the infectious chains of HIV/AIDS. The promise of Mother Nature to protect humans from microbes is still unshaken. The healing of people with HIV/AIDS innately flows from this base pharmacy of natural products. Anti-HIV natural products should be incorporated into teas to be taken as medicinal beverages. This is more so urgent in Africa which, in terms of this new realization to utilize anti-HIV natural products, is lagging behind Asian countries like China where medicinal teas are a common part of officially recognized natural pharmacopoeias.

Every cloud has a silver lining. And when one looks at the dark cloud of HIV/AIDS, that silver lining is mainly made up of plants and other natural products that outdo HIV and related opportunistic infections. Here is the point: Everything we need to fight HIV/AIDS is at our disposal; it is all present in the garden of Mother Nature. All around us, there is a garden of abundant natural products for treating and managing HIV/AIDS and related opportunistic diseases. If only we can harness this garden, we could defeat HIV/AIDS. The available treasure of natural products is a comprehensive life insurance cover against HIV. Nature has destined humanity to defeat AIDS.

References

Abd-Elazem, I.S., Chen, H.S., Bates, R.B., & Huang, R.C.C. (2002). Isolation of two highly potent and non-toxic inhibitors of human immunodeficiency virus type 1 (HIV-1) integrase from *Salvia miltiorrhiza*. *Antiviral Research*, *55*(1), 91-106.

Abdelgadir, H.A., & van Staden, J. (2013). Ethnobotany, ethnopharmacology and toxicity of *Jatropha curcas* L. (Euphorbiaceae): A review. *South African Journal of Botany*, *88*, 204-218.

Ali, H., König, G.M., Khalid, S.A., Wright, A.D., & Kaminsky, R. (2002). Evaluation of selected Sudanese medicinal plants for their in vitro activity against hemoflagellates, selected bacteria, HIV-1-RT and tyrosine kinase inhibitory, and for cytotoxicity. *Journal of Ethnopharmacology*, *83*(3), 219-228.

Artan, M., Li, Y., Karadeniz, F., Lee, S.H., Kim, M.M., & Kim, S.K. (2008). Anti-HIV-1 activity of phloroglucinol derivative, 6, 6'-bieckol, from *Ecklonia cava*. *Bioorganic and Medicinal Chemistry*, *16*(17), 7921-7926.

Asada, Y., Sukemori, A., Watanabe, T., Malla, K.J., Yoshikawa, T., Li, W., ... & Lee, K.H. (2013). Isolation, structure determination, and anti-HIV evaluation of tigliane-type diterpenes and biflavonoid from *Stellera chamaejasme*. *Journal of Natural Products*, *76*(5), 852-857.

Asres, K., & Bucar, F. (2005). Anti-HIV activity against immunodeficiency virus type 1 (HIV-I) and type II (HIV-II) of compounds isolated from the stem bark of Combretum molle. *Ethiopian Medical Journal*, *43*(1), 15-20.

Bashyal, B.P., Wellensiek, B.P., Ramakrishnan, R., Faeth, S.H., Ahmad, N., & Gunatilaka, A.L. (2014). Altertoxins with potent anti-HIV activity from *Alternaria tenuissima* QUE1Se, a fungal endophyte of *Quercus emoryi*. *Bioorganic and Medicinal Chemistry*.

Bedoya, L.M., Abad, M.J., Sánchez-Palomino, S., Alcami, J., & Bermejo, P. (2010). Ellagitannins from *Tuberaria lignosa* as entry inhibitors of HIV. *Phytomedicine*, *17*(1), 69-74.

Bedoya, L.M., Márquez, N., Martínez, N., Gutiérrez-Eisman, S., Álvarez, A., Calzado, M.A., ... & Alcamí, J. (2009). SJ23B, a jatrophane diterpene activates classical PKCs and displays strong activity against HIV *in vitro*. *Biochemical Pharmacology*, *77*(6), 965-978.

Bedoya, L.M., Álvarez, A., Bermejo, M., González, N., Beltrán, M., Sánchez-Palomino, S., ... & Alcamí, J. (2008). Guatemalan plants extracts as virucides against HIV-1 infection. *Phytomedicine*, *15*(6), 520-524.

Bedoya, L.M., Sanchez-Palomino, S., Abad, M.J., Bermejo, P., & Alcami, J. (2001). Anti-HIV activity of medicinal plant extracts. *Journal of Ethnopharmacology*, *77*(1), 113-116.

Bessong, P.O., Obi, C.L., Andréola, M.L., Rojas, L.B., Pouységu, L., Igumbor, E., ... & Litvak, S. (2005). Evaluation of selected South African medicinal plants for inhibitory properties against human immunodeficiency virus type 1 reverse transcriptase and integrase. *Journal of Ethnopharmacology*, *99*(1), 83-91.

Bessong, P.O., Obi, C.L., Igumbor, E., Andreola, M.L., & Litvak, S. (2004). In vitro activity of three selected South African medicinal plants against human immunodeficiency virus type 1 reverse transcriptase. *African Journal of Biotechnology*, *3*(10), 555-559.

Bonn-Miller, M.O., Oser, M.L., Bucossi, M.M., & Trafton, J.A. (2014). Cannabis use and HIV antiretroviral therapy adherence and HIV-related symptoms. *Journal of Behavioral Medicine*, *37*(1), 1-10.

Bot, Y.S., Mgbojikwe, L.O., Nwosu, C., Abimiku, A., Dadik, J., & Damshak, D. (2007). Screening of the fruit pulp extract of *Momordica balsamina* for anti HIV property. *African Journal of Biotechnology*, *6*(1), 47-52.

Chang, C.W., Lin, M.T., Lee, S.S., Liu, K., Hsu, F.L., & Lin, J.Y. (1995). Differential inhibition of reverse transcriptase and cellular DNA polymerase-α activities by lignans isolated from Chinese herbs, *Phyllanthus myrtifolius* Moon, and tannins from *Lonicera japonica* Thunb and *Castanopsis hystrix*. *Antiviral Research*, *27*(4), 367-374.

Cheng, M.J., Lee, K.H., Tsai, I.L., & Chen, I.S. (2005). Two new sesquiterpenoids and anti-HIV principles from the root bark of *Zanthoxylum ailanthoides*. *Bioorganic and Medicinal Chemistry*, *13*(21), 5915-5920.

Cheng, Y.Y., Chen, H., He, H.P., Zhang, Y., Li, S.F., Tang, G.H., ... & Hao, X.J. (2013). Anti-HIV active daphnane diterpenoids from *Trigonostemon thyrsoideum*. *Phytochemistry*, *96*, 360-369.

Chinnaiyan, S.K., Subramanian, M.R., Vinoth Kumar, S., Chandu, A.N., & Deivasigamani, K. (2013). Antimicrobial and anti-HIV activity of extracts of *Canthium coromandelicum* (Burm. f.) Alston leaves. *Journal of Pharmacy Research*, *7*(7), 588-594.

Chinsembu, K.C., & Hedimbi, M. (2010). Ethnomedicinal plants and other natural products with anti-HIV active compounds and their putative modes of action. *International Journal of Biotechnology and Molecular Biology Research*, *1*(6), 74-91.

Chukwujekwu, J.C., Ndhlala, A.R., De Kock, C.A., Smith, P.J., & van Staden, J. (2014). Antiplasmodial, HIV-1 reverse transcriptase inhibitory and cytotoxicity properties of *Centratherum punctatum* Cass. and its fractions. *South African Journal of Botany*, *90*, 17-19.

Chung, C.Y., Hwang, T.L., Kuo, L.M., Kuo, W.L., Cheng, M.J., Wu, Y. H., ... & Chen, J.J. (2013). New benzo [c] phenanthridine and benzenoid derivatives, and other constituents from *Zanthoxylum ailanthoides*: Effects on neutrophil pro-inflammatory responses. *International Journal of Molecular Sciences*, *14*(11), 22395-22408.

Cirne-Santos, C.C., Souza, T.M. L., Teixeira, V.L., Fontes, C.F.L., Rebello, M.A., Castello-Branco, L.R.R., ... & Bou-Habib, D.C. (2008). The dolabellane diterpene Dolabelladienetriol is a typical noncompetitive inhibitor of HIV-1 reverse transcriptase enzyme. *Antiviral Research*, *77*(1), 64-71.

Ding, J., Bao, J., Zhu, D., Zhang, Y., & Wang, D.C. (2010). Crystal structures of a novel anti-HIV mannose-binding lectin from *Polygonatum cyrtonema* Hua with unique ligand-binding property and super-structure. *Journal of Structural Biology*, *171*(3), 309-317.

Ding, L., Münch, J., Goerls, H., Maier, A., Fiebig, H.H., Lin, W.H., & Hertweck, C. (2010). Xiamycin, a pentacyclic indolosesquiterpene with selective anti-HIV activity from a bacterial mangrove endophyte. *Bioorganic and Medicinal Chemistry Letters*, *20*(22), 6685-6687.

Eldeen, I.M.S., Seow, E.M., Abdullah, R., & Sulaiman, S.F. (2011). *In vitro* antibacterial, antioxidant, total phenolic contents and anti-HIV-1 reverse transcriptase activities of extracts of seven *Phyllanthus* sp. *South African Journal of Botany*, *77*(1), 75-79.

Eldeen, I., Elgorashi, E.E., Mulholland, D.A., & van Staden, J. (2006). Anolignan B: A bioactive compound from the roots of *Terminalia sericea*. *Journal of Ethnopharmacology*, *103*(1), 135-138.

Ellithey, M.S., Lall, N., Hussein, A.A., & Meyer, D. (2013). Cytotoxic, cytostatic and HIV-1 PR inhibitory activities of the soft coral *Litophyton arboreum*. *Marine drugs*, *11*(12), 4917-4936.

Ellithey, M.S., Lall, N., Hussein, A.A., & Meyer, D. (2014). Cytotoxic and HIV-1 enzyme inhibitory activities of Red Sea marine organisms. *BMC Complementary and Alternative Medicine*, *14*(1), 77.

El-Mekkawy, S., Meselhy, M.R., Nakamura, N., Hattori, M., Kawahata, T., & Otake, T. (2000). Anti-HIV-1 phorbol esters from the seeds of *Croton tiglium*. *Phytochemistry*, *53*(4), 457-464.

Eshwarappa, R.S.B., Iyer, R.S., Subbaramaiah, S.R., Richard, S.A., & Dhananjaya, B.L. (2014). Antioxidant activity of *Syzygium cumini* leaf gall extracts. *BioImpacts: BI*, *4*(2), 101-107.

Férir, G., Hänchen, A., François, K.O., Hoorelbeke, B., Huskens, D., Dettner, F., ... & Schols, D. (2012). Feglymycin, a unique natural bacterial antibiotic peptide, inhibits HIV entry by targeting the viral envelope protein gp120. *Virology*, *433*(2), 308-319.

Gambari, R., & Lampronti, I. (2006). Inhibition of immunodeficiency type-1 virus (HIV-1) life cycle by medicinal plant extracts and plant-derived compounds. *Advances in Phytomedicine*, *2*, 299-311.

Gangwar, M., Goel, R.K., & Nath, G. (2014). *Mallotus philippinensis* Muell. Arg (Euphorbiaceae): Ethnopharmacology and phytochemistry review. BioMed Research International, Volume 2014, Article ID 213973, 13 pages http://dx.doi.org/10.1155/ 2014/213973.

Guo, J., Xu, X., Rasheed, T.K., Yoder, A., Yu, D., Liang, H., ... & Wu, Y. (2013). Genistein interferes with SDF-1-and HIV-mediated actin dynamics and inhibits HIV infection of resting CD4 T cells. *Retrovirology, 10*(1), 62.

Hajiaghaalipour, F., Kanthimathi, M.S., Sanusi, J., & Rajarajeswaran, J. (2014). White tea (*Camellia sinensis*) inhibits proliferation of the colon cancer cell line, HT-29, activates caspases and protects DNA of normal cells against oxidative damage. *Food Chemistry (in press)*.

Helfer, M., Koppensteiner, H., Schneider, M., Rebensburg, S., Forcisi, S., Müller, C., ... & Brack-Werner, R. (2014). The root extract of the medicinal plant *Pelargonium sidoides* is a potent HIV-1 attachment inhibitor. *PloS One, 9*(1), e87487.

Hong, K.J., Lee, H.S., Kim, Y.S., & Kim, S.S. (2011). Ingenol protects human T cells from HIV-1 infection. *Osong Public Health and Research Perspectives, 2*(2), 109-114.

Huang, N., Wu, M.Y., Zheng, C.B., Zhu, L., Zhao, J.H., & Zheng, Y.T. (2013). The depolymerized fucosylated chondroitin sulfate from sea cucumber potently inhibits HIV replication via interfering with virus entry. *Carbohydrate Research, 380,* 64-69.

Huang, N., Yang, L.M., Li, X.L., Zheng, C.B., Wang, R.R., Yang, Y.P., & Zheng, Y. T. (2012). Anti-HIV activities of extracts from Pu-erh tea. *Chinese Journal of Natural Medicines, 10*(5), 347-352.

Huang, S. Z., Zhang, X. J., Li, X. Y., Kong, L. M., Jiang, H. Z., Ma, Q. Y., ... & Zhao, Y. X. (2012). Daphnane-type diterpene esters with cytotoxic and anti-HIV-1 activities from *Daphne acutiloba* Rehd. *Phytochemistry, 75,* 99-107.

Huang, S.Z., Zhang, X., Ma, Q.Y., Peng, H., Zheng, Y.T., Hu, J.M., ... & Zhao, Y.X. (2014). Anti-HIV-1 tigliane diterpenoids from *Excoecaria acertiflia* Didr. *Fitoterapia, 95,* 34-41.

Huang, S.Z., Zhang, X., Ma, Q.Y., Zheng, Y.T., Xu, F.Q., Peng, H., ... & Zhao, Y.X. (2013). Terpenoids and their anti-HIV-1 activities from *Excoecaria acerifolia. Fitoterapia, 91,* 224-230.

Hurinanthan, V. (2013). *Anti-HIV activity of selected South African medicinal plants* (Doctoral dissertation). Durban University of Technology: South Africa.

Jiang, Y., Ng, T.B., Wang, C.R., Zhang, D., Cheng, Z.K., Liu, Z., ... & Liu, F. (2010). Inhibitors from natural products to HIV-1 reverse transcriptase, protease and integrase. *Mini Reviews in Medicinal Chemistry, 10*(14), 1331-1344.

Jiang, Y., Wong, J.H., Fu, M., Ng, T.B., Liu, Z.K., Wang, C.R., ... & Liu, F. (2011). Isolation of adenosine, iso-sinensetin and dimethylguanosine with antioxidant and HIV-1 protease inhibiting activities from fruiting bodies of *Cordyceps militaris. Phytomedicine, 18*(2), 189-193.

Kalidas, C., & Mohan, V.R. (2009). *In vitro* rapid clonal propagation of *Phyllanthus urinaria* Linn. (Euphorbiaceae)- a medicinal plant. *The Researcher, 4,* 61–65.

Kapewangolo, P., Hussein, A.A., & Meyer, D. (2013). Inhibition of HIV-1 enzymes, antioxidant and anti-inflammatory activities of *Plectranthus barbatus*. *Journal of Ethnopharmacology, 149*(1), 184-190.

Khazir, J., Mir, B.A., Pilcher, L., & Riley, D.L. (2014). Role of plants in anticancer drug discovery. *Phytochemistry Letters, 7*, 173-181.

Killinger, B., Shah, M., & Moszczynska, A. (2014). Co-administration of betulinic acid and methamphetamine causes toxicity to dopaminergic and serotonergic nerve terminals in the striatum of late adolescent rats. *Journal of Neurochemistry, 128*(5), 764-775.

Klos, M., Van de Venter, M., Milne, P.J., Traore, H.N., Meyer, D., & Oosthuizen, V. (2009). *In vitro* anti-HIV activity of five selected South African medicinal plant extracts. *Journal of Ethnopharmacology, 124*(2), 182-188.

Kongkum, N., Tuchinda, P., Pohmakotr, M., Reutrakul, V., Piyachaturawat, P., Jariyawat, S., ... & Napaswad, C. (2012). DNA topoisomerase IIα inhibitory and anti-HIV-1 flavones from leaves and twigs of *Gardenia carinata*. *Fitoterapia, 83*(2), 368-372.

Kostova, I., Raleva, S., Genova, P., & Argirova, R. (2006). Structure-activity relationships of synthetic coumarins as HIV-1 inhibitors. *Bioionorg. Chem. Applic., 1*(9), doi 10.1155/BCA/2006/68274.

Kuete, V., Metuno, R., Keilah, P.L., Tshikalange, E.T., & Ngadjui, B.T. (2010). Evaluation of the genus *Treculia* for antimycobacterial, anti-reverse transcriptase, radical scavenging and antitumor activities. *South African Journal of Botany, 76*(3), 530-535.

Kuete, V., Voukeng, I.K., Tsobou, R., Mbaveng, A.T., Wiench, B., Beng, V.P., & Efferth, T. (2013). Cytotoxicity of *Elaoephorbia drupifera* and other Cameroonian medicinal plants against drug sensitive and multidrug resistant cancer cells. *BMC Complementary and Alternative Medicine, 13*(1), 250.

Kumar, S., & Pandey, A.K. (2014). Medicinal attributes of *Solanum xanthocarpum* fruit consumed by several tribal communities as food: an in vitro antioxidant, anticancer and anti HIV perspective. *BMC Complementary and Alternative medicine, 14*(1), 112.

Kumar, S., Chashoo, G., Saxena, A.K., & Pandey, A.K. (2013). Parthenium hysterophorus: a probable source of anticancer, antioxidant and anti-HIV agents. *BioMed Research International, 2013*.

Kuo, R.Y., Qian, K., Morris-Natschke, S.L., & Lee, K.H. (2009). Plant-derived triterpenoids and analogues as antitumor and anti-HIV agents. *Natural Product Reports, 26*(10), 1321-1344.

Lam, S.K., & Ng, T.B. (2010). A dimeric high-molecular-weight chymotrypsin inhibitor with antitumor and HIV-1 reverse transcriptase inhibitory activities from seeds of *Acacia confusa*. *Phytomedicine, 17*(8), 621-625.

Laure, F., Raharivelomanana, P., Butaud, J.F., Bianchini, J.P., & Gaydou, E.M. (2008). Screening of anti-HIV-1 inophyllums by HPLC–DAD of

Calophyllum inophyllum leaf extracts from French Polynesia Islands. *Analytica Chimica Acta, 624*(1), 147-153.

Lee, J., Huh, M.S., Kim, Y.C., Hattori, M., & Otake, T. (2010). Lignan, sesquilignans and dilignans, novel HIV-1 protease and cytopathic effect inhibitors purified from the rhizomes of *Saururus chinensis. Antiviral Research, 85*(2), 425-428.

Leteane, M.M., Ngwenya, B.N., Muzila, M., Namushe, A., Mwinga, J., Musonda, R., ... & Andrae-Marobela, K. (2012). Old plants newly discovered: *Cassia sieberiana* DC and *Cassia abbreviata* Oliv. Oliv. root extracts inhibit in vitro HIV-1c replication in peripheral blood mononuclear cells (PBMCs) by different modes of action. *Journal of Ethnopharmacology, 141*(1), 48-56.

Li, S.F., Zhang, Y., Huang, N., Zheng, Y.T., Di, Y.T., Li, S.L., ... & Hao, X.J. (2013). Daphnane diterpenoids from the stems of *Trigonostemon lii* and their anti-HIV-1 activity. *Phytochemistry, 93*, 216-221.

Liang, J., Chen, J., Tan, Z., Peng, J., Zheng, X., Nishiura, K., ... & Liu, L. (2013). Extracts of the medicinal herb *Sanguisorba officinalis* inhibit the entry of human immunodeficiency virus-1. *Journal of Food and Drug Analysis, 21*(4), S52-S58.

Liang, J., Li, Y., Liu, X., Huang, Y., Shen, Y., Wang, J., ... & Zhao, Y. (2014). *In vivo* and *in vitro* antimalarial activity of bergenin. *Biomedical Reports, 2*(2), 260-264.

Lin, L.T., Hsu, W.C., & Lin, C.C. (2014). Antiviral natural products and herbal medicines. *Journal of Traditional and Complementary Medicine, 4*(1), 24.

Liu, H.T., Liu, J.S., Zhang, J., Guo, Y.J., Qi, Y. D., Jia, X.G., ... & Xiao, P. G. (2014). Chemical constituents in plants of genus *Kadsura* Kaempf. ex Juss. *Chinese Herbal Medicines, 6*(3), 172-197.

Liu, S., Lu, H., Zhao, Q., He, Y., Niu, J., Debnath, A.K., ... & Jiang, S. (2005). Theaflavin derivatives in black tea and catechin derivatives in green tea inhibit HIV-1 entry by targeting gp41. *Biochimica et Biophysica Acta (BBA)-General Subjects, 1723*(1), 270-281.

Louvel, S., Moodley, N., Seibert, I., Steenkamp, P., Nthambeleni, R., Vidal, V., ... & Klimkait, T. (2013). Identification of compounds from the plant species *Alepidea amatymbica* active against HIV. *South African Journal of Botany, 86*, 9-14.

Lubbe, A., Seibert, I., Klimkait, T., & Van der Kooy, F. (2012). Ethnopharmacology in overdrive: The remarkable anti-HIV activity of *Artemisia annua. Journal of Ethnopharmacology, 141*(3), 854-859.

Lv, C., Zheng, Z.L., Miao, F., Geng, H.L., Zhou, L., & Liu, L.P. (2014). New Dihydro-β-agarofuran Sesquiterpenes from Parnassia wightiana Wall: Isolation, Identification and Cytotoxicity against Cancer Cells. *International Journal of Molecular Sciences, 15*(6), 11111-11125.

Lv, H., Kong, Y., Yao, Q., Zhang, B., Leng, F.W., Bian, H.J., ... & Bao, J. K. (2009). Nebrodeolysin, a novel hemolytic protein from mushroom *Pleurotus nebrodensis* with apoptosis-inducing and anti-HIV-1 effects. *Phytomedicine*, *16*(2), 198-205.

Matsuse, I.T., Lim, Y.A., Hattori, M., Correa, M., & Gupta, M.P. (1998). A search for anti-viral properties in Panamanian medicinal plants.: The effects on HIV and its essential enzymes. *Journal of Ethnopharmacology*, *64*(1), 15-22.

Mazimba, O. (2014). Pharmacology and phytochemistry studies in *Peltophorum africanum*. *Bulletin of Faculty of Pharmacy, Cairo University. Bulletin of Faculty of Pharmacy*, 52, 145–153.

Mbaveng, A.T., Kuete, V., Mapunya, B.M., Beng, V.P., Nkengfack, A.E., Meyer, J.J.M., & Lall, N. (2011). Evaluation of four Cameroonian medicinal plants for anticancer, antigonorrheal and antireverse transcriptase activities. *Environmental Toxicology and Pharmacology*, *32*(2), 162-167.

Mehbub, M.F., Lei, J., Franco, C., & Zhang, W. (2014). Marine Sponge Derived Natural Products between 2001 and 2010: Trends and Opportunities for Discovery of Bioactives. *Marine Drugs*, *12*(8), 4539-4577.

Modi, M., Dezzutti, C.S., Kulshreshtha, S., Rawat, A.K.S., Srivastava, S. K., Malhotra, S., ... & Gupta, S.K. (2013). Extracts from *Acacia catechu* suppress HIV-1 replication by inhibiting the activities of the viral protease and Tat. *Virology Journal*, *10*(1), 309.

Modi, M., Pancholi, B., Kulshrestha, S., Rawat, A.K., Malhotra, S., & Gupta, S.K. (2013). Anti-HIV-1 activity, protease inhibition and safety profile of extracts prepared from Rhus parviflora. *BMC Complementary and Alternative Medicine*, *13*(1), 158.

Molchanova, V., Chikalovets, I., Chernikov, O., Belogortseva, N., Li, W., Wang, J.H., ... & Lukyanov, P. (2007). A new lectin from the sea worm *Serpula vermicularis*: Isolation, characterization and anti-HIV activity. *Comparative Biochemistry and Physiology Part C: Toxicology and Pharmacology*, *145*(2), 184-193.

Moshi, M.J., & Mbwambo, Z.H. (2005). Some pharmacological properties of extracts of *Terminalia sericea* roots. *Journal of Ethnopharmacology*, *97*(1), 43-47.

Mukhtar, M., Arshad, M., Ahmad, M., Pomerantz, R.J., Wigdahl, B., & Parveen, Z. (2008). Antiviral potentials of medicinal plants. *Virus Research*, *131*(2), 111-120.

Mushi, N.F., Mbwambo, Z.H., Innocent, E., & Tewtrakul, S. (2012). Antibacterial, anti-HIV-1 protease and cytotoxic activities of aqueous ethanolic extracts from *Combretum adenogonium* Steud. Ex A. Rich (Combretaceae). *BMC Complementary and Alternative Medicine*, *12*(1), 163.

Nance, C.L., Siwak, E.B., & Shearer, W.T. (2009). Preclinical development of the green tea catechin, epigallocatechin gallate, as an HIV-1 therapy. *Journal of Allergy and Clinical Immunology*, *123*(2), 459-465.

Narayan, L.C., Rai, V.R., & Tewtrakul, S. (2013). Emerging need to use phytopharmaceuticals in the treatment of HIV. *Journal of Pharmacy Research*, *6*(1), 218-223.

Narayan, V., Ravindra, K.C., Chiaro, C., Cary, D., Aggarwal, B.B., Henderson, A.J., & Prabhu, K.S. (2011). Celastrol inhibits tat-mediated human immunodeficiency virus (HIV) transcription and replication. *Journal of Molecular Biology*, *410*(5), 972-983.

Ncube, B., van Staden, J., Okem, A., & Ndhlala, A. R. (2013). Hypoxis (Hypoxidaceae) in African traditional medicine. *Journal of Ethnopharmacology*, *50*(3), 818-827.

Ndhlala, A.R., Ncube, B., Okem, A., Mulaudzi, R.B., & van Staden, J. (2013). Toxicology of some important medicinal plants in southern Africa. *Food and Chemical Toxicology*, *62*, 609-621.

Ng, Y.M., Yang, Y., Sze, K.H., Zhang, X., Zheng, Y.T., & Shaw, P.C. (2011). Structural characterization and anti-HIV-1 activities of arginine/glutamate-rich polypeptide luffin P1 from the seeds of sponge gourd (*Luffa cylindrica*). *Journal of Structural Biology*, *174*(1), 164-172.

Nutan, M.M., Goel, T., Das, T., Malik, S., Suri, S., Rawat, A.K.S., ... & Gupta, S.K. (2013). Ellagic acid & gallic acid from *Lagerstroemia speciosa* L. inhibit HIV-1 infection through inhibition of HIV-1 protease & reverse transcriptase activity. *The Indian Journal of Medical Research*, *137*(3), 540.

Ogata, T., Higuchi, H., Mochida, S., Matsumoto, H., Kato, A., Endo, T., ... & Kaji, H. (1992). HIV-1 reverse transcriptase inhibitor from *Phyllanthus niruri*. *AIDS Research and Human Retroviruses*, *8*(11), 1937-1944.

Palamthodi, S., & Lele, S.S. (2014). Nutraceutical applications of gourd family vegetables: *Benincasa hispida*, *Lagenaria siceraria* and *Momordica charantia*. *Biomedicine and Preventive Nutrition*, *4*(1), 15-21.

Pandey, V.C., Singh, K., Singh, J.S., Kumar, A., Singh, B., & Singh, R.P. (2012). *Jatropha curcas*: A potential biofuel plant for sustainable environmental development. *Renewable and Sustainable Energy Reviews*, *16*(5), 2870-2883.

Park, I.W., Han, C., Song, X., Green, L.A., Wang, T., Liu, Y., ... & He, J.J. (2009). Inhibition of HIV-1 entry by extracts derived from traditional Chinese medicinal herbal plants. *BMC Complementary and Alternative Medicine*, *9*(1), 29.

Peng, W., Qin, R., Li, X., & Zhou, H. (2013). Botany, phytochemistry, pharmacology, and potential application of *Polygonum cuspidatum* Sieb. et Zucc.: A review. *Journal of Ethnopharmacology*, *148*(3), 729-745.

Perera, T., Berna, A., Scott, K., Lemaitre-Guillier, C., & Bernier, F. (2008). Proteins related to St. John's Wort p27SJ, a suppressor of HIV-1 expression, are ubiquitous in plants. *Phytochemistry*, *69*(4), 865-872.

Queiroz, K.C.S., Medeiros, V.P., Queiroz, L.S., Abreu, L.R.D., Rocha, H. A.O., Ferreira, C.V., ... & Leite, E.L. (2008). Inhibition of reverse transcriptase activity of HIV by polysaccharides of brown algae. *Biomedicine and Pharmacotherapy, 62*(5), 303-307.

Remoli, A. L., Marsili, G., Battistini, A., & Sgarbanti, M. (2012). The development of immune-modulating compounds to disrupt HIV latency. *Cytokine and Growth Factor Reviews, 23*(4), 159-172.

Sánchez-Duffhues, G., Calzado, M.A., de Vinuesa, A.G., Caballero, F.J., Ech-Chahad, A., Appendino, G., ... & Muñoz, E. (2008). Denbinobin, a naturally occurring 1, 4-phenanthrenequinone, inhibits HIV-1 replication through an NF-κB-dependent pathway. *Biochemical Pharmacology, 76*(10), 1240-1250.

Seca, A.M., Grigore, A., Pinto, D.C., & Silva, A. (2014). The genus *Inula* and their metabolites: From ethnopharmacological to medicinal uses. *Journal of Ethnopharmacology, 154*(2), 286-310.

Selvam, P., Maddali, K., & Pommier, Y. (2010). Studies of HIV-1 integrase inhibitory activity of *Wrightia tinctoria. Antiviral Research, 86*(1), A28.

Selvam, P., Maddali, K., Marchand, C., & Pommier, Y. (2010). Studies of HIV integrase inhibitory activity of *Morinda citrifolia* L non-fruit extracts. *Antiviral Research, 86*(1), A45-A46.

Semenya, S.S., Potgieter, M.J., & Erasmus, L.J.C. (2013). Indigenous plant species used by Bapedi healers to treat sexually transmitted infections: Their distribution, harvesting, conservation and threats. *South African Journal of Botany, 87*, 66-75.

Serafini, M., Del Rio, D., Yao, D.N., Bettuzzi, S., & Peluso, I. (2011). Health benefits of tea. CRC Press, Boca Raton (Florida).

Singh, G., & Pai, R.S. (2014). Recent advances of resveratrol in nanostructured based delivery systems and in the management of HIV/AIDS. *Journal of Controlled Release, 194* (2014), 178-188.

Singh, N., Shaik, S., Dewir, Y., Khanyile, Z., Smith, M., Shode, F., ... & Nicholas, A. (2009). Detection of L-canavanine in the cancer bush (*Lessertia frutescens* L.), a reputed anti-HIV/AIDS medicinal plant. *South African Journal of Botany, 75*(2), 440.

Singh, S., Shenoy, S., Nehete, P.N., Yang, P., Nehete, B., Fontenot, D., ... & Sastry, K.J. (2013). *Nerium oleander* derived cardiac glycoside oleandrin is a novel inhibitor of HIV infectivity. *Fitoterapia, 84*, 32-39.

Srivastava, R. (2014). A review on phytochemical, pharmacological, and pharmacognostical profile of *Wrightia tinctoria*: Adulterant of kurchi. *Pharmacognosy Reviews, 8*(15), 36.

Sun, R., Song, H.C., Wang, C.R., Shen, K.Z., Xu, Y.B., Gao, Y.X., ... & Dong, J.Y. (2011). Compounds from *Kadsura angustifolia* with anti-HIV activity. *Bioorganic and Medicinal Chemistry Letters, 21*(3), 961-965.

Tewtrakul, S., Itharat, A., & Rattanasuwan, P. (2006). Anti-HIV-1 protease-and HIV-1 integrase activities of Thai medicinal plants known as Hua-Khao-Yen. *Journal of Ethnopharmacology, 105*(1), 312-315.

Theo, A., Masebe, T., Suzuki, Y., Kikuchi, H., Wada, S., Obi, C.L., ... Hattori, T., 2009. *Peltophorum africanum*, a traditional South African medicinal plant, contains an anti HIV-1 constituent, betulinic acid. *The Tohoku Journal of Experimental Medicine, 217*(2), 93-99.

Tian, R.R., Chen, J.C., Zhang, G.H., Qiu, M.H., Wang, Y.H., Du, L., ... & Zheng, Y.T. (2008). Anti-HIV-1 activities of hemslecins A and B. *Chinese Journal of Natural Medicines, 6*(3), 214-218.

Tshikalange, T.E., Meyer, J.J.M., Lall, N., Munoz, E., Sancho, R., Van de Venter, M., & Oosthuizen, V. (2008). In vitro anti-HIV-1 properties of ethnobotanically selected South African plants used in the treatment of sexually transmitted diseases. *Journal of Ethnopharmacology, 119*(3), 478-481.

Vo, T.S., & Kim, S.K. (2010). Potential anti-HIV agents from marine resources: an overview. *Marine Drugs, 8*(12), 2871-2892.

Wan, Z., Lu, Y., Liao, Q., Wu, Y., & Chen, X. (2012). Fangchinoline inhibits human immunodeficiency virus type 1 replication by interfering with gp160 proteolytic processing. *PloS One, 7*(6), e39225.

Wang, C.R., Zhou, R., Ng, T.B., Wong, J.H., Qiao, W.T., & Liu, F. (2014). First report on isolation of methyl gallate with antioxidant, anti-HIV-1 and HIV-1 enzyme inhibitory activities from a mushroom (*Pholiota adiposa*). *Environmental Toxicology and Pharmacology, 37*(2), 626-637.

Wang, J.H., Kong, J., Li, W., Molchanova, V., Chikalovets, I., Belogortseva, N., ... & Zheng, Y.T. (2006). A β-galactose-specific lectin isolated from the marine worm *Chaetopterus variopedatus* possesses anti-HIV-1 activity. *Comparative Biochemistry and Physiology Part C: Toxicology and Pharmacology, 142*(1), 111-117.

Wang, R.R., Gu, Q., Wang, Y.H., Zhang, X.M., Yang, L.M., Zhou, J., ... & Zheng, Y.T. (2008). Anti-HIV-1 activities of compounds isolated from the medicinal plant *Rhus chinensis*. *Journal of Ethnopharmacology, 117*(2), 249-256.

Wang, R.R., Gu, Q., Yang, L.M., Chen, J.J., Li, S. Y., & Zheng, Y.T. (2006). Anti-HIV-1 activities of extracts from the medicinal plant *Rhus chinensis*. *Journal of Ethnopharmacology, 105*(1), 269-273.

Wang, S.X., Liu, Y., Zhang, G.Q., Zhao, S., Xu, F., Geng, X.L., & Wang, H.X. (2012). Cordysobin, a novel alkaline serine protease with HIV-1 reverse transcriptase inhibitory activity from the medicinal mushroom *Cordyceps sobolifera*. *Journal of Bioscience and Bioengineering, 113*(1), 42-47.

Wei, Y., Ma, C.M., & Hattori, M. (2009). Anti-HIV protease triterpenoids from the acid hydrolysate of *Panax ginseng*. *Phytochemistry Letters, 2*(2), 63-66.

Wei, Y., Ma, C.M., Chen, D.Y., & Hattori, M. (2008). Anti-HIV-1 protease triterpenoids from *Stauntonia obovatifoliola* Hayata subsp. *intermedia*. *Phytochemistry, 69*(9), 1875-1879.

Williams, J.C., Appelberg, S., Goldberger, B.A., Klein, T.W., Sleasman, J. W., & Goodenow, M.M. (2014). Δ9-Tetrahydrocannabinol treatment during human monocyte differentiation reduces macrophage susceptibility to HIV-1 infection. *Journal of Neuroimmune Pharmacology, 9*(3), 369-379.

Wink, M., & Van Wyk, B.E. (2008). Mind-altering and poisonous plants of the world. Briza Publications, Pretoria.

Wintola, O.A., & Afolayan, A.J. (2014). *Alepidea amatymbica* Eckl. & Zeyh.: A review of its traditional uses, phytochemistry, pharmacology, and toxicology. *Evidence-Based Complementary and Alternative Medicine, 2014.*

Woradulayapinij, W., Soonthornchareonnon, N., & Wiwat, C. (2005). In vitro HIV type 1 reverse transcriptase inhibitory activities of Thai medicinal plants and *Canna indica* L. rhizomes. *Journal of Ethnopharmacology, 101*(1), 84-89.

Wu, T.S., Su, C.R., & Lee, K.H. (2012). Cytotoxic and Anti-HIV Phenanthroindolizidine Alkaloids from *Cryptocarya chinensis*. *Natural Product Communications, 7*(6), 725.

Xue, Y. Q., Di, J.M., Luo, Y., Cheng, K.J., Wei, X., & Shi, Z. (2014). Resveratrol oligomers for the prevention and treatment of cancers. *Oxidative Medicine and Cellular Longevity, 2014 (in press).*

Yadav, I.K., Jaiswal, D., Singh, H.P., Mishra, A., & Jain, D.A. (2009). Anti-HIV drugs from natural sources. *Pharmaceutical Research, 1*(2), 93-109.

Yang, J., Li, L., Tan, S., Jin, H., Qiu, J., Mao, Q., ... & Liu, S. (2012). A natural theaflavins preparation inhibits HIV-1 infection by targeting the entry step: Potential applications for preventing HIV-1 infection. *Fitoterapia, 83*(2), 348-355.

Yu, D., Morris-Natschke, S.L., & Lee, K.H. (2007). New developments in natural products-based anti-AIDS research. *Medicinal Research Reviews, 27*(1), 108-132.

Yusa, K., Oh-hara, T., Tsukahara, S., Baba, K., Taniguchi, M., Kozawa, M., ... & Tsuruo, T. (1994). Inhibition of human immunodeficiency virus type 1 (HIV-1) replication by daphnodorins. *Antiviral Research, 25*(1), 57-66.

Zampella, A., Sepe, V., Luciano, P., Bellotta, F., Monti, M.C., D'Auria, M.V., ... & Homophymine, A. (2008). An anti-HIV cyclodepsipeptide from the sponge *Homophymia* sp. *Journal of Organic Chemistry, 73*, 5319–5327.

Zhang, G.H., Wang, Q., Chen, J.J., Zhang, X.M., Tam, S.C., & Zheng, Y. T. (2005). The anti-HIV-1 effect of scutellarin. *Biochemical and Biophysical Research Communications, 334*(3), 812-816.

Zhang, X., Huang, S.Z., Gu, W.G., Yang, L.M., Chen, H., Zheng, C.B., ... & Zheng, Y.T. (2014). Wikstroelide M potently inhibits HIV replication by targeting reverse transcriptase and integrase nuclear translocation. *Chinese Journal of Natural Medicines, 12*(3), 186-193.

Zhang, X., Yang, L.M., Liu, G.M., Liu, Y.J., Zheng, C.B., Lv, Y.J., ... & Zheng, Y.T. (2012). Potent anti-HIV activities and mechanisms of action of a pine cone extract from *Pinus yunnanensis*. *Molecules, 17*(6), 6916-6929.

Zhao, W.L., Feng, D., Wu, J., & Sui, S.F. (2010). Trichosanthin inhibits integration of human immunodeficiency virus type 1 through depurinating the long-terminal repeats. *Molecular Biology Reports, 37*(4), 2093-2098.

Zhao, W.L., Zhang, F., Feng, D., Wu, J., Chen, S., & Sui, S.F. (2009). A novel sorting strategy of trichosanthin for hijacking human immunodeficiency virus type 1. *Biochemical and Biophysical Research Communications, 384*(3), 347-351.

Zhao, Y., Jiang, F., Liu, P., Chen, W., & Yi, K. (2012). Catechins containing a galloyl moiety as potential anti-HIV-1 compounds. *Drug Discovery Today, 17*(11), 630-635.

Zhou, X., Liu, J., Yang, B., Lin, X., Yang, X.W., & Liu, Y. (2013). Marine natural products with anti-HIV activities in the last decade. *Current Medicinal Chemistry, 20*(7), 953-973.

Table 2.1: Anti-HIV natural products with known active compounds and modes of action

Species	Active compounds	Mode of action
Andrographis paniculata	Aqueous extracts of leaves	Inhibition of HIV protease and reverse transcriptase
	Diterpene lactones (andrographolide)	Inhibit HIV-infected cells from arresting in G2 phase in which viral replication is optimal. Inhibit cell-to-cell transmission, viral replication and syncytia formation in HIV-infected cells
Acer okamotoanum	Flavonoid gallate ester	Anti-HIV-1 integrase activity
Lentinus edodes	Sulfated lentinan	Prevent HIV-induced cytopathic effect
Galanthus nivalis	Plant lectins: *G. nivalis* agglutinin (GNA)	Potent inhibitors that stop the spread of HIV among lymphocytes by targeting gp120 envelope glycoprotein; most prominent anti-HIV activity is found among MBLs; GNA has specificity for terminal α(1-3)-linked mannose residues
Hippeastrum hybrids	*Hippeastrum* hybrid agglutinin (HHA), and monocot mannose-binding lectins (MBLs)	HHA recognizes both terminal and internal α(1-3)- and α(1-6)-linked mannose residues
Rhus succedanea	Biflavonoids, robustaflavone and hinokiflavone	Strong inhibition of the polymerase of HIV-1 reverse transcriptase
Ancistrocladus korupensis	Michellamines A and B	Anti-HIV -1 and anti-HIV-2 activities Act at early stage of the HIV life cycle by inhibiting reverse transcriptase and at later stages by inhibiting cellular fusion and syncytium formation
Polyalthia suberosa	Lanostane-type triterpene, suberosol	Anti-HIV replication activity in H9 lymphocytes cells *in vitro*
Lomatium suksdorfii	Suksdorfin	Suppress HIV-1 viral replication in H9 lymphocyte cells
Panax ginseng	Unknown	Increases CD4/8 cells; has serious side effects
Agardhiella tenera	Sulfonated polysaccharides	Inhibit the cytopathic effect of human immunodeficiency virus type 1 (HIV-1) and type 2 (HIV-2) in MT-4 cells
Bulbine alooides	Aqueous and ethanol extracts	Extracts of *B. alooides*, *H. sobolifera*, Extracts of *B. alooides* retained HIV-1 protease inhibition after dereplication to remove non-specific tannins/ polysaccharides
Achyrocline satureioides *Arctium lappa*	Two dicaffeoylquinic acids: 3,5-dicaffeoylquinic acid, and 1-methoxyoxalyl-3,5-dicaffeoylquinic acid Wedelolactone (a coumarin	Potent and irreversible inhibition of HIV-1 integrase Inhibit HIV-1 replication, block cell-to-cell transmission of HIV-1

	derivative); orobol (an isoflavone derivative).	
Arnebia euchroma	Monosodium and monopotassium salts of isomeric caffeic acid tetramer	Inhibitory activity against HIV replication in acutely infected H9 cells
Humulus lupulus	Xanthohumol	HIV-1 inhibitory activity as well as HIV-1-induced cytopathic effects, production of viral p24 antigen and reverse transcriptase in C8166 lymphocytes
Tripterygium hypoglaucum	Triptonine A and Triptonine B	Exhibit potent in vitro anti-HIV activity
Celastrus hindsii	Celasdin B Diterpene lactones (nortripterifordin)	Anti-HIV replication activity in H9 lymphocytes cells in vitro
Tripterygium wilfordii		Inhibit HIV replication in H9 lymphocytes
Callophyllum cordato-oblongum	Cordatolide A and B	Inhibitory activity against HIV-1 replication
	(+)-calanolide A	Inhibit cytopathic effects of HIV-1 in T-cell lines, including both CEM-SS cells and MT-2 cells
Marila laxiflora	Laxofloranone	Novel non-nucleoside reverse transcriptase inhibitor with potent anti-HIV-1 activity
Symphonia globulifera	Guttiferone A	Inhibition of the cytopathic effects of in vitro HIV infection Cytoprotection of CEM-SS cells from HIV-1 infection; Inhibition of
Hypericum perforatum	Hypericin, 3-hydroxy lauric acid	HIV-1 replication; anti-HIV activity with little or no cytotoxicity
Combretum molle	Gallotannin	Inhibits RNA-dependent-DNA polymerase activity of HIV-1 reverse transcriptase
Terminalia chebula	Gallic acid and galloyl glucose	Inhibits ribonuclease activity of reverse transcriptase; also has HIV integrase inhibitory activity
Monotes africanus	Prenylated flavonoids,	HIV-inhibitory activity in XTT-based, whole cell screen
Vatica astrotricha	6,8-diprenylaromadendrin 6,8-diprenylkaempferol Prostratin, a 12-deoxyphorbol	Inhibition of HIV-1 entry; Blocks HIV-1 replication at the entry step.
Homalanthus nutan	Prostratin, a 12-deoxyphorbol	Putative mechanisms are: down regulation of CD4 expression in CEM and MT-2 cells, interference in protein kinase C enzyme pathway. Prostratin is a potent activator of HIV replication and expression in latently infected T-cells; hence it is used to flush out latent HIV from lymph nodes during antiretroviral therapy.
Acacia auriculiformis	Saponins, alkaloids	Anti-HIV activity.
Peltophorum africanum	Gallotannin	Inhibits RNA-dependent-DNA polymerase activity of HIV-1 reverse transcriptase; inhibits ribonuclease H activity of reverse transcriptase.
Ganoderma lucidum	Ganoderiol and Ganodermanontriol, Ganoderic acid Several triterpenes such as	Inhibition of HIV-1 induced cytopathic effect in MT-4 cells. Inhibit HIV-1 protease;

Ganoderma species including *G. lucidum, G. frondosa,* and *G. pfeifferi*	ganoderiol F (6a), ganodermanontriol (7a), and ganoderic acid B (8a); immunomodulators such as (1-6)-β-D-glucan, heteropolysaccharides, polysaccharide-protein complex, glycoproteins, (1-3)-β-D-glucan with (1-6)-β-D-glucosyl branches, complex mixture of polysaccharides and lignin, heteroglucans, glucoronoxylomannans, and lectins	Antiviral agents against HIV-1: ganoderiol F (6a) and ganodermanontriol (7a) inhibit HIV-1 induced cytopathic effect; ganoderic acid B (8a) inhibits HIV-1 protease Lignins inhibit HIV protease; Sulfated (1-3)-β-D-glucan with (1-6)-β-D-glucosyl branches prevent HIV-induced cytopathic effect; polysaccharide-protein complexes inhibit HIV-1 gp120 binding to CD4 receptors and reverse transcriptase.
Swertia franchetiana	Flavonone-xanthone glucoside	Inhibits HIV-1 reverse transcriptase.
Calophyllum teysmannii	(-)-calanolide B	Less activity than the A form.
Inonotus obliquus	Water-soluble lignins	Inhibit HIV-1 protease.
Garcinia speciosa	Protostanes, garcisaterpenes A and C	Inhibitory activity against HIV-1 reverse transcriptase.
Melissa officinalis	Rosmarinic acid	Inhibit HIV-1 virions carrying different X4 and R5 HIV-1 Envs as well as the heterologous VSV-G, interfers with MoMLV infection; inhibit fusion of HIV-1 particles with cells. Inhibit HIV-1 particles carrying R5 Envs; inhibit HIV-1 replication; target HIV-1 virion (virucidal)
Mentha piperita L. *Prunella vulgaris* L.	Sulfonated polysaccharides	Anti-HIV replication in H9 lymphocyte cells
Sideritis akmanii	Linearol	
Detarium microcarpum	Catechins 1-5	Inhibit HIV-1 reverse transcriptase activity in a non-specific way.
Magnolia spp.	Neolignans e.g. magnolol 1 and honokiol 2	Antioxidant, anti-depressant, induces apoptosis in tumor cells, weak anti-HIV-1 activity.
Epinetrum villosum	Cycleanine, a bisbenzylisoquinoline alkaloid	Acts against HIV-2 but is 10-times less active against HIV-1.
Stephania cepharantha	Cepharanthine	Potently inhibit HIV replication.
Musa acuminata	BanLec, a jacalin-related lectin	Binds to glycosylated viral envelopes and blocks viral entry, hence is a good microbicide; potent inhibitor of HIV-1 replication.
Myrothamnus flabellifolius	Polyphenols	Polyphenols protect cell membranes against free radical-induced damage.
	Gallotannins, 3,4,5-tri-O-galloylquinic acids	Anti-burn properties; 3,4,5-tri-O-galloylquinic acids have anti-HIV reverse transcriptase activity.
Nostoc ellipsosporum	Cyanovirin-N, an 11 KDa anti-HIV-1 protein	Inhibits HIV-1 replication through its vivid binding to HIV-1 gp120 and as a result, inactivates the viruses and blocks the fusion of viruses to the cell membrane.
Phyllanthus niruri	Niruriside	Specific inhibitor of REV protein/RRE RNA.
Flammulina velutipes	Velutin	Inhibition of HIV-1 reverse transcriptase.
Phytolacca americana	Pokeweed antiviral protein (PAP)	PAP has broad-spectrum antiviral activity against HIV; it is used as an antiviral microbicide; its anti-HIV-1 activity is superior *in vitro* compared to zidovudine (AZT).
Pinus parviflora	PC6, an extract from cones, has potent immune modulatory activities.	Inhibits replication of HIV-1 via reverse transcriptase and modification of microenvironment.

Punica granatum	PJ-S21	PJ-S21 inhibits binding of gp120 III-CD4 complexes to cells expressing CXCR4; inhibitor of X4 and R5 virus binding to the cellular receptor CD4 and co-receptors CXCR4/CCR5
Crataegus pinatifida	Uvaol and ursolic acid	Inhibitory activity against HIV-1 protease
Geum japonicum	Maslinic acid	Inhibitory activity against HIV-1 protease
Oldenlandia affinis	Circulins	Anti-HIV activity
Palicourea condensata	Palicourein	Inhibits the *in vitro* cytopathic effects of HIV-1 infection of CEM-SS cells.
Citrus paradisi	6',7'-dihydroxy-bergamottin	Enhances bioavailability of HIV protease inhibitor (e.g. saquinavar) by inhibiting cytochrome P450 iso-enzyme 3A4 in liver and gut.
Citrus spp.	Limonin and nomilin	Inhibit HIV-1 protease. Inhibit the production of HIV-1 p-24 antigen in infected monocytes and macrophages
Clausena excavate	Limonoid (clausenolide-1-ethyl ether)	HIV inhibitory activity in 1A2 cell line in syncytium assay
Euodia roxburghiana	Buchapine	Protect CEM-SS cells from cytopathic effects of HIV-1 *in vitro*
Toddalia asiatica	Itidine	Inhibit HIV-reverse transcriptase
Xanthoceras sorbifolia	Oleanolic acid	Inhibit HIV-1 replication in acutely infected H9 cells.
Schisandra sphaerandra	Nigranoic acid	Inhibit HIV-1/2 reverse transcriptase.
Schizymenia pacifica	Sulfated polysaccharide	Inhibit reverse transcriptase.
Kadsura lancilimba	Triterpene lactone, lancilactone	Inhibitory activity against HIV replication in H9 lymphocytes.
Symplocos setchuensis	Harmine	Inhibit HIV replication in H9 lymphocyte cells.
Camellia japonica	Camellia-tannin H	HIV-1 protease inhibitory activity.
Camellia sinensis	Polyphenol; epigallocatechin-3-gallate	Inhibit semen-derived enhancer of virus infection (SEVI) activity and abrogates semen-mediated enhancement of HIV-1 infection.
Curcuma longa	Curcumin	Inhibits HIV-1 integrase, HIV-1 and HIV-2 protease, and HIV-1 Long Terminal Repeat-directed gene expression.

Adapted from Chinsembu and Hedimbi (2010)

Table 2.2: Other natural products with unknown anti-HIV active compounds

Species	Active constituents	Mechanism of action
Baccharis dracunculifolia	Brazilian propolis called Alecrim propolis and red coloured propolis from	Anti-HIV-1 activity against integrase
Eclipta prostrata	Cuba and Venezuela: contain phenolics, triterepenoids, isoflavonoids,	

	prenylated benzophenones and a naphthoquinone epoxide; 3-methyl-3-butenyl is the active anti-HIV principle	
Thonningia sanguinea	Unknown	Stops HIV/AIDS-related diarrhoea, skin diseases and mycoses
Alnus viridis *Betula alleghaniensis*	Unknown	Anti-yeast activity
Jatropha curcas	Unknown	Inhibits HIV induced cytopathic effect; moderate cytoprotective effect against HIV
Trigonostema xyphophylloides		Inhibition of HIV-1 entry
Pelargonium sidoides *Pelargonium reniforme*	Unknown	Anecdotal ethnomedicinal uses reported for management of HIV/AIDS-related opportunistic infections in Southern Africa
Castanospermum australe	Castanospermine	Blocks glycoprotein processing via inhibition of glucosidase I located in the endoplasmic reticulum
Peltophorum africanum	(+)-Catechin (flavonoid), bergenin (a C-galloyl-glycoside), betulinic acid	Used to treat diarrhoea, dysentery, sore throat wounds, HIV/AIDS, STIs,; betulinic acid had highest anti-HIV activity
Sutherlandia frutescens	L-canavanine, GABA, and D-pinitol	L-canavanine has anti-viral activity against HIV and interacts with efflux of nevirapine; D-pinitol has been suggested as a treatment for wasting in cancer and AIDS patients though evidence is scanty
Garcinia kola	Biflavonoids, xanthones, benzophenones	Anti-inflammatory, anti-microbial, antihepatotoxic, and antiviral activities
Hypericum chinense	Biyouyanagin A, which contains sesquiterpene, cyclobutane and spirolactone moieties	Significant activity against HIV
Hypoxis hemerocallidea *H. colchicifolia*	Hypoxoside, sterols, and glycosides	Used by persons with moderate or advanced AIDS
Hypoxis rooperi		
Melissa officinalis	Aqueous extracts	Exhibits a high and concentration-dependent activity against HIV-1 infection in immune cells; active against virions carrying diverse envelopes
Leonotis leonurus	Aqueous and ethanol extracts	Ethanol extract of *L. leonurus* inhibit HIV-1 by 33%; and *L. leonurus* inhibit HIV-1 reverse transcriptase and protease

Adapted from Chinsembu and Hedimbi (2010)

Table 2.3: Agents that inhibit general HIV replication

Species	Active compounds	Mode of action	References
Alepidea amatymbica	Rosmarinic acid	Moderate anti-HIV replication activity	Louvel, Moodley, Seibert, Steenkamp, Nthambeleni, & Vidal et al.. (2013)
Cassia sieberiana	Tannins, sterols, anthraquinones and polyphenols	Block HIV replication	Leteane, Ngwenya, Muzila, Namushe, Mwinga, & Musonda et al.. (2012)
Excoecaria acerifolia	Diterpenoids known as excocarinols A–E	Reduce HIV-1 replication	Huang, Zhang, Ma, Zheng, Xu, & Peng et al.. (2013) Huang, Zhang, Ma, Peng, Zheng, & Hu et al.. (2014)
Kadsura spp.	Lignans and triterpenoids	Work against HIV replication	Liu, Liu, Zhang, Guo, Qi, & Jia et al.. (2014)
Pleurotus nebrodensis	Hemolysin (nebrodeolysin)	Inhibits replication of HIV-1	Lv, Kong, Yao, Zhang, Leng, & Bian (2009).
Polyalthia suberosa	Lanostane-type triterpene	Suppress HIV replication	Narayan, Rai, & Tewtrakul (2013)
Streptomyces	Feglymycin	Inhibits HIV replication and cell-to-cell transfer between HIV-infected and uninfected CD4 cells	Férir, Hänchen, François, Hoorelbeke, Huskens, & Dettner et al.. (2012)
Thelenota ananas	Fucosylated chondroitin sulfate	Blocks HIV replication even in drug-resistant strains	Huang, Wu, Zheng, Zhu, Zhao, & Zheng (2013)
Trichosanthes kirilowii	Trichosanthin, a protein extracted from the root tuber	Inhibits HIV replication	Zhao, Zhang, Feng, Wu, Chen, & Sui (2009).

Table 2.4: Inhibitors of HIV entry and spread

Species	Active compounds	Mode of action	References
Camellia sinensis	Theaflavins	Targets the viral entry step through the disruption of gp41 6-HB core structure; can be developed into cheaper topical microbicide for preventing sexual trans-	Yang, Li, Tan, Jin, Qiu, & Mao et al. (2012)

		mission of HIV	
Cassia abbreviata	Tannins, sterols, anthraqui-nones and polyphenols	Inhibits HIV binding/entry, and also inhibits alpha-glucosidase, an enzyme whose inhibition decreases infectivity of HIV	Leteane, Ngwenya, Muzila, Namushe, Mwinga, & Musonda et al. (2012)
Galanthus nivalis	Plant lectin *Galanthus nivalis* agglutinin (GNA)	A potent inhibitor that stops the spread of HIV among lymphocytes by targeting gp 120 envelope glycoprotein	Narayan, Rai, & Tewtrakul (2013)
Hemsleya jinfushanen-sis	Hemslecins A and B	Inhibit HIV entry and syn-cytia formation	Tian, Chen, Zhang, Qiu, Wang, & Du (2008)
Nerium oleander	Oleandrin	Reduces expression of the envelope glycoprotein gp120	Singh, Shenoy, Ne-hete, Yang, Nehete, & Fontenot et al. (2013)
Polygonatum cyrtonema	Lectins	Bind HIV gp120 and stop entry of HIV into cells	Ding, Bao, Zhu, Zhang, & Wang (2010)
Sanguisorba officinalis	Unknown	Blocks entry by acting on the viral envelope directly	Liang, Chen, Tan, Peng, Zheng, & Nishiura (2013)
Streptomyces	Feglymycin	Inhibits HIV cell-to-cell transfer between HIV-infected and uninfected CD4 cells	Férir, Hänchen, François, Hoo-relbeke, Huskens, & Dettner et al. (2012)
Streptomyces pre-sent in an endophyte from the mangrove plant *Bruguiera gymnorrhiza*	Xiamycin, a novel pentacy-clic indolosesquiterpene	Blocks CCR5 tropic HIV-1 infection	Ding, Münch, Goerls, Maier, Fie-big, Lin, & Hertweck (2010)
Thelenota ananas	Fucosylated chondroitin sulfate	Blocks HIV entry even in drug-resistant strains	Huang, Wu, Zheng, Zhu, Zhao, & Zheng (2013)

Table 2.5: Inhibitors of HIV reverse transcriptase

Species	Active compounds	Mode of action	References
Acacia auriculiform-is	Saponins, alkaloids	Inhibit HIV-1 reverse transcriptase	Narayan, Rai, & Tewtrakul (2013)
Acacia confusa	Chymotrypsin inhibitor in seeds	Stops activity of HIV-1 reverse transcriptase; IC50 of 871.5 mM	Lam, & Ng (2010)
Ancistrocladus korupensis	Michellamines A and B	Inhibit HIV reverse tran-scriptase	Narayan, Rai, & Tewtrakul (2013)
Andrographis paniculata	Unknown	Inhibits HIV reverse transcriptase	Narayan, Rai, & Tewtrakul (2013)
Bersama engleriana	Unknown	Blocks HIV reverse tran-	Mbaveng, Kuete, Mapunya,

		scriptase	Beng, Nkengfack, Meyer, & Lall (2011)
Callophyllum inophyllum	Pyranocoumarins such as (+)-inophyllum B	Inhibit HIV-1 reverse transcriptase	Laure, Raharivelomanana, Butaud, Bianchini, & Gaydou (2008)
Canthium coromandelicum	Unknown ingredient in methanolic extract	Blocks HIV reverse transcriptase	Chinnaiyan, Subramanian, Vinoth Kumar, Chandu, & Deivasigamani (2013)
Combretum molle	Gallotannin and gallic acid	Inhibit HIV-1 reverse transcriptase	Narayan, Rai, & Tewtrakul (2013)
Cordyceps sobolifera	Cordysobin, a serine protease	Blocks HIV-1 reverse transctiptase	Wang, Liu, Zhang, Zhao, Xu, Geng, & Wang (2012)
Garcinia speciosa	Protostanes and garcisaterpenes A and C	Blocks HIV-1 reverse transcriptase	Narayan, Rai, & Tewtrakul (2013)
Gardenia carinata	Flavones	Anti-HIV-1 reverse transcriptase activity. Active compounds inhibit human DNA topoisomerase IIα; thus cytotoxic to humans	Kongkum, Tuchinda, Pohmakotr, Reutrakul, Piyachaturawat, Jariyawat et al. (2012)
Hypoxis sobolifera	Hypoxoside, rooperol	Inhibit HIV reverse transcriptase	Ncube, van Staden, Okem, & Ndhlala (2013)
Momordica charantia	Alpha-and beta-momorcharin; Momordica anti-HIV protein(MAP30); lectins	Alpha-and beta-momorcharin are inhibitors of HIV-1 integrase; lectins inhibit reverse transcriptase; MAP30 inhibits core protein synthesis, reverse transcription, integration and syncytium formation	Palamthodi, & Lele (2014)
Pholiota adiposa	Methyl gallate; also rich in proteins, essential amino acids, dietary fiber, trace elements, vitamins, and carbohydrates	Methyl gallate inhibits HIV-1 reverse transcriptase	Wang, Zhou, Ng, Wong, Qiao, & Liu (2014)
Phyllanthus niruri	Gallic acid, flavonoids, alkaloids, terpenes and lignans	Inhibits HIV reverse transcriptase	Ogata, Higuchi, Mochida, Matsumoto, Kato, & Endo et al. (1992)
Phyllanthus pulcher, P. urinaria and *P. myrtifolius*	Unknown	Inhibit HIV reverse transcriptase	Eldeen et al. (2011)
Plectranthus barbatus	Unknown	Poor inhibition of HIV-1 reverse transcriptase	Kapewangolo, Hussein, & Meyer (2013)
Rhus succedanea	Biflavonoids, robustaflavone and hinokiflavone	Stops HIV reverse transcriptase	Narayan, Rai, & Tewtrakul (2013)
Sanguisorba officinalis	Unknown	Inhibits reverse transcriptase in resistant HIV strains	Liang, Chen, Tan, Peng, Zheng, & Nishiura (2013)
Swertia franchetiana	Flavones-xanthone glycoside	Inhibits HIV-1 reverse transcriptase	Narayan, Rai, & Tewtrakul (2013)
Terminalia chebula	Galloyl glucose	Inhibits HIV-1 reverse transcriptase	Narayan, Rai, & Tewtrakul (2013)

Treculia obovoidea, Treculia africana, Treculia acuminata	Triterpenes, coumarins, saponins, phenols, and flavonoids	Possess anti-HIV reverse transcriptase activity	Kuete, Metuno, Keilah, Tshikalange, & Ngadjui (2010)

Table 2.6: Inhibitors of HIV integrase

Species	Active compounds	Mode of action	References
Achyrocline satureioides	Dicaffeoylquinic acids: 3,5-dicaffeoylquinic acid, and 1- methoxyoxalyl-3,5-dicaffeoylquinic acid	Potent and irreversible inhibition of HIV-1 integrase	Narayan, Rai, & Tewtrakul (2013)
Camellia sinensis	Catechins with the galloyl moiety	Inhibit HIV integrase	Jiang, Ng, Wang, Zhang, Cheng, & Liu et al. (2010)
Dioscorea birmanica	Unknown	Inhibit HIV integrase	Tewtrakul, Itharat, & Rattanasuwan (2006)
Inula crithmoides	1,5-di-O-caffeoylquinicacid	Potent HIV-1 integrase inhibitor	Seca, Grigore, Pinto, & Silva (2014)
Smilax corbularia	Unknown	Inhibit HIV integrase	Tewtrakul, Itharat, & Rattanasuwan (2006)
Trichosanthes kirilowii	Trichosanthin	Inhibits integration through depurinating long-terminal repeats	Zhao, Feng, Wu, & Sui (2010)

Table 2.7: Inhibitors of HIV protease

Species	Active compounds	Mode of action	References
Andrographis paniculata	Unknown	Inhibits HIV protease	Narayan, Rai, & Tewtrakul (2013)
Cordyceps militaris, an entomopathogenic fungus	Adenosines such as pentamethoxyflavone, dimethylguanosine, and pentamethoxyflavone	Inhibits HIV-1 protease	Jiang, Wong, Fu, Ng, Liu, & Wang et al. (2011).
Hypoxis sobolifera Bulbine alooides Leonotis leonurus	Unknown parts of aqueous and ethanol extracts	Inhibit HIV-1 protease	Klos, Van de Venter, Milne, Traore, Meyer, & Oosthuizen (2009)
Inonotus obliquus	Water soluble lignins	Inhibit HIV-1 protease	Narayan, Rai, & Tewtrakul (2013)
Leonotis leonurus Bulbine alooides	Tannins and sulfated polysaccharides- have low bioavailability	Mild inhibition of HIV-1 protease	Klos, Van de Venter, Milne, Traore, Meyer, & Oosthuizen (2009)
Panax ginseng	Triterpenes	Inhibit HIV protease	Wei, Ma, & Hattori (2009)
Pholiota adipose, an edible mushroom widely cultivated in China	Methyl gallate; also rich in proteins, essential amino acids, dietary fiber, trace elements, vitamins, and carbohydrates	Methyl gallate inhibits protease activity	Wang, Zhou, Ng, Wong, Qiao, & Liu (2014)
Plectranthus barbatus	Unknown	Poor inhibition of protease	Kapewangolo, Hussein, & Meyer (2013)
Saururus chinensis	Lignan (saururin B), dilignan (manassantin A),	Saururin B and manassantin A are novel HIV-1	Lee, Huh, Kim, Hattori, & Otake (2010)

81

	sesquilignans (manassantins A, B and saucerneol B)	protease inhibitors	
Stauntonia obovatifoliola Hayata subsp. *intermedia*	Triterpenoids and triterpenes	Inhibitory activity against HIV-1 protease	Wei, Ma, Chen, & Hattori (2008)

Table 2.8: Inhibitors of HIV cytopathic effect

Species	Active compounds	Mode of action	References
Daphne acutiloba	Daphnane-type diterpene esters named acutilobins A–G	Inhibit cytopathic effects of HIV-1 (EC50); 12 compounds showed more activity than AZT	Huang, Zhang, Li, Kong, Jiang, & Ma et al. (2012)
Euphorbia ingens	Ingenol	Helps T cells to survive longer against viremia after HIV-1 infection, without exerting cytotoxic effects; also reactivates HIV in cell reservoirs by inducing HIV replication	Hong, Lee, Kim, & Kim (2011)
Jatropha curcas	Diterpenes, coumarins, flavonoids	Potent inhibition of HIV-induced cytopathic effects with low cytotoxicity; cycloprotective activity against HIV	Pandey, Singh, Singh, Kumar, Singh, & Singh (2012); Abdelgadir, & van Staden (2013)
Kadsura angustifolia	Cycloartane triterpenoids such as angustific acid A	Inhibit cytopathic effects of HIV	Sun, Song, Wang, Shen, Xu, & Gao (2011)
Luffa cylindrical	Luffin P1 (a peptide from the seeds)	Inhibition of HIV cytopathogenic effect and capture of the HIV-1 p24 protein	Ng, Yang, Sze, Zhang, Zheng, & Shaw (2011)
Saururus chinensis	Lignan (saururin B), dilignan (manassantin A), sesquilignans (manassantins A, B and saucerneol B)	Manassantins A, B and saucerneol B are novel classes of HIV-1-induced cytopathic effect inhibitors	Lee, Huh, Kim, Hattori, & Otake (2010)
Trigonostemon thyrsoideum	Daphnane diterpenoids and trigothysoids;	Inhibit cytopathic effects of HIV-1	Cheng, Chen, He, Zhang, Li, & Tang et al. (2013)

Table 2.9: Natural products with other modes of action on HIV

Species	Anti-HIV active compounds	Mode of action	References
Celastrus hindsii	Celasdin B	Inhibits HIV through an unknown mechanism	Narayan, Rai, & Tewtrakul (2013)
Dendrobium nobile Dendrobium moniliforme Ephemerantha lonchophylla Cannabis sativa	A new anthraquinone called denbinobin	Denbinobin inhibits HIV-1 reactivation, HIV-1-LTR activity, prevents the binding of NF-kB to DNA, and has antioxidation and anti-inflammation actions	Sánchez-Duffhues, Calzado, de Vinuesa, Caballero, Ech-Chahad, & Appendino (2008)
Euphorbia hyberna	Jatrophane diterpenes	Antagonist of HIV-1 latency in resting CD4 cell reservoirs i.e. induces HIV replication	Bedoya, Márquez, Martínez, Gutiérrez-Eisman, Álvarez, & Calzado (2009)
Euphorbia ingens	Ingenol	Reactivates HIV in cell reservoirs by inducing HIV replication	Hong, Lee, Kim, & Kim (2011)
Homalanthus nutans Pimelea prostrata	Prostratin	Reactivates transcription in latent HIV-1 provirus in T cells	Remoli, Marsili, Battistini, & Sgarbanti (2012)
Lessertia frutescens	L-canavanine	Unknown	Singh, Shaik, Dewir, Khanyile, Smith, & Shode et al. (2009)
Mauritiana rugosa Mauritiana oenoplia	Betulinic acid	Exhibits unknown biological activities against HIV but development of betulinic acid derivatives for clinical use has been hampered by adverse pharmacological and physicochemical characteristics of this class of compounds	Khazir, Mir, Pilcher, & Riley (2014)
Peltophorum africanum	Betunilic acid, flavonoids, coumarins	Unknown	Mazimba (2014)
Polygonum cuspidatum	5,7-dimethoxyphthalide, catechin, emodin8-O-β-D-glucopyranoside and resveratrol	Exhibited fairly strong antiviral effect against HIV-1; resveratrol attenuated Tat-induced HIV-1 trans-activation	Peng, Qin, Li, & Zhou (2013)
Tripterygium hypoglaucum	Triptonine A and Triptonine B	Inhibit HIV through an unknown mechanism	Narayan, Rai, & Tewtrakul (2013)
Tripterygium wilfordii	Diterpene lactones	Inhibit HIV through an unknown mechanism	Narayan, Rai, & Tewtrakul (2013)
Tripterygium wilfordii	Celastrol, a triterpenoid	Exhibits highest inhibitory activity against Tat	Narayan, Ravindra, Chiaro, Cary, Aggarwal, Henderson, & Prabhu (2011)

Table 2.10: Anti-HIV agents- Part 3

Species	Active compound	Mode of action	References
Acacia catechu	Unknown compounds in n-butanol fraction	Potent inhibitory activity against HIV-1 protease (IC_{50} = 12.9 µg/ml), but no action against reverse transcriptase or integrase	Modi, Dezzutti, Kulshreshtha, Rawat, Srivastava, & Malhotra et al. (2013)
Alepidea amatymbica	Diterpenoids, phenolic acids, rosmarinic acid	Moderate activity against HIV replication	Wintola & Afolayan (2014)
Ancistrocladus heyneanus diospyros leucomelas Syzygium formosanum Tetracera boliviana Tryphyllum peltatum Ziziphus vulgaris	Betulinic acid, a naturally occurring pentacyclic triterpene belonging to the lupane family	Inhibits HIV-1 replication with an EC_{50} value of 1.4 µM	Kuo, Qian, Morris-Natschke, & Lee (2009)
Combretum adenogonium	Unknown	Blocks HIV-1 protease with IC_{50} value of 26.5 µg/ml,	Mushi, Mbwambo, Innocent, & Tewtrakul (2012)
Corticium simplex	Natural steroidal alkaloid named Cortistatin A	Potently suppresses Tat-dependent HIV transcription	Mehbub, Lei, Franco, & Zhang (2014)
Cryptocarya chinensis	Phenanthroindolizidine alkaloids	Significantly suppresses growth of HIV-infected H9 cells with an EC_{50} value of 1.88 µg/mL	Wu, Su, & Lee (2012)
Dictyota mertensii Lobophora variegata, Spatoglossum schroederi Fucus vesiculosus	Sulfated fucans	Inhibit HIV reverse transcriptase	Queiroz, Medeiros, Queiroz, Abreu, Rocha, & Ferreira et al. (2008)
Ecklonia cava	8,8'-bieckol and 8,4'''-dieckol	Inhibit effect of HIV-1 reverse transcriptase and protease	Artan, Li, Karadeniz, Lee, Kim, & Kim (2008)
Elaoephorbia drupifera	Euphol, tirucallol, euphorbol, ingenol, elaeophorbate, epitaraxerol, taraxerone, friedelin, lupenone, lupeol, olean-12-ene-3-one, olean-12-ene-3-ol, elaeophorbate	Moderately inhibit HIV-1 and HIV-2 proviral DNA copying	Kuete, Voukeng, Tsobou, Mbaveng, Wiench, Beng, & Efferth (2013)
Ganoderma colossum	Colossolactones, new lanostane triterpenes	Anti-protease activity	Kuo, Qian, Morris-Natschke, & Lee (2009)
Homophymia sp.	Cyclodepsipeptide called homophymine A	Exhibits cytoprotective activity against HIV-1 infection with a IC50 of 75 nM	Zampella, Sepe, Luciano, Bellotta, Monti, & D'Auria, (2008)
Lagerstroemia speciosa	Gallic acid and ellagic acid	Inhibit reverse transcriptase and HIV protease, respectively	Nutan, Goel, Das, Malik, Suri, & Rawat et al. (2013)

Litophyton arboretum	Sarcophytol M, chimyl alcohol and erythro-*N*-dodecanoyl-docosasphinga-(4*E*,8*E*)-dienine	Strong HIV-1 protease inhibitory activity (IC50 12 ± 1.3 µg/mL).	Ellithey, Lall, Hussein, & Meyer (2014)
Cassiopia andromeda			
Galaxura filamentosa			Ellithey, Lall, Hussein, & Meyer (2013)
Mallotus philippinensis	Mallotojaponin	Inhibits reverse transcriptase	Gangwar, Goel, & Nath (2014)
Momordica charantia	Kuguacins A–E, belong to family of cucurbitacins	Anti-HIV activity possibly through blocking the transmission of virus through cell-to-cell fusion	Kuo, Qian, Morris-Natschke, & Lee (2009)
Parnassia wightiana	Dihydro-β-agarofuran sesquiterpene polyesters	General anti-HIV activity	Lv, Zheng, Miao, Geng, Zhou, & Liu (2014)
Parthenium hysterophorus	Unknown	40% inhibition of HIV-1 reverse transcriptase	Kumar, Chashoo, Saxena, & Pandey (2013)
Pelargonium sidoides	Unknown	Potent HIV-1 attachment inhibitor	Helfer, Koppensteiner, Schneider, Rebensburg, Forcisi, & Müller (2014)
Rhus parviflora	Unknown	Inhibition of HIV-1 protease activity.	Modi, Pancholi, Kulshrestha, Rawat, Malhotra, & Gupta (2013)
Rodgersia aesculifolia	Bergenin, a sesquiterpene lactone compound	Anti-HIV replication	Liang, Li, Liu, Huang, Shen, & Wang et al. (2014)
Sanguisorba officinalis	Unknown	Entry inhibitor with significant ability against CCR5 and CXCR4 tropic HIV-1; works against strains resistant to anti- reverse transcriptase and anti-protease drugs	Liang, Chen, Tan, Peng, Zheng, & Nishiura (2013)
Solanum xanthocarpum	Flavonoids	Low inhibition of HIV-1 reverse transcriptase	Kumar, & Pandey (2014)
Spathodea campanulata	Ajugol, p-hydroxybenzoic acid, methyl p-hydroxybenzoate	Unknown	Kuete, Voukeng, Tsobou, Mbaveng, Wiench, Beng, & Efferth (2013)
Stellera Chamaejasme	Stelleracins, tigliane-type diterpenes, 12-*O*-benzoylphorbol 13-octanoate	Inhibit HIV-1 replication; potent anti-HIV with EC$_{90}$ values of less than 1 nM	Asada, Sukemori, Watanabe, Malla, Yoshikawa, & Li et al. (2013)
Stephaniae tetrandrae	Fangchinoline, a bisbenzyl-isoquinoline alkaloid	Inhibits HIV-1 gp160 processing, resulting in reduced envelope glycoprotein incorporation into nascent virions	Wan, Lu, Liao, Wu, & Chen (2012)
Syzygium cumini	Phenolics, flavonoids, phytosterols, terpenoids,	General anti-HIV effect	Eshwarappa, Iyer, Subbaramaiah, Richard, & Dhananjaya (2014)

Trigonostema xyphophyl-loides	Unknown	Inhibits HIV-1 replication and syncytia formation; inhibits	Park, Han, Song, Green, Wang, & Liu et al. (2009)
Vatica astrotricha		HIV-1 replication by blocking HIV-1 interaction with target cells like CD4/CCR5	
Wrightia tinctoria	Unknown	Anti-HIV replication	Srivastava (2014)
Zanthoxylum ailanthoides	Coumarins, lignans, flavonoids, quinolines, benzenoids, and triterpenoids	General anti-HIV properties	Chung, Hwang, Kuo, Kuo, Cheng, & Wu (2013)

3

Pharmacopoeia of Natural Remedies for Skin Diseases

Introduction

The skin is the first part of the body that people see. It gives the first impression of an individual's state of health or sickness. A healthful human body begins with a wholesome skin. Unfortunately, biological organisms and particles such as viruses as well many external chemical and physical agents that cause infection, oxidation and inflammation induce skin diseases. And in this age of HIV/AIDS, skin diseases are on the upswing. In fact, skin diseases are one of the earliest signs and clinical manifestations of AIDS. To cope with this increasing incidence and severity of skin diseases, people all over the world use natural products for daily skin care and management of skin disorders.

This chapter is a modest quest for the different pharmacopoeias of natural products used to manage skin diseases. Starting with an overview of the skin barrier, the chapter immediately delves into the association between skin diseases and HIV/AIDS. Then the chapter makes an interesting exposition of the ancient, religious and modern-day data on the use of natural products to reduce oxidation, inflammation and microbial infections of the skin.

Three important questions about skin diseases are confronted in this chapter:

1. What natural products heal skin diseases caused by free radicals and oxidation?
2. What natural products alleviate inflammatory skin diseases?
3. What natural products help combat microbial infections of the skin?

By the end of this chapter, answers to these questions will become clear. Since treatises on African natural products used in the management of skin diseases are few and far between, the overarching aim of this chapter is to explore and document natural pharmacopoeias for skin diseases in Africa. Still, natural products used to manage skin diseases in other parts of the world are revealed. Although the chapter is by no means exhaustive, it is systematically premised on peer-reviewed records, thus guaranteeing validity and reliability.

Skin Barrier

The human skin is the body's punch bag. It feels the heat from the sun. It takes the full brunt of environmental attacks and microbial slurs. Without a functional and intact skin barrier, the human body would be open to external attacks emanating from the many biological, chemical and physical agents twenty-four-seven. The skin is a protective fence around the body. The point is this: Either the skin is resilient to microbial pathogens and chemical and physical intruders. Or, the skin is porous and allows these intruders to penetrate and sneak into the body at will, provoking diseases.

In terms of area, the skin is the largest organ of the body, covering about 1.5 to $2m^2$ in adult humans. It serves many important functions: protection, percutaneous absorption, temperature regulation, fluid maintenance, sensory and disease control (Abbasi, Khan, Ahmad, Zafar, Jahan, & Sultana, 2010). According to Nicolaou (2013), the skin constitutes a physical barrier that protects the body from injury, infection, water and electrolyte loss, as well as playing an important role in immune function.

Lall and Kishore (2014) reiterate the fact that the skin is the most extensive organ in the body which protects the internal environment from the external one. It also contributes to human beauty - a quality that gives desirable pleasure and aesthetic value to human senses. Tsai, Lin, Liang, Yen, Chiang and Lee (2014) repeat that as the largest organ of the human body, the skin shields against environmental threats, including bacteria, fungi, viruses, ultraviolet (UV) radiation and air pollution. The skin also plays a crucial role in the rapid cellular response enacted by resident immune cells that recognize a variety of pathogenic structures and induces a cascade of pro-inflammatory responses.

The skin consists of different layers of cells which support the formation of a highly keratinized outer epidermal permeability barrier, whilst the epidermis and dermis host a number of primary cells including epidermal keratinocytes, melanocytes, Langerhans cells, dermal fibroblasts, mast cells and infiltrating leukocytes. Keratinocytes are the predominant cell type in the epidermis and act as a barrier against environmental and microbial assaults. They are also involved in the progression of numerous inflammatory skin diseases such as psoriasis and contact dermatitis.

As stated by Haag, Tscherch, Arndt, Kleemann, Gersonde and Lademann et al. (2014), the chief function of the skin is to act as the primary barrier against external biotic and abiotic agents and to prevent massive water loss from the body. Indeed, the skin shields the human body from hazards such as chemicals, microorganisms, environmental pollutants and allergens. The skin's barrier is situated in the stratum corneum which consists of cross-linked corneocytes surrounded by a continuous lipid matrix, mainly composed of ceramides, cholesterol and free fatty acids.

The stratum corneum is the outermost layer of the skin. It consists of dead and flattened cells (corneocytes). This tough and horny layer of keratin is mixed with lipids which help maintain the skin's hydration, elasticity and effective barrier functions. Changes in the lipid profile impair the barrier function of the skin and promote skin diseases including xerosis cutis, the medical term for abnormally dry skin. Patients suffering from atopic dermatitis exhibit low levels of stratum corneum ceramides.

Microbial Skin Diseases

Chiller, Selkin and Murakawa (2001) describe the skin as a milieu for controlled microbial growth. But the skin also supports the growth of commensal bacteria which protect the host from pathogenic bacteria. According to Chiller et al. (2001), resident gram-positive bacteria include *Staphylococcus, Micrococcus* and *Corynebacterium* species. *Staphylococcus aureus* and *Streptococcus pyogenes* are notoriously pathogenic to the skin causing epidermal infections such as impetigo and ecthyma. *S. aureus* infection of hair follicles (folliculitis) causes tiny whiteheaded spots surrounded by small red pimples. Dermal infections consist of erysipelas, cellulitis and necrotizing fasciitis. The pilosebaceous section is involved in folliculitis, furunculosis and carbunculosis. *Tinea pedis* (athletes' foot) and *Tinea corporsis* (ringworm) are also common skin infections.

Moreover, *S. aureus* and *S. pyogenes* produce toxins that may elicit a superantigen response, causing massive release of cytokines (Chiller et al., 2001). Staphylococcal scalded skin syndrome, toxic shock syndrome, and scarlet fever are all superantigen-mediated disorders. Gram-negative organisms such as *Pseudomonas aeruginosa, Pasteurella multocida, Capnocytophaga canimorsus, Bartonella* sp., *Klebsiella rhinoscleromatis* and *Vibrio vulnificus* are not typical resident skin microflora but may cause cutaneous infections (Chiller et al., 2001).

Skin and mucosal infections are common in populations living in habitats with poor sanitation, areas that lack treated potable water, and persons with insufficient awareness of hygienic habits. Jong, Ermuth and Augustin (2013) explain that many factors may contribute to the cause, development and burden of chronic skin diseases, such as genetic, immunologic, environmental and psychological factors. These authors give the example of eczema, a skin disease which involves a genetic component in the form of a general allergic oversensitivity (atopic dermatitis) or an environmental component caused by irritants or other allergens (contact dermatitis).

Psoriasis, another common chronic skin disease, is a multi-genetic condition which causes a strong disturbance of the immune system with inflammatory skin manifestation (Jong et al., 2013). Standard care for eczema and psoriasis consists of topical ointments with corticosteroids or calcineurin inhibitors, phototherapy or systemic immuno-modifying agents. Since chronic skin diseases have an enormous impact on the quality of life, patients frequently seek new treatment options including natural products, which are in high demand in recent years.

Skin Diseases during HIV Infection

Skin diseases are a major health burden in both developed and developing countries. These diseases tend to be chronic and persistent, in some cases transmittable from person to person, and often linked to immunosuppression in HIV/AIDS patients. Skin diseases are one of the diagnostic criteria for HIV/AIDS. Abbasi et al. (2010) reckon that, in general, skin infections account for about 34% of all the human diseases worldwide. They affect people of all ages and constitute a major concern for doctor consultations.

Oftentimes, the starting point for HIV/AIDS-related stigma is the skin, because it is what people can see. When people notice skin infections like boils, eczema and herpes zoster, their foremost perception is that the skin infections are a manifestation of HIV/AIDS. Skin diseases are the face of AIDS. Because they are very difficult to hide, skin infections unfortunately become the focus of stigma in people living with HIV/AIDS.

Although some skin diseases are persistent and difficult to treat, the mortality rate for skin diseases is relatively low. The aetiology of skin disorders clearly shows the close interface and association that exists between an individual's health and their natural and sociocultural environment (Martínez and Barboza, 2010). Inflammation contributes to skin healing and repair, especially during injury, and is also a central feature in a number of dermatoses and cancer (Nicolaou, 2013).

Skin diseases are now a major concern because they are part of the battery of opportunistic infections in HIV/AIDS. Skin manifestations are usually the first sign of HIV infection and conversion to AIDS as more than 90% of HIV-infected individuals develop skin and mucosal complications at some stage during HIV infection (Njoronge and Bussmann, 2007). In Sub-Saharan Africa, estimates suggest that over 78 million people are infected with tinea capitis, a fungal infection of the scalp (ringworm of the scalp), mostly prevalent in HIV-positive individuals.

According to Ramos-e-Silva, Lima, Schechtman, Trope and Carneiro (2012), skin diseases are a good clinical indicator for predicting the individual's immune status. While the normal CD4 count in adults ranges from 500 to 1,500 cells per mm^3, the CD4 count progressively decreases with evolution of

AIDS. Skin diseases often influence the individual's general condition and point to a poor prognosis. An association of skin diseases with HIV infection serves as an indicator of advanced HIV infection heralding AIDS.

In Rundu, Namibia, microbial skin diseases (acnes, boils, eczema, herpes zoster, sores, leprosy, mycoses, psoriasis, rashes, wounds, and general skin infections) account for 25% of all ethnomedicinal plants used to manage HIV/AIDS-related opportunistic infections. In the neighbouring town of Katima Mulilo, Zambezi Region, microbial skin diseases account for 21% of all plants used as HIV/AIDS medications. This demonstrates that skin diseases are a chronic and major HIV/AIDS challenge that is usually managed by the use of natural products.

Skin Diseases in Ancient Times and Religious Faiths

The traditional practice of topically treating dermatological conditions with plant-derived medicines predates the cultures of ancient Egypt and remains vital today in both civilized and uncivilized societies. In ancient civilisation, Egyptians were apparently the first to use the whipped ostrich eggs, olive oil, and resin mixed with milk for the treatment of a range of skin conditions. Humans have suffered skin infections since time immemorial, even during biblical times when Job was inflicted with sores and boils. Al-Gammal (1998) documents that the plant Elecampane, whose botanical name is *Inula campana* - sometimes referred to as *Inula helenium* - is famous for its successful use as a medication by Job who had chronic sore boils.

Skin diseases lie at the centre of religious dogma in both Christian and Islamic faiths. Indeed, the use of natural products including plants to treat skin diseases such as boils is well documented in the Bible, see 2 Kings 20:7 where a poultice of common figs (*Ficus* sp.) was applied to heal boils.

The Bible makes several references to skin diseases: "Skin for skin!" Satan replied... So Satan went out from the presence of the Lord and afflicted Job with painful sores from the soles of his feet to the crown of his head (Job 2: 4-7). The Lord will afflict your knees and legs with painful boils that cannot be cured, spreading from the soles of your feet to the top of your head (Deuteronomy 28: 35). "Prepare a poultice of figs." They did so and applied it to the boil, and he recovered (2 Kings 20:7).

In the Bible, skin diseases are so horrendous that they prompt punishment, shame and isolation. In Exodus 9:10, the Bible says:

> So they took soot from a furnace and stood before Pharaoh. Moses tossed it into the air, and festering boils broke out on people and animals.

Deuteronomy 28:27 also talks of skin diseases: The Lord will afflict you with the boils of Egypt and with tumours, festering sores and the itch, from which you cannot be cured.

Skin diseases like sores are also a symbol of poverty and destitution, as in the New Testament story of Lazarus. In Luke 16:19-21, the Bible says:

> There was a rich man who was dressed in purple and fine linen and lived in luxury every day. At his gate was laid a beggar named Lazarus, covered with sores and longing to eat what fell from the rich man's table. Even the dogs came and licked his sores.

In the biblical stories about Lazarus and Job, skin diseases such as boils, sores and ulcers are a graphic illustration of a human condition that is repugnant and repulsive. People with skin diseases such as leprosy were unclean and ostracized.

Leviticus 13:1-5 says:

> The Lord said to Moses and Aaron, "When anyone has a swelling or a rash or a bright spot on his skin that may become an infectious skin disease, he must be brought to Aaron the priest or to one of his sons who is a priest. The priest is to examine the sore on his skin, and if the hair in the sore has turned white and the sore appears to be more than skin deep, it is an infectious skin disease. When the priest examines him, he shall pronounce him ceremonially unclean.
>
> If the spot on his skin is white but does not appear to more than skin deep and the hair in it has not turned white, the priest is to put the infected person in isolation for seven days. On the seventh day the priest is to examine him, and if he sees that the sore is unchanged and has not spread in the skin, he is to keep him in isolation another seven days.

Thus, even in biblical times, skin diseases were so awful that the first person that Jesus healed was a man suffering from a skin disease - leprosy.

Matthew 8:1-4 says:

> When Jesus came down from the mountain-
> side, large crowds followed him. A man with
> leprosy came and knelt before him and said, "Lord,
> if you are willing, you can make me clean." Jesus
> reached out his hand and touched the man. "I am
> willing," he said. "Be clean!" Immediately he was
> cleansed of his leprosy. Then Jesus said to him, "See
> that you don't tell anyone. But go, show yourself to
> the priest and offer the gift Moses commanded, as a
> testimony to them."

AlGhamdi, AlHomoudi and Khurram (2013) propound that the recommendations for skin care practices in Islamic teachings are analogous to current
medical guidelines. According to these Islamic scholars, sun avoidance - which
is recommended by Islam, is mandatory for diseases such as systemic lupus
erythematosus, melasma and skin cancers. They insist that skin care and hygienic practices are recommended in Islam, an important principle for reducing
the transmission of infections in modern medicine. AlGhamdi and co-workers
claim that even the removal of the penis' foreskin during male circumcision,
which is now a proven method to protect against sexually transmitted infections including HIV, is supported by Islamic practice.

In Zambia, communities of the Lunda and Luvale people of North-
Western Province, who since time immemorial have removed the penis' fore-
skin during the traditional ritual of *Mukanda* or male circumcision, have low
HIV infection rates.

Natural Products as Agents of Skin Care and Therapy

Natural products especially plants are widely used to treat skin diseases.
Nowadays, many people would rather apply natural cosmetics because of increased awareness of side effects from synthetic chemicals and petroleum by-
products in many commercial skin care formulations. In fact, this is the main
reason skin care products based on natural products registered a 21% global
increase in revenue between 2006 and 2011. Currently, the most common examples of natural skin care ingredients include palm oil, sesame seed oil,
linseed, jojoba oil, sandalwood, witch hazel, tea tree oil and chamomile. Natural
products now play a major role in the treatment of various skin disorders in

many countries around the world; thus natural products significantly contribute to the healthcare of the skin.

Globally, hundreds of medicinal plant species are used as traditional medicines for the treatment and management of skin diseases caused by bacteria, fungi and viruses. Even in developed countries like Germany, plant-based skin care products containing *Mahonia aquifolium* and *Cardiospermum halicacabum* significantly lessen chronic skin disease severity and improve patient satisfaction and quality of life in a very comparable way to patients on standard skin treatment (Jong et al., 2013). The efficacy of plants such as *Matricaria recutita*, *Hamamelis virginiana*, *Arnica montana* and *Calendula officinalis* has been established in pre-clinical and clinical studies.

Lall and Kishore (2014) acknowledge the long history in the use of plants to heal skin diseases and improve skin care. In their review of 117 plant species used for skin care in South Africa, Lall and Kishore (2014) note that the use of natural ingredients for skin care is very popular. Skin care products based on medicinal plant preparations are coming back to take over dermatological therapy. We now live in an era of bullish interest in natural products as skin care products and dermatological medicines. In any case, thousands of current pharmaceutical drugs were first isolated from natural sources including ethnomedicinal plants.

Plants and other natural products serve beneficial cosmetic functions for the care of the human skin. Their natural ingredients improve the biological functions of the skin and supply excellent nutrients necessary for a healthy skin. Many scientists concur that botanical products are a rich source of vitamins, antioxidants, various oils, essential oils, hydrocolloids, proteins, terpenoids and other bioactive molecules. Natural products confer beneficial functions to the skin, mainly due to their antimicrobial, anti-protozoal, anti-inflammatory and antioxidant properties. Antioxidant functions are derived from carotenoids, flavonoids and polyphenols.

Teshome, Gebre-Mariam, Asres, Perry and Engidawork (2008) opine that skin disorders are among the major diseases for which traditional medicines are personally utilized at a much larger scale. There is hardly any community in the world where there is no knowledge of a local plant suitable for treating a skin disease or condition such as a sore. Therefore, it is not at all astonishing that in most communities plant remedies form the first line of treatment for skin diseases.

Some studies claim that compounds which protect plants from abiotic and environmental stress, such as UV rays, drought, salinity, freezing and high temperature, produce similar protective effects on human skin, because such compounds act via the activation of basic signal transduction mechanisms that are conserved in all eukaryotic cells (Apone, Tito, Carola, Arciello, Tortora, &

Filippini et al., 2010). Activation of defense response genes responsible for the protection and repair of damage caused by stress agents has analogous mechanisms in both plant and human cells.

Take the case of *Ximenia americana*, a plant with many medicinal benefits to the skin. Studies now show that abiotic stress genes of *X. americana* are constitutively expressed in natural conditions. Continuous transcription of abiotic stress genes is perhaps the reason this plant produces phytochemicals that 'kill two birds with one stone': While the chemicals are naturally designed to protect the plant from environmental stressors, they also have many beneficial effects on the skin. The same applies to jojoba (*Simmondsia chinensis*), a plant that thrives in the desert. Since its genes induce products that enable the plant to tolerate drought and fight off free oxygen radicals, jojoba oil has now found wide applications in skin care products with antioxidant and sunscreen properties.

There is evidence that phytonutrients such as plant sugars and protein molecules attenuate skin ageing through the increase of collagen synthesis, or the reduction of collagen degradation caused by matrix proteases. For example, skin ageing can also be reduced and corrected by resveratrol (3,5,4'-trihydroxy-*trans*-stilbene), a naturally occurring polyphenolic compound found in red wine, red grapes, peanuts and many plants (Lephart, Sommerfeldt, & Andrus, 2014). Since resveratrol stimulates the expression of the sirtuin activator gene, an anti-ageing factor, it has the potential to be used in products to maintain and improve human skin health. Many studies have also elucidated the anti-HIV activity of resveratrol, capable of reducing HIV infection by 20-30%.

Dermatophytes are fungi that cause skin, hair, and nail infections. Plant extracts are commonly utilized in dermatological and cosmetic formulations to treat dermatophytes. Functional extracts are made through pressing (e.g. *Aloe vera*) or prepared by aqueous or ethanolic isolations. At home, many plant extracts are used for wound healing and skin regeneration. This traditional usage of natural products is being replaced by more sophisticated cosmetic and dermopharmaceutical formulations.

Skin, Oxidative Radicals and Natural Products

Haag et al. (2014) maintain that because the skin is the outermost organ of the human body, it is continuously exposed to pro-oxidative agents like radiation, nitrogen oxides, and ozone. Free radical formation in the skin is predominantly due to sun irradiation, which is one of the most important environmental hazards leading to a higher risk of skin cancer, accelerated skin ageing, and inflammation. Chronic exposure to the sun's radiation induces in the human body various skin conditions including cancer and premature ageing characterzed by wrinkles, scaling, dryness, dilatation of blood vessel and loss of collagen.

According to Ziegler, Jonason, Leffellt, Simon, Sharma and Kimmelman et al. (1994), sunlight acts as a carcinogen because sunlight mutates the p53 tumour-suppressor gene. The p53 mutations induced by ultraviolet radiation (in sunlight) are found in >90% of human squamous cell carcinoma of the skin. Inactivating p53 reduces the appearance of sunburn cells, apoptotic keratinocytes generated by overexposure to ultraviolet radiation. These authors claim the skin possess a p53-dependent 'guardian-of-the-tissue' response to DNA damage which aborts precancerous cells. If this response is reduced in a single cell by a prior p53 mutation, sunburn can select for clonal expansion of the p53-mutated cell into the disordered keratinocytes that lead to actinic keratosis. Sunlight can act twice: as tumour initiator and tumour promoter.

Exposure to ultraviolet B (UVB) radiation, an environmental carcinogen in its own right, provokes oxidative and inflammatory skin damage, thus magnifying the risk of skin cancer. Excessive contact with UVB also increases immunosuppression, adverse skin reactions, and skin photo-ageing. Obviously, in HIV-infected persons, increased exposure to UVB quickens progression to AIDS.

Due to increases in the number of skin cancers diagnosed every year, adverse effects of UV rays are progressively being recognized, and public health education is now directed at measures that increase photoprotection, including the use of sunscreens. Several natural products offer protection against the sun and are being developed or incorporated into sunscreens. An optimal sunscreen should contain all elements which reflect, absorb and scatter UV radiation in order to provide a broad-spectrum of protection throughout the whole UV range (290–400 nm) of the solar radiation reaching the Earth's surface.

Consistent with Lall and Kishore (2014), preparations of plants rich in phenolics protect the skin from UV radiation. Proteins, absorbing lipids, and nucleotides are also used as the skin's natural sun blockers. Seed oils are ideally suited to perform the role of sunscreens because fatty acids have been shown to be natural sun blockers when applied onto the skin. Natural oils are some of the most efficient sunscreens, offering 20-30% resistance to UV rays. Castor oil has a natural sun protection factor (SPF) of 5.6 and jojoba oil has SPF of 4. Other SPF values for natural oils are: red raspberry seed oil (30-50), carrot seed oil (30), wheat germ oil (20), soybean oil (10), cocoa butter (10), olive oil (7.5), coconut oil (7.1), avocado (4), eucalyptus oil (2.6), sesame oil (1.7), and tea tree oil (1.7) (Kaur & Saraf, 2010).

Jojoba oil, which has natural sun blocking properties, is included in a commercial sunscreen called *Desert Sun*, a product of Fabupharm- a pharmaceutical company in Otjiwarongo, Namibia. *Desert Sun* has an SPF of 30. Manu-factured in South Africa, *Everysun* sunscreen lotion-with SPF of 50, consists of natural products like castor oil and *Vitis vinifera* (grape) seed extracts. Grape seed oil contains oligometric procyanidins, 20-times more efficacious than vit-amin C in scavenging and removing dangerous free radicals from the skin. It also slows down ageing.

The natural antagonist of free radicals is the antioxidant network of the skin- enzymatic as well as non-enzymatic antioxidants. The skin barricade against oxidative stress is mainly located in the epidermis where there are high-er concentrations of antioxidants than in the dermis. The main protective system in the human skin is the natural pigment melanin- which absorbs and scatters UV radiation, and the skin's antioxidant enzymes: catalase, superoxide dismutase and glutathione peroxidase. In addition, the tumour suppressor pro-tein p53 plays an important role in UVB protection, acting as a transcription factor that controls genes involved in the cell cycle, programmed cell death and DNA repair.

Chaudhari, Kawade and Funne (2011) explored common plants employed in skin care and conclude that oxidative stress and the formation of radicals is one of the major mechanisms that mediates skin diseases and ageing. Lall and Kishore (2014) also emphasize that plants used in skin care have wound heal-ing, antioxidant and anti-inflammatory actions. These authors explain that antioxidants are radical scavengers which protect the human body from free radicals by inhibiting various oxidizing chain reactions. Several studies reveal that reactive oxygen species (ROS) generated in the skin promote the for-mation of many skin disorders.

Continuous exposure to environmental factors such as UV radiation is dangerous to the skin. It leads to changes in skin connective tissues emanating from the formation of lipid peroxides, enzymes and reactive oxygen species; overall this leads to various skin diseases. As HIV infection progresses to AIDS, production of ROS and oxidative stress take a heavier toll on the body, bringing forth an eruption of a myriad of skin diseases like eczema, boils, pso-riasis, herpes zoster, tumours, and etc. Owing to their antioxidant and anti-inflammatory properties and functions, a wide variety of natural products are used to treat and manage these skin conditions.

Lall and Kishore (2014) echo the point that plant extracts contain numer-ous naturally occurring compounds useful as antioxidants. Natural antioxidants like alpha-tocopherol, beta-carotene and phenolic compounds promote the good health of the skin. A wide variety of plant polyphenols have been report-ed to possess anti-oxidative and anti-inflammatory properties, thereby protecting the skin from photo-damage (Choi, Kundu, Chun, Na, & Surh 2014). Flavonoids, which represent the most common and widely distributed group of plant phenolics abundant in foods, also have beneficial effects on the skin.

Other antioxidant phenolics which underwrite excellent benefits to the skin are: rosmarinic acid, p-coumaric acid, caffeic acid, ferulic acid, chlorogenic acid, luteolin, apigenin, genkwanin, quercitrin, rutin, epicatechin and catechin. These antioxidants are mainly found in plant species belonging to the family Lamiaceae. Studies show that rosmarinic acid, a phenolic acid derivative, the isoflavone genistein and silibin from milk thistle have skin protective effects against UVB-induced ROS through p53 activation and decreased DNA damage. Rosemary (*Rosmarinus officinalis*) diterpenes also display strong antioxidant, anti-inflammatory and skin-protective actions.

Rutin (3- rhamnosyl-glucosylquercetin), a polyphenol present in many edible plants such as onions and apples, and drinks including tea and red wine, grants beneficial pharmacological actions to the skin e.g. antibacterial, antioxidant, anti-inflammatory, anti-mutagenic and anticancer (Choi et al., 2014). What do these studies tell us about rutin? Eating foods rich in rutin can fend off skin diseases and improve skin health. Eating onions and apples and drinking tea and moderate amounts of red wine can improve the health of your skin. Topical application of rutin to the skin also inhibits oxidation caused by dangerous UVB radiation.

Another good example is that of myconoside, a glycoside abundantly present in extracts of the European resurrection plant *Haberlea rhodopensis* which strongly stimulates antioxidant skin defences and extracellular matrix protein synthesis (Gechev, Hille, Woerdenbag, Benina, Mehterov, & Toneva et al., 2014). Like many other resurrection plants, *Haberlea* extracts also protect the skin against oxidation by UV radiation and microbial infections. Natural antioxidants prevent ROS formation by scavenging them out of cells, or completely destroying them; thus ultimately arresting skin disorders. Other plant antioxidants stop the initiation or propagation of oxidative pathways, and repair oxidative damage done to skin cells by ROS. Unsurprisingly, antioxidants derived from natural sources have attracted much interest in herbal preparations for skin disorders.

Deters, Meyer and Stintzing (2012) admit that the antioxidant potential of phenolic ingredients and their moisturizing effects are two well-known properties of cosmetic formulations. They give the examples of two xerophytic plants that possess beneficial effects on human skin: the common ice plant, *Mesembryanthemum crystallinum*, and the cactus pear, *Opuntia ficus-indica*. Both plants are used traditionally in dermatologic and cosmetic preparations. Cactus pear is a prominent nutritional, medicinal and cosmetical plant in Mexico, Italy, Spain, Brazil, Chile, Argentina and California. *Opuntia* species are used as ethnoremedies for many diseases by the indigenous people of Mexico and Peru.

Deters et al. (2012) note that *M. crystallinum*, a facultative halophyte, is adapted to extreme environmental conditions by synthesis of protective substances (osmolytes) and antioxidants such as betacyanins, mesembryanthin and other flavonoids. Their experiments show that the beneficial effects of common ice plant and cactus pear extracts on the skin are mainly due to the antioxidant and moisturizing molecules produced by the plants. The plants' chemical compounds also promote the growth of fibroblasts and keratinocytes especially during wound healing and skin regeneration. It goes without saying that the vitality and antioxidant functions of the skin barrier may be strengthened by the application of special skin care products rich in antioxidants.

Haag et al. (2014) assert that one promising natural antioxidant is the substance hyperforin, a major constituent of the plant St. John's Wort (*Hypericum perforatum*) which is a well-known treatment of atopic dermatitis (eczema) in addition to providing anti-inflammatory, anti-tumour, antibacterial and antioxidant properties. Experiments reveal that a cream rich in hyperforin improves the skin's protection against free oxygen radicals. Plus, radical formation due to irradiation is reduced and important skin lipids which are responsible for the barrier function of the skin are increased. Hyperforin also aids the differentiation and proliferation of the keratinocytes and thus may be an auspicious treatment for skin diseases such as atopic dermatitis and psoriasis.

Rodrigues, Palmeira-de-Oliveira, das Neves, Sarmento, Amaral and Oliveira (2013) emphasize that free radicals inflict oxidative damage to biological molecules while phenolic compounds- due to their antioxidant activity, are able to neutralize their adverse action. Several studies now attest to the fact that topical application of natural antioxidants is useful in preventing photo-ageing and ameliorating skin diseases mediated by oxidative stress. In addition, plant extracts may contain compounds with antimicrobial and other beneficial properties. Rodrigues and co-workers argue that although many herbal agents used in cosmetics have been selected by a process of trial and error, or through human experience rather than experimental investigation, growing scientific evidence points to a vast and complex arsenal of plant active ingredients able to calm, smooth, actively restore, heal and protect the human skin.

Plant polyphenols exhibit potent antioxidant properties. In animal models and *in vitro* cells, plant polyphenols show potent immuno-modulatory and beneficial effects in inflammation and photoprotection. Green tea (*Camellia sinensis*) and cocoa beans (*Theobroma cacao*) contain polyphenols called catechins, natural agents that slow skin ageing, improve skin health, and ameliorate skin diseases such as psoriasis and atopic dermatitis. Numerous skin cosmetic products are now manufactured from tea and cocoa.

Cocoa butter, also called theobroma oil, is an edible vegetable fat extracted from the cocoa bean. It is used to make chocolate, as well as skin lotions, creams and pharmaceuticals. The reason cocoa butter improves skin health and care is that it contains antioxidants which fight off ROS, and fatty acids (oleic, stearic and palmitic acids) which hydrate and moisturise dry skin. Thus, cocoa butter helps alleviate symptoms of dermatitis and eczema. Likewise, cocoa butter contains cocoa mass polyphenol, a natural antioxidant that prevents carcinogenesis of skin cells and slows the production of IgE antibodies, known to worsen symptoms of dermatitis and eczema.

Catechins in green tea slow down the ageing process and protect the skin from sun damage and help remove free radicals from the skin. Specifically, epigallocatechin-3-gallate is a potent phytochemical that guards the skin against the ravages of UV exposure and DNA damage. In the skin, free radicals damage cells and speed up the progression of cancer, ageing, and many other skin diseases. Washing with green tea is a cheaper way to restore and enhance the overall health condition of the skin. Thus, green tea is now available in many commercial face wash products. Catechins may alleviate skin cancer, sun damage, wrinkles, and skin photo-ageing (dermatoheliosis).

Scurvy is a disease that occurs when a person lacks adequate amounts of vitamin C. The disease is characterzed by body weakness, low blood count, gum disease and skin haemorrhages (bleeding). Although topical application of vitamin C (ascorbic acid) improves collagen production and removes free radicals from the skin by 20 times compared to ingestion, it goes without saying that eating fruits rich in vitamin C can reduce incidences of scurvy and help maintain a healthy skin. Vitamin C contributes to a smooth skin, reduces skin photo-ageing and helps alleviate acne lesions. Experiments show that vitamin C helps improve skin health by at least 60%.

Natural Products for Healing Inflammatory Skin Diseases

Katiyar (2005) contends that many environmental factors like sunlight cause injuries and inflammation of the skin. Sunburn, for example, can cause the production of highly grievous ROS, leading to acute or chronic skin inflammation. Acute inflammation results from exposure to UV radiation or from contact with chemical irritants while chronic inflammation results from a sustained immune cell mediated inflammatory response within the skin itself (Lall & Kishore, 2014). Skin inflammation presents as redness, heat and swelling, mainly due to alterations in the blood vessels in the injured skin.

Many studies show that inflammatory skin diseases are the most common problem in dermatology. They present in many different forms, from occasional skin rashes accompanied by skin itching and redness, to chronic conditions such as dermatitis (eczema), rosacea, seborrheic dermatitis, and psoriasis. Skin inflammation can be characterized as acute or chronic.

Acute inflammation can result from exposure to ultraviolent radiation, ionizing radiation, allergens, or to contact with chemical irritants like soaps and hair dyes. This type of inflammation is typically resolved within 1 to 2 weeks with little accompanying tissue destruction. In contrast, chronic inflammation results from a prolonged and extra-ordinarily strong and provocative cellular immune response within the skin itself. This inflammation is long-lasting and causes serious tissue destruction, like the one which presents as cold sores on the lips.

Inflammatory skin diseases include eczema, psoriasis, and acne. Fungal infections, too, usually cause eczema. For these diseases, most therapeutic options rely on the use of glucocorticoseteroids. Although most glucocorticoseteroids are anti-inflammatory, they also unfortunately cause immune suppression. For this reason, we are turning to the use of natural products that are anti-inflammatory without being immuno-suppressive. Indeed, many natural products act as anti-inflammatory agents. For example, phyto-flavonoids such as quercetin thwart biochemical pathways for pro-inflammatory prostaglandins and leukotrienes.

Psoriasis is a relatively common chronic inflammatory and proliferative skin disease, with genetic and environmental aetiologies characterized by abnormalities in skin lipids and increased production of inflammatory mediators. Atopic dermatitis is a common chronic allergic inflammatory skin disease. It is caused by genetic and environmental factors and is characterized by abnormal skin barrier formation (Nicolaou, 2013). Through different pathways, pro-inflammatory chemical mediators like leukotrienes activate the pathobiochemical and clinical presentation of psoriasis and atopic dermatitis.

Curcumin, one of the most potent natural anti-inflammatory substances, is a yellow phenolic compound present in the rhizomes of the Indian curry spice plant turmeric whose scientific name is *Curcuma longa*; a herbaceous perennial plant of the ginger family, Zingiberaceae. Curry powder contains turmeric and therefore contains curcumin, an effective scavenger of ROS and reactive nitrogen species. Therefore, eating foods spiced with natural turmeric and curry is good for the skin; it reduces inflammatory skin diseases.

Apple fruits are rich in quercetin, a natural bioflavonoid with very effective anti-inflammatory properties. Quercetin switches off the synthesis of inflammatory leukotrienes, which are a thousand-fold more potent than histamines in promoting inflammation. Quercetin therefore fights skin inflammation in a very powerful way. Consumption of foods and other natural products rich in quercetin is recommended in the management of inflammatory skin diseases such as eczema and psoriasis.

Another important natural anti-inflammatory compound is alpha-bisabolol, a natural monocyclic sesquiterpene first isolated from the plant

101

commonly known as chamomile, *Matricaria chamomilla*, family Asteraceae. Other plants that contain alpha-bisabolol are *Eremanthus erythropappus*, *Smyrniopsis aucheri*, *Salvia runcinata* and *Vanillosmopsis* species. Alpha-bisabolol is present in essential oils and ameliorates skin inflammation and cancer.

Alpha-bisabolol is now being ubiquitously added to cosmetic products like aftershave creams, hand and body lotions, deodorants, lipsticks, sun-protective products, baby care products and sports creams. Dried and fresh chamomile is made into teas which are a good supply of alpha-bisabolol. Chamomile tea is one of the world's most popular herbal teas. Apart improving the anti-inflammatory properties of the skin, chamomile also boosts the immune system, induces sleep and fights flu and colds. Hence, chamomile is used in traditional medicine in many cultures of the world.

Natural Products for Treating Microbial Skin Diseases

Many natural products treat microbial infections of the skin in humans. In Ethiopia, for example, Tadeg, Mohammed, Asres and Gebre-Mariam (2005) documented that eight species of plants traditionally used to treat various human skin diseases have antimicrobial properties. These plants are: *Acokanthera schimperi* (Apocynaceae), *Calpurnia aurea* (Leguminosae), *Kalanchoe petitiana* (Crassulaceae), *Lippia adoensis* (Verbenaceae), *Malva parviflora* (Malvaceae), *Olinia rochetiana* (Oliniaceae), *Phytolacca dodecandra* (Phytolaccaceae) and *Verbascum sinaiticum* (Scrophulariaceae).

Tadeg et al. (2005) found that extracts of *Lippia adoensis* and *Olinia rochetiana* are the most active against bacterial and fungal strains, respectively. In addition, almost all species of plants were found to have activity on at least one microbial strain. The antimicrobial activity profile also showed that *S. aureus* and *Trichophyton mentagrophytes* were the most susceptible bacterial and fungal strains, respectively (Tadeg et al., 2005). Their results demonstrate the power of natural products to combat microbial infections of the skin, thus, justifying their claimed traditional uses in the management of various microbial skin diseases.

A small corpus of empirical studies supports the antimicrobial activities of plant extracts traditionally used in treating skin diseases. On the authority of Mabona, Viljoen, Shikanga, Marston and Van Vuuren (2013), *Elephantorrhiza elephantina*, an ethnomedicinal plant for acne vulgaris, has remarkable antimicrobial activity against *Propionibacterium acnes*. *Diospyros mespiliformis*, a well-known anti-HIV plant remedy, is also used to manage skin mycoses especially ringworm. In addition, *D. mespiliformis* exhibits antifungal activity against *Trichophyton mentagrophytes* and *Microsporum canis*.

Mabona et al. (2013) describe that the aqueous root extracts of *Pentanisia prunelloides* mixed in a 1:1 ratio with *E. elephantina* exhibit synergistic interactions against skin pathogens *S. aureus*, gentamycin–methicillin resistant *S. aureus*, *Staphylococcus epidermidis* and *Candida albicans*. After fractionating extracts of the plant *Aristea ecklonii*, which is traditionally used to treat skin diseases, the South African scientists isolated plumbagin, a known anti-HIV bioactive compound with significant antimicrobial actions, minimum inhibitory concentrations from 2 to 16 μg/ml. Studies have also shown the antibacterial and antifungal effects of resveratrol, a phytoalexin that belongs to the group of compounds known as stilbenes.

Natural Pharmacopoeias for Skin Diseases in Southern Africa

South Africa

Afolayan, Grierson and Mbeng (2014) aver that among the Xhosa people of Amathole District in Eastern Cape, South Africa, 25 skin disorders are managed using 106 medicinal plant species. In the survey, Afolayan et al. (2014) document that the most widely used plant species to treat skin infections is *Aloe ferox*, family Xanthorrhoeaceae, locally known as *Umhlaba*. This is followed by *Carpobrotus edulis*, also known as *Unomatyum-tyum*. The leaf juice is known to destroy germs; hence it is used to treat eczema, wounds, burns and skin ulcers. Besides, the plant has strong antioxidant activity as it removes dangerous hydrogen peroxide radicals from skin cells (Omoruyi, Bradley, & Afolayan, 2012).

Skin hygiene and cosmetics are part and parcel of Xhosa traditional medicine. The Xhosa people use crushed avocado (*Persea americana*) seeds to treat pimples, wrinkles and protect facial skin from sun damage. The ethnomedicinal application of avocados to maintain skin health among the Xhosa people is justified and rational given the current biochemical knowledge of avocados. *Persea americana* is now increasingly recognized as one of the most nutrient-rich fruits due to its abundance of monounsaturated fatty acids, dietary fibre, proteins, vitamins, antioxidants and minerals.

Wang, Bostic and Gu (2010) mention several studies which show that avocados are rich in unsaturated fatty acids, fibre, vitamins B and E, and other nutrients. Avocados also contain lipophilic carotenoids that are anti-carcinogenic. The lipophilic extract of avocado inhibits prostate cancer cell growth (Lu, Arteaga, Zhang, Huerta, Go, & Heber, 2005), induces apoptosis in human breast cancer cells (Ding, Chin, Kinghorn, & D'Ambrosio, 2007), and attenuates liver injury (Kawagishi, Fukumoto, Hatakeyama, He, Arimoto, & Matsuzawa et al., 2001).

A fresh avocado consists of about 18% peel and 13% seed. During industrial processing of avocado, peels and seeds form part of the industrial waste. In their analysis, Wang et al. (2010) found that avocado seeds and peels contribute 57% and 38% of the antioxidant capacities of the whole fruit. Avocado skins have chlorophylls and carotenoids - these two pigments are well known antioxidants. Avocado seeds and peels contain procyanidins, including catechins and epicatechins. Chemically, it is these procyanidins that are the main compounds that contribute to the antioxidant valour of avocados. Antioxidant action reduces sun damage to skin cells, slows the progression of skin cancer, ageing, and ameliorates many other skin diseases. Washing the face with extracts of avocado seeds and peels is an inexpensive method to improve skin health and beauty.

Procyanidins from grape seeds and cocoa also offer many health benefits such as preventing cancers and other chronic diseases. Obviously, eating good quantities of avocados, besides harnessing avocado seeds and peels generated from avocado processing, could be great sources of phenolic nutraceuticals- these are foods that have health-giving additives and medicinal benefits including the prevention and treatment of skin diseases.

The following eight species were recorded for the first time in the management of skin disorders in South Africa: *Acalypha glabrata*, *Albuca setosa*, *Capsicum annuum*, *Pseudocrossidium crinitum*, *Behnia reticulate*, *Buddleja saligna*, *Buxus natalensis*, and *Cymbopogon marginatus* (Afolayan et al., 2014). The leaf paste of *Buddleja saligna* is used for the treatment of skin rashes in children. The plant *Gasteria obliqua* known locally as *Intelezi* is widely distributed in the Eastern Cape (Dold & Cocks, 2000). A decoction of *G. obliqua* leaves is locally used as a bath to cleanse the skin and for the treatment of skin irritations. Other plants used to treat and manage skin diseases in South Africa are shown in Table 3.1.

In another study, Ncube, Ndhlala, Okem and van Staden (2013) observe that *Hypoxis hemerocallidea*, a Southern African anti-HIV medicinal plant known to have phytosterol glucosides (β-sitosterol), diglucoside hypoxoside, aglycone rooperol, sterols and sterolins, has ethnomedicinal applications in the treatment of pimples, wounds, skin rashes and dermatitis. Capsules and powders of *Hypoxis* are marketed under the name *African Potato*, mostly for their immune enhancing potentialities. Some of the skin formulations containing *Hypoxis* include a cream called *Down To Earth* and a tonic named *Stameta*. These natural products are sold in health shops and pharmacies in South Africa.

The bulbs of the plant *Boophone disticha*, also known as *Incotho* in Xhosa, have been used as a hunting arrow poison and narcotic by the Khoi-San people as early as 2,000 years ago. But, the bulbs are also applied in the treatment of skin rashes, wounds, boils and swellings (Nair & van Staden, 2014). Phytochemical investigations by Cheesman, Nair and van Staden (2012) identified two known crinane alkaloids (buphanidrine and distichamine) in *B. disticha*; both of these compounds are broad-spectrum antibacterial agents that help in healing various skin infections. Extracts of *B. disticha* are active against methicillin-sensitive *S. aureus* with a minimum inhibitory concentration of 7.25 mg/ml. The plant also has excellent activities against skin pathogens such as *Bacillus subtilis*, *Escherichia coli*, *Klebsiella pneumonia* and *C. albicans*.

Maroyi (2014) revealed that extracts from the roots of the tree *Elaedendron transvaalense*, a treatment for skin rashes, also block HIV-1 reverse transcriptase. He also writes that *Bulbine alooides*, a herbal treatment for skin rashes, has anti-HIV activity. Other studies have documented the use of *Senna petersiana* in the treatment of skin infections. Some of the traditionally used anti-HIV/AIDS plants like *Aloe ferox*, *Cassia occidentalis* and *Terminalia sericea* are also remedies for opportunistic skin diseases and genital sores.

An important appraisal of Southern African medicinal plants of dermatological relevance is provided by Mabona and Van Vuuren (2013). They explore fundamental knowledge available on the antimicrobial, anti-inflammatory, and wound healing properties of medicinal plants used to treat skin ailments. Table 3.2 and Table 3.3 show plants used to manage skin diseases in Southern Africa. Other plant remedies for antimicrobial infections of the skin are shown in Table 3.4.

Betsie Rood, in her book *Nature's Own Pharmacy* (Rood, 2013), says eczema is managed through the application of extracts from *Cichorium intybus* (chicory), *Oncosiphon glabratum*, *Brassica oleracea* (common cabbage), *Nasturtium officinale* (watercress), *Chenopodium ambrosioides* (called *buchu* in South Africa), *Lablab purpureus*, *Fumaria officinalis* (fumitory), and *Salvinia officinalis* (common name is sage; in Latin *salvare* means sage, to save or to heal, also a Latin name denoting drug). Other plants for eczema treatment are *Linum usitatissimum* (flax), *Carpobrotus edulis* (sour fig), *Sorghum bicolor* (sorghum), and *Hermannia hyssopifolia*.

Botswana

In Botswana, Okatch, Ngwenya, Raletamo and Andrae-Marobela (2012) documented that traditional healers use several plants to manage skin diseases (rashes, sores or thrush) related to HIV infection: *Dichrostachys cinerea (Moselesele)*, *Maerua angolensis (Moretete/Moreketi)*, *Plumbago zeylanica (Masigomabe)*, *Combretum imberbe (Motswiri)*, *Indigofera flavicans (Tshikadithata)*, *Clerodendrum ternatum (Legonyana)*, *Capparis tomentosa (Motawana)*, and *Terminalia sericea (Mogonono)*. *C. tomentosa* shows activity against bacteria, hence is well suited to treat bacterial skin diseases.

In relation to their study of Botswana plants that inhibit HIV replication, Leteane, Ngwenya, Muzila, Namushe, Mwinga and Musonda et al. (2012) disclose that *Cassia sieberiana* (*Mororwe*) heals skin rashes and body sores; *Combretum albopanctum* (*Moriri wa tau*) treats skin rashes, thrush and herpes; *P. zeylanica* (*Masigomabe*) lessens symptoms of sores, external rashes, thrush and herpes; *Spermacoce deserti* (*Makgonatsotlhe*) remedies skin rashes, thrush and herpes; and *Ximenia caffra* (*Moretologa wa kgomo*) relieves thrush, herpes and general skin diseases.

Namibia

Among the Ovambo people of northern Namibia, *Salvadora persica*, known as *Omunkwavu*, is used to manage skin rashes. This ethnomedicinal usage is consistent with reports that the aqueous extracts of *S. persica* have an inhibitory effect on the growth of *C. albicans*, *Enterococcus faecalis*, *Streptococcus* and *S. aureus* (Halawany, 2012). The bark and roots of *Garcinia buchananii*, known as *Mukononga* in the siLozi language of the Zambezi Region, is used to treat skin infections in Namibia. The plant also has HIV-1 protease inhibitory action (Maroyi, 2014).

Abrus precatorius, known as *Mupitipiti* in siLozi, has activity against clinically important bacteria, and is used to treat oral candidiasis and syphilitic ulcers; it also inhibits HIV-1 reverse transcriptase. Some of its active chemical compounds are abrusoside (a cycloartane glycoside) and flavonol glycoside. Well known plants *Moringa oleifera* and *Ximenia americana* also heal skin infections and possess anti-HIV activities, respectively. Chinsembu has documented anti-HIV plants used to treat skin diseases in Namibia, see Table 3.5.

Kigelia africana is a remedy for skin infections, removes sun spots (solar keratosis) and is now included in skin creams and shampoos. In our research group at the University of Namibia, we have shown the antibacterial activities of extracts of different *K. africana* genotypes. Extracts of a *K. africana* genotype found in the Parliament Gardens were more potent than those from Kavango Region and Rocky Crest suburb in Windhoek.

Saini, Kaur, Verma, Ripudaman and Singh (2009) point out that extracts of *K. africana* contain irridoids, naphthoquinone, meroterpenoid naphthoquinones, coumarin derivatves, lignans, sterols and flavonoids. These chemical substances bequeath *K. africana* with a plethora of medicinal properties. For example, extracts of *K. africana* are used to treat skin diseases such as boils, wounds, psoriasis, ringworms, eczema and fungal infections. Known as the sausage tree, *K. africana* is harnessed in the management of malaria, pneumonia, dysentery, syphilis, gonorrhoea and tapeworms. Maroyi (2014) quotes a study in Kenya by Rukanga and co-workers which reported the HIV-1 reverse transcriptase inhibitory activity of *K. africana*.

Among the Topnaar people, *Pechuel-loeschea leubnitziae* plant extract is also used for the treatment of measles, sores and skin disorders and for the disinfection of wounds (Van Damme, Van Den Eynden, & Vernemmen, 1922). This ethnomedicinal usage of *P. leubnitziae* is warranted given that the plant has activity against several gram-positive and gram- negative bacteria. The Himba mix roasted and powdered roots of *P. leubnitziae* with fat; they rub this formulation onto their necks as a skin cosmetic. They also drink an extract of the roots to treat gonorrhoea or use it cutaneously for STIs and skin infections.

Maerua schinzii is a treatment for skin acnes. *Acanthosicyos horridus* (nara bush), contains anti-cancer and anti-inflammatory compounds called cucurbitacins as well as oils that hydrate the skin and protect against sun burn and acnes. *Ricinus communis* (castor bean) oil and leaf poultices heal wounds and skin diseases.

Zambia

Kigelia africana is termed *Muvung'uvung'u* among the Lunda people of northwestern Zambia where young women smear fruit extracts to enlarge breasts. In many parts of Africa, men use the plant's extracts to enlarge the penis to sausage proportions. The Tonga women in the Zambezi Valley of Zambia apply cosmetic formulations of *K. africana* fruits to their faces to ensure a blemish free complexion. Extracts of *K. africana* contain broad-spectrum antimicrobial activities which support their ethnomedicinal applications to treat skin diseases such as acnes and eczema.

Ziziphus mauritiana, also known as *Masau* in Nyanja, is a wild fruit plant very rich in vitamin C. It contains 20 to 30% sugar, up to 2.5% protein and 12.8% carbohydrates. Aqueous extracts and powders have broad-spectrum antibacterial activity and are therefore used as dressing to prevent bacterial infections and to aid in wound healing during male circumcision among the Lunda and Luvale people of Zambia. With reference to *Z. mauritiana*, Kennedy Kazeza, a graduate of the *Mukanda* (male circumcision) initiation ceremony of Zambezi, North-Western Province, Zambia, said:

> It has taken me down memory lane to my own initiation (*Mukanda*). I was 12 years old when I was circumcised. I vividly remember one of the medicines used on my wound was *Akasongole* or in my tribe *Likolo* (*Makolo* for plural) - a hard wild fruit, green when unripe and golden yellow when fully ripe.

For two weeks this green unripe fruit was my wife! They made a hole in it, the size of my manhood and every morning I would dip my member in it for 30 minutes or so. That's all the penicillin I ever needed for my wound! In just two weeks, I was able to climb trees and sleep freely without worries of having to '*kulitalukunya ku chilonda*' (scratching the wound) in the night.

East African Pharmacopoeia

Ethiopia

In Ethiopia, *P. zeylanica* is a medicinal plant commonly used to treat skin diseases (Teshome et al., 2008). It is locally known as *Amera* in the Amharic tribe. The plant is widely distributed in the west and north-western parts of Ethiopia at 1500–2200m above sea level. Apart from Africa, *P. zeylanica* is also found in tropical and subtropical regions of Asia and Australia. In ethnobotanical surveys, *P. zeylanica* is used for the management of wounds, eczema, scabies, and leprosy (Teshome et al., 2008). *Dodonaea viscosa*, a treatment for skin infections in Ethiopia, also inhibits HIV replication (Maroyi, 2014).

Many studies show that *P. zeylanica* has several phytochemicals including plumbagin, linoleic acid, palmitic acid, nonylnonanoate, stigmasterol acetate, lupeol acetate, friedelinol, lupeol, lupanone, sitosterone and stigmasterol. Plumbagin is the main active chemical compound in the root of this plant whose uses in dermatological therapy are attributable to its antimicrobial, antiprotozoal and pesticidal properties.

Inula confertiflora is used in Ethiopia to treat skin diseases of viral origin, wounds and eczematous lesions (Seca, Grigore, Pinto, & Silva, 2014). At Addis Abba University, Bruck Messele, while studying the role of *I. confertiflora* in treating dermatological disorders in Ethiopia, observed good antifungal activity against *Trichophyton mentagrophytes*, mostly due to the presence of sesquiterpene lactones and flavonoids.

Kenya

In the East African country of Kenya, Ochwang'i, Kimwele, Oduma, Gathumbi, Mbaria and Kiama (2014) acknowledge different plant species applied by local communities in the management of skin tumours. The plants are presented in Table 3.6. What chemical constituents in these plants support ethnomedicinal claims for treating skin cancer?

Many skin cancer ethnomedicinal plants listed in Table 3.6 have known biological activities. For instance, the activity of *Justicia betonica* is partly due to the presence of alkaloids (jusbetonin, 10H-quindoline), triterpenes and lignans. *Rhus vulgaris* has antimicrobial activity. A leaf decoction of the plant *Phyllanthus fischeri* is used to manage HIV/AIDS. *Abrus precatorius* secretes a lectin called abrin, with antitumour properties, in addition to its isoflavan quinones and hydroquinones that confer antiprotozoal activity.

An anti-HIV plant *Spathodea campanulata* contains ursolic acid, a natural pentacyclic triterpene acid used in skin cosmetics that also inhibits various skin cancer cells. Ursolic acid is abundant in apple peels, several foods, and many herbs. Apart from being an anti-inflammatory agent, ursolic acid interferes with carcinogenesis by inhibiting the signal transducer and activator of transcription 3 (STAT3) protein, hence ursolic acid is considered a natural remedy for many cancers, especially skin cancer.

Yu, Pardoll and Jove (2009) found that activation of STAT3 increases tumour cell proliferation, survival and invasion while suppressing anti-tumour immunity. The persistent activation of STAT3 also mediates tumour-promoting inflammation. Yu et al. (2009) suggest that STAT3 is a promising target to redirect inflammation for cancer therapy. Due to these pharmacological actions against skin cancer, ursolic acid is included in health products for topical application to the skin.

Grace, Simmonds, Smith and Van Wyk (2008) document the therapeutic uses of *Aloe* species in Southern Africa. *Aloe volkensii* exudates contain a mixture of the stereoisomers aloin A (barbaloin) and aloin B (isobarbaloin) and roots have anthraquinones which together heal skin lesions and jiggers (Ochwang'i et al., 2014). The annual herb *Bidens pilosa* confers antibacterial, antioxidant, antiprotozoal, and anticancer activities. Stem bark decoction of *Bridelia micrantha* contains phytochemicals including alkaloids, flavonoids, steroids, tannins and saponins which are useful in managing skin ailments and venereal diseases. A leaf decoction of *Cyphostemma serpens* is applied to arrest abscesses, boils, and other skin diseases.

Several studies submit that *Harungana madagascariensis* - a natural source for dermatological agents and cosmetics - contains phenols, alkaloids, flavonoids, tannins, and saponins. Its antibacterial action has found medicinal uses in staving off skin diseases and wounds, sore throat, diarrhoea, and STIs. Roots are also used to accelerate breast development in young women, while a root and bark infusion interrupts menstruation. *Melia azedarach* consists of anti-inflammatory alkaloids with broad-spectrum antibiotic activities valuable in ameliorating skin diseases. Other studies show that extracts of the plants *Calodendrum capense*, *Warburgia salutaris*, *Croton sylvaticus*, *Zantedeschia aethiopica*, *T. sericea* and *Withania somnifera* deter fungal infections of the skin.

Among the Luo and Suba people of Kenya, the following plant species are harvested for use as skin remedies: *Commiphora africana* (boils, skin rash), *Thevetia peruviana* (skin rash), *Lannea schweinfurthii* (boils, skin rash), *Azadirachta indica* (boils, skin rash), *Cocos nucifera* (skin rash), *Euclea divinorum* (boils, skin rash), *Aloe* sp. (boils), and *X. americana* (skin rash) (Nagata, Jew, Kimeu, Salmen, Bukusi, & Cohen, 2011). In Uganda, the most important plant species used for skin diseases in HIV/AIDS patients is *Zehneria scabra* and *Psorospermum febrifugum* (Mugisha, Asiimwe, Namutebi, Borg-Karlson, & Kakudidi, 2014).

Rwanda

Plants that modulate melanogenesis are used for voluntary depigmentation of the facial skin. In Sub-Saharan Africa, lighter skin is sometimes associated with more beauty and women bleach their skins before weddings. Now, in order to lure men who are mesmerized by lighter skin tone, women bleach or whiten their skins using products containing the chemicals hydroquinone or mercury. Skin bleaching is very common in countries like Rwanda, Democratic Republic of the Congo, Kenya and Zambia - where more than 70% of women have bleached faces. These skin lightening chemicals may cause skin cancer, leukaemia, liver problems and thyroid disorders. But the use of natural plant products to lighten skin circumvents side-effects attributable to hydroquinone and mercury.

West African Pharmacopoeia

In Cameroon, three plants *Dissotis perkinsiae*, *Adenocarpus mannii* and *Barteria fistulosa*, are used for the treatment of skin diseases including wounds. Studies reveal that many species of *Adenocarpus*, which contain flavonoids, alkaloids, and polyphenols, are used for the treatment of skin diseases such as leprosy, scabies and acne. *Barteria fistulosa*, family Passifloraceae, is widely used for the treatment of wounds and rheumatism. This plant contains tannins, alkaloids, terpenoids, flavonoids, iridoids and cyanoheterosides. The anti-HIV plant *Zingiber officinale* (ginger) is used to manage skin infections (Maroyi, 2014).

The Ghanaian people utilize many plants to manage skin disorders, this according to a study by Pesewu, Cutler and Humber (2008). Some of the plants are: *Alstonia boonei* (cleaning wounds), *Rauwolfia vomitoria* (parasitic skin diseases), *Parquetina nigrescens* (candidiasis), *Balanites aegyptica* (herpes zoster), *Cassia alata* (herpes zoster, eczema and mycosis), *Crateva religiosa* (leprosy), *Combretum micranthium* (wounds), *Terminalia avicennoides* (boils), *Momordica charantia* (measles), *Persea americana* (skin ulcers), *Psidium guajava* (measles or herpes zoster), and *Gardenia ternifolia* (body itching or syphilis). All these plants have proven antibacterial effects. Extracts of *Alchornea cordifolia*, also used to treat wounds, display the widest spectrum of antibacterial activity.

In Nigeria, a mixture of *Nigella sativa* and honey is called *alpha-Zam*, an effective nutraceutical used by HIV patients. In one study, a *N. sativa* remedy increased body weight from 53 to 63 kg, decreased HIV viral load from 42,300 copies to less than 50 copies of RNA per millilitre and increased CD4 cell count from an average of 227 to 680 mm^3 per litre at 4 months post-therapy (Onifade, Jewell, Ajadi, Rahamon, & Ogunrin, 2013). *N. sativa* alleviates other signs of HIV infection such as diarrhoea, fever, cough, oral thrush and skin rashes.

Asian Pharmacopoeia

India

It is estimated that in India, traditional healers use roughly 2,500 plant species in the preparation of herbal medicines (Pei, 2001). Skin diseases like eczema, leucoerma, ringworm, scabies and many other conditions are usually treated with herbal drugs. In one survey, Policepatel and Manikrao (2013) document 60 plant species, belonging to 34 families, which are used for the treatment of common skin diseases. A paste made from the bark of *A. indica*, locally known as *Bevu*, is applied to heal many skin diseases.

Clerodendrum serratum has many medicinal uses such as being hepatoprotective, antioxidant, anti-inflammatory and anticancer, mainly due to the presence of saponins (terpenoids and steroids), flavonoids and phenolics (Patel, Acharya, & Acharya, 2014). *C. serratum* is used to treat skin diseases in Indian traditional medicine. Because of its flavonoids and phenolics, the plant also diminishes the occurrence and severity of skin papilloma. *Clerodendrum trichotomum* inhibits HIV-1 integrase.

The fresh latex of *Euphorbia tirucalli*, also known as Kolkalli, heals eczema while a leaf decoction of the same plant heals skin infected by ringworms. Leaf extracts of *Lantana camara* and *Mangifera indica* are separately used as treatments for wounds. Juice from the aerial parts of *Carica papaya*, *M. charantia* and *P. zeylanica* is applied to remedy skin affected by ringworms. A *Tephrosia purpurea* leaf extract is rubbed into the skin to relieve itching. *Acanthus ilicifolius*, a mangrove shrub along the Indian coast, is a remedy for skin diseases such as boils and wounds; it has activity against several bacteria and fungi (Govindasamy & Arulpriya, 2013). *M. charantia* is also applied as a therapy for skin cancer (Palamthodi & Lele, 2014).

Bhat, Hegde, Hegde and Mulgund (2014) list plants used to treat skin diseases in Ghats, India. Some of the plants and skin diseases are: *Acacia catechu* (pruritus), *Aloe vera* (all types of skin diseases), *A. indica* (ringworm or scabies), *Diospyros montana* (eczema or skin sores), *Ficus exasperata* (eczema, pruritus, ringworm or scabies), *Jatropha curcas* (eczema), *M. indica* (pruritus, scabies or septic due to skin allergies), *Mimosa pudica* (dermatitis or ringworms), *Moringa oleifera* (sores on the penis), *Plumbago indica* and *P. zeylanica* (eczema), *Ziziphus rugosa* and *Ziziphus xylopyrus* (boils) and *Terminalia chebula* (is a remedy for intertrigo, an inflammation or rash on the skin which tends to occur in warm, moist areas of the body where two skin surfaces or 'skin folds' rub or press against each other). Use values for the following plants are high: *Pongamia pinnata* (pruritus, scabies or herpes), *Naregamia alata* (eczema, pruritus or scabies), *Randia dumetorum* (herpes, pruritus or scabies) and *Girardinia diversifolia* (herpes, pruritus or scabies).

In India, the medicinal plant *Berberis aristata*, family Berberidaceae, is an Ayurvedic and multi-medicinal herb used since ancient times (Potdar, Hirwani, & Dhulap, 2012). It is also named *Indian berberi, Daruharidra, Daruhaldi, Darvi* and *Chitra*. Potdar et al. (2012) assert that *B. aristata* is a useful anti-pyretic, antimicrobial, anti-hepatotoxic, anti-hyperglycaemic, anticancer, antioxidant and anti-lipidemic agent. Because *B. aristata* has activity against the bacterium *Helicobacter pylori*, it is used to manage ulcers and other gastrointestinal disorders. These authors submit that extracts of *B. aristata* are useful in the treatment of diarrhoea, haemorrhoids, gynaecological disorders, HIV/AIDS, osteoporosis, diabetes, eye and ear infections, wounds, jaundice, malaria fever and a host of skin diseases. In their review, Potdar et al. (2012) found that several patents of *B. aristata* were registered as anti-HIV agents.

Potdar et al. (2012) note that *B. aristata* is one of the 73 plants applied against traditional skin diseases in Nepal. They observe that the Malani tribal societies in Himachal Pradesh, India, also utilize *B. aristata* to cure skin diseases. Studies illustrate that a herbal gel formulation containing this plant extract has activity against resistant strains of microbes such as *S. aureus, Pseudomonas aeruginosa* and *Corynebacterium*. Little wonder a formulation of *B. aristata* is an effective prescription for skin infections. *B. aristata* is now included in cosmetic preparations for skin care, treating alopecia, chronic skin disorders and as an agent to slow the ageing process.

Duraipandiyan and Ignacimuthu (2011) tested 45 Indian plants used in the treatment of dermatophytes. They found that the following plants have broad-spectrum antifungal activity: *Albizzia procera, Atalantia monophylla, Asclepias curassavica, Azima tetracantha, Cassia fistula, Cinnomomum verum, Costus speciosus, Nymphaea stellata, Osbeckia chinensis, Piper argyrophyllum, Punica granatum, Tinospora cordifolia* and *Toddalia asiatica*. The plant *Cassia auriculata*, used to treat skin diseases, contains triterpenoids and glycosides. Another plant remedy for skin disorders, *C. fistula*, has active compounds such as anthraquinone, glycosides, fistulic acids and benzoic acid. The stem bark of *P. zeylanica*, which contains an active ingredient called plumbagin, heals bacterial and fungal skin infections in India. *Sphaeranthus indicus*, a plant remedy for leprosy, consists of chemical compounds such as cinnamaldehyde, geraniol and geranyl acetate.

Okhuarobo, Ehizogie Falodun, Erharuyi, Imieje, Falodun and Langer (2014) reviewed that the plant *Andrographis paniculata* is used in many Asian countries to treat various skin diseases. In English, *A. paniculata* is nicknamed the 'king of bitters'. Phytochemical analysis shows that *A. paniculata* contains various compounds including labdane diterpenoid lactones and flavonoids which confer antimicrobial, anti-inflammatory and antioxidant activities. The major active constituent of *A. paniculata* is termed andrographolide, an awesome pharmacophore with anticancer and immunomodulatory activities (Rajagopal, Kumar, Deevi, Satyanarayana, & Rajagopalan, 2003).

Inula, family Asteraceae, is a large genus in the tribe Inuleae with more than one hundred species. This genus is found mainly in Africa, Asia (20 species are distributed in China) and in Europe, predominantly in the Mediterranean area. In Ayurvedic medicine - one of the world's oldest medical systems which originated in India more than 3,000 years ago - the plant *Inula racemosa*, known as *Pushkarmool* by the Indian people, is used as a treatment for tuberculosis and topically applied in the treatment of various skin diseases (Seca et al., 2014).

Hippocrates described *Inula campana*, sometimes referred to as *Inula helenium*, as a good and effective cure for chronic skin eruptions and itching. In temperate Europe and Asia, *Inula viscosa* is also included in the large palette of herbs used against psoriasis (Seca et al., 2014). Extracts of *I. helenium* are topically applied to treat wounds, freckles and dandruff. Most of the biological actions of *Inula* plant species such as anticancer, anti-inflammatory and antioxidant activities are attributable to the presence of flavonoids (Seca et al., 2014). *Inula* species also possess many antimicrobial and antiprotozoal properties, hence their use for the treatment of skin infections.

Interestingly, compounds isolated from *Inula* are also effective in plant protection where they inhibit several pathogens or pests. For example, the oily paste extract of *I. viscosa* leaves is not only helpful in the management of downy mildew caused by *Plasmopara viticola* in grapes but also used in other fungicidal preparations against foliar diseases caused by pathogens belonging to the families Oomycetes, Ascomycetes and Basidiomycetes. The active antifungal agent in *Inula* species is tomentosin, an active ingredient which also blocks proliferation of cancer cells and induces apoptosis of aggressive skin melanoma. Melanocytes, the natural photo-protectors of the skin, secrete melanin which protects the skin's epidermal cells from DNA damage caused by UV radiation.

Tomentosin derived from *Inula* plants is very useful in natural product formulations for treating skin diseases.

Pakistan and Philippines

Abbasi et al. (2010) conducted an ethnopharmacological study of medicinal plants used to manage skin diseases in Pakistan. The following plants are utilized in the amelioration of skin diseases in Pakistan: *Berberis lyceum*, *Bergenia ciliata*, *Melia azedarach*, *Otostegia limbata*, *Phyla nodiflora*, *Prunus persica* and *Zingiber officinale* (ginger). *Ajuga bracteosa* is applied to remove pimples; *Allium cepa* (onions) is used to treat boils and warts; *Aloe vera* is a remedy for boils; and *Arisaema speciosum* heals boils, carbuncle and warts.

Other plants used to treat skin diseases in Pakistan are: *Brassica campestris* is a remedy for boils and warts; *Calotropis procera* is applied to manage eczema and ringworms; *Cedrela toona* treats scabies and pimples; *Clematis grata* relieves eczema and warts; *Dalbergia sissoo* works as an anti-dandruff; *Datura stramonium* alleviates boils and warts; *M. azedarach* is a remedy for boils, pimples and scabies; *Nerium oleander* eases boils, leprosy and warts; and *Rhus chinensis* heals pimples and boils.

In the Philippines, *Hibiscus rosa-sinensis* is a treatment for boils and skin eruptions, and *Cocos nucifera* and *Gliricidia sepium* separately soothe scabies (Abe & Ohtani, 2013).

Traditional Chinese medicine

Among the Hakka people of Guangdong province in China, several plants are ethnodrugs for skin diseases. A study by Au, Wu, Jiang, Chen, Lu and Zhao (2008) revealed that a decoction of the whole plant of *Solidago decurrens* (*Id'ziwongfa*) treats eczema and skin ulcers. *Viola inconspicua* (*Hiongtidangcao'iab*) leaf decoction heals ulcerative carbuncle (abscesses, boils or sores) and skin ulcers, and *Xanthium sibiricum* (*Cong'ngizi*) root and leaf decoctions cure itchy skin, abscess bleeding and skin ulcers. Other medicinal plants for rectifying skin disorders are: *Portulaca oleracea*, a remedy for skin inflammation and *Impatiens balsamina* cures athlete's foot, pruritus (intense itching) and abscess bleeding. The Chinese medicinal plant *Hemsleya jinfushanensis* produces two moderate anti-HIV agents, hemslecins A and B, which interfere with HIV entry. Hemslecin A works against infectious diseases and hemslecin B reduces skin cancer.

Polygonum perfoliatum treats athlete's foot, and *Hibiscus mutabilis* cures furunculosis, a medical condition whereby large areas of the skin are covered in persistent boils. *Lolangoik* in Hakka dialect is a disease of scabies on the foot that is difficult to cure, and, even when healed, easily recurs. This syndrome is very common among HIV patients, diabetic individuals and the elderly. The Hakka people treat *Lolangoik* by using aloe creams that they apply onto the wounds. Using a few of these plants, external treatment of skin diseases is occasionally undertaken during medicinal baths - which also wash away bad luck accumulated throughout the year; hence medicinal baths are common on the eve of the Chinese New Year.

Several species of *Inula* are used in traditional medicine throughout the world, although more common in Traditional Chinese Medicine. The major component of *Inula crithmoides* roots extract, 1,5-di-O-caffeoylquinic acid, is a potent HIV-1 integrase inhibitor; it has undergone evaluation as a promising novel HIV therapeutic agent. Chinese scientists have initiated clinical trials of this compound to test its efficacy in the treatment of HIV/AIDS and hepatitis B.

According to Tsai et al. (2014), *Phyla nodiflora* is used in traditional Chinese herbal medicine to treat ulcers and skin inflammation. Its medicinal properties are aligned to the effect of eupafolin (6-methoxy 5,7,3',4'-tetrahydroxyflavone), which has antioxidant, anti-inflammatory and anticancer activities. *Rhododendron brachycarpum* (contains the active compound rhododenrin) has been used to treat skin inflammatory diseases in traditional oriental medicine (Jeon, Kim, Kim, Oh, Lee, Shin, & Kim, 2013). Since topically applied rhododendron alleviates skin inflammation in mice, it can therefore be potentially used to treat inflammatory skin diseases such as psoriasis in humans.

Other Pharmacopoeias

Even in modern-day Russia, phytotherapy is a recognized and distinct field of medicine, meaning herbal formulations are allowed by government authorities to be administered as medicines to patients. Shikov, Pozharitskaya, Makarov, Wagner, Verpoorte and Heinrich (2014) show that extracts from the dried roots and rhizomes of *Rhodiola rosea* inhibit HIV-1 protease by 70%. But *R. rosea*, commonly known as roseroot, also has phytochemicals that enrich the antioxidant functions of human skin cells, in addition to healing severe skin disorders.

Other phytoremedies for skin conditions are: *Alnus incana*, which increases antioxidant enzymes and skin healing and has radioprotective and anti-inflammatory properties; *Bidens tripartita* reduces desquamation of the skin; *Tanacetum vulgare* poultices contain flavonoids and phenolcarbonic acids, and are used to heal skin eruptions, kill lice and fleas, and treat scabies; and *Polemonium caeruleum* reduces fat levels in the skin.

Pine buds (*Pinus silvestris*) are widely used in Russian traditional medicine as an expectorant and a weak diuretic for the treatment of chronic bronchitis and tuberculosis. Pine buds can be used for aromatic baths that improve skin conditions and support the treatment of arthritis. Another Russian skin treatment is *Gemmae Betulae* which consists of the buds of *Betula pendula* and *Betula pubescens*.

Birch buds are widely used in Russian traditional medicine as a diuretic, expectorant, diaphoretic, blood-purifier, and analgesic, as an anti-infective agent and an antiseptic for wound healing, to treat furunculosis, and as a wash to remove skin spots (Shikov et al., 2014). Infusions and decoctions of birch buds are used in stomatology and otolaryngology for their anti-inflammatory properties, to treat stomatitis, gingivitis, periodontitis, glossitis, sore throat, chronic tonsillitis, acute respiratory diseases and as a rinse applied to gauze pads, which are moistened with infusions or decoctions (Shikov et al., 2014).

In Portugal, Rodrigues et al. (2013) describe seven species of *Medicago* (*Medicago minima, Medicago tornata, Medicago truncatula, Medicago rigidula, Medicago scutelata, Medicago segitalis* and *Medicago sativa*) as a potential source of natural compounds with high levels of antioxidant activity, low cytotoxicity for skin cells and the ability to potentially prevent microbial infections of the skin. As a consequence, there is an increasing demand for plant extracts to be included into cosmetics, either as fragrances or for their medicinal properties.

Rodrigues et al. (2013) explain that herbal extracts are used by cosmetic industry to beautify and maintain the physiological balance of the human skin. According to these authors, the desirable features of cosmetic ingredients are efficacy, safety, novelty, formulation stability, easy metabolism in the skin and low cost. These important characteristics are also found in herbal cosmetics, causing a huge public demand. Still, compared to synthetic cosmetic products, herbal products are mild and biodegradable and simultaneously present low toxicity.

At the University of Ghent in Belgium, De Spiegeleer, Boonen, Malysheva, Mavungu, De Saeger and Roche et al. (2013) describe preparations of *Spilanthes acmella* which are used to treat skin diseases like swimmers eczema and are also used as anti-wrinkle agents. Moreover, dermatological formulations with *Echinaceae purpurea* reduce wrinkles, improve skin hydration and wound healing. Part of the natural pharmacopoeia used in traditional Toba medicine, Argentina, for the treatment of skin disorders is shown in Table 3.7.

A Closer Look at Natural Products for Skin Care

It would seem the skin is an index of the body's health and wellbeing, a structure at the cross-roads of either allowing the body's invasion by or defence against infective and harmful agents. The skin lies at the intersection of 'beauty and the beast'. This means that the integrity, strength and formidability of the skin are the key pillars for a healthy and disease-free body. A healthy skin is the starting point for a healthy body. This narrative is helped by many chemical agents in plants.

There are three basic antagonists to a healthy skin: free radicals and oxidation, inflammation and microbial pathogens. Microbial infections of the skin (acnes, boils, eczema, herpes zoster, sores, leprosy, mycoses, psoriasis, rashes, wounds, and general skin infections) are on the increase due to HIV/AIDS. Persons suffering from microbial skin infections use many different natural products. In Namibia, microbial skin diseases account for a quarter of all ethnomedicinal plants used to manage HIV/AIDS.

The efficacy of natural products to treat skin diseases has been practiced since ancient times. Both Christianity and Islam acknowledge the importance of skin diseases in their faiths. Natural products contain chemical compounds with antimicrobial, anti-protozoal, anti-inflammatory and antioxidant activities. Hence, they confer beneficial functions to the skin. Exposure of the skin to the sun and its harmful UV radiation - much like HIV infection - causes oxidation (the formation of reactive oxygen species in cells). Oxidation makes the skin susceptible to microbial infections and cancer.

Oxidization is synonymous to decay, deterioration and decomposition. Look at what happens when you leave a piece of apple in the sun. It starts to decompose, to rot and deteriorate. It begins to change its colour to brown. This is similar to what happens when human cells undergo oxidation. Cells undergoing oxidation do decay, decompose and deteriorate; they eventually turn into dead inorganic matter. Given this understanding, oxidation due to the sun or HIV infection makes body cells to rot, deteriorate and decompose at a much faster rate, leading to a myriad of diseases like cancer or AIDS.

Reactive oxygen species (free radicals) which are produced by various metabolic processes and biochemical pathways, UV radiation or oxidizers may damage cells, initiating pro-inflammatory reactions. In using natural products to enhance the health of the skin and protect it from microbial diseases, the principle is simple: Appropriately formulated skin care natural products help maintain skin barrier integrity and enrich its protective capacity. Without a doubt, natural products help prevent and treat microbial infections and inflammatory conditions of the skin.

Free radicals often injure skin cells, damage the skin cells' DNA and trigger the chain reaction for skin diseases. Yes, normal cells also produce free radicals but such free radicals are few and easily controlled by natural antioxidants that the skin produces. Eating foods rich in antioxidants helps maintain a healthy and disease-free skin. Drinking copious amounts of alcohol leads to substantial production of free radicals, increased oxidation of the skin and ultimately it increases the manifestation of skin diseases. People who drink too much alcohol have pale skins and are prone to many skin diseases. Many people who indulge in excessive drinking of alcohol also develop red lips.

In some Black people, there is progressive loss of melanin on the lips, eventually leading to red lips. In countries such as Zambia, red lips invite HIV/AIDS stigma. Other than being a genetically designed substructure, red lips may physiologically signal a breach in the antioxidant protocols of the skin. Such breaches may be due to exposure to oxidising radiation from the sun, lack of adequate natural antioxidants in the diet and perhaps disorders and infections (including HIV) that cumulatively increase the production of reactive oxygen species in the body. Excessive consumption of alcohol produces free radicals and reduces the antioxidant functions of the body leading to red lips.

On the flip-side, there are many foods that are good for the skin. These foods are rich in antioxidants. Eating adequate amounts of foods rich in antioxidants helps quench free radicals thereby improving the texture and health of the skin. Green tea and cocoa contain antioxidant phytochemicals such as polyphenols that remove free radicals from the skin. Corollary, drinking green tea and cocoa, or eating chocolate, helps improve the health of the skin. Washing the skin with water extracts of green tea removes the oxidizing sting from the skin (free radicals); it gives the skin a 'calming effect' which produces a strong healthy skin.

Therefore, oxidation of the skin is the tragic foundation of many skin disorders and diseases. Exposure to the sun should be avoided or the harmful effects of radiation from the sun should be reduced by applying sunscreens and other ointments. This is because the sun oxidizes the human skin, leading to many skin disorders and diseases. Excessive exposure to the sun also diminishes the body's immune functions. It causes immune suppression, which in turn makes the body to succumb to microbial infection. Consequently, many extracts of natural products with antioxidant and sunscreen activities are now part of skin care products; many of them ameliorate infections such as eczema, rosacea, dermatitis and psoriasis.

Natural products are useful sunscreens that prevent skin oxidation due to the sun. The concept of using sunscreens is not new to Africans. Many African people traditionally apply natural products and chemical dyes to protect their skins from the harmful effects of the sun. In many parts of Africa, indigenous people smear on their exposed skin natural oils extracted from castor beans, groundnuts, cocoa, and etc., to block the sun's harmful rays and protect themselves from photo-damage. The Himba people of Opuwo, northern Namibia, protect themselves against the harsh and harmful rays of the sun by applying red ochre (hydrated iron oxide) compounds all over their exposed bodies. Yet ochre - in use since the African Middle Stone Age - also softens the skin, protects against the cold, insect bites and is taken as an iron supplement.

Among the Lunda people of North-Western Province in Zambia, for example, ochre - a brown natural earth pigment containing hydrated iron oxide - is mixed with castor oil, locally known as *Imonu*, and applied onto the exposed bodies of adolescent girls during initiation ceremonies to mark their puberty. Apart from imparting natural brown earth pigmentation, the formulation also moisturizes and protects the girls' exposed skins from the harsh tropical sun. After 3-4 days of rigorous dancing in the hot sun, the ochre-castor oil natural sunscreen, known as *Ing'ula*, ensures that the skins of the girls - now fully initialized into adulthood - are unscathed, hence looking succulent, emollient, beautiful and ready for marriage. Castor oil has SPF of 5.6 (Kaur & Saraf, 2010).

Palmer's Cocoa Butter Formula, a cosmetic lotion which smoothes and tones skin, is made by E.T. Browne Drug Co., Inc., USA. It contains *Theobroma cacao* (cocoa) extract and vitamin E. According to the product label, the lotion absorbs quickly, creating a protective barrier that locks in moisture. Medically, *Palmer's Cocoa Butter* lotion is loaded with antioxidants and suitable for eczema prone skin, soothes skin after sun exposure and provides a soft, youthful appearance. Other natural ingredients in the lotion are *Elaeis guineensis* (palm) oil, *Cocos nucifera* (coconut) oil, cellulose, and cocoa seed butter. The SPF for this product is not indicated.

Apart from being an antioxidant, palm oil is also a potent natural product against skin microorganisms. It is non-toxic and useful in wound healing. In Nigeria, palm oil is a constituent of traditional soaps used to treat several skin infections as well as drinks used to treat gonorrhoea and respiratory infections. Coconut oil detoxifies, moisturizes and helps fight microbial infections and cancer of the skin. It also removes dead cells, leaving the skin smoother. Biodegradable cellulose from natural sources hydrates dry skin by locking in moisture, thus allowing a deeper penetration of the other active ingredients.

A cocoa butter lotion manufactured by SFL (abbreviation is not explained) and marketed by Nyati Cosmetics in Primrose, South Africa, has SPF of 5. According to the product label, application of this 'light and bright' body lotion ensures a lovely, moisturized and even body and hand skin tone. Natural products in this lotion include cocoa butter and *Glycyrrhiza glabra* root extract, the latter inhibits acne-causing bacteria. Due to its antioxidant and anti-inflammatory properties, *G. glabra* (licorice) extracts act synergistically to treat skin conditions such as rosacea, dermatitis and psoriasis.

Finally, water melons are also good for the skin. Water melons are mild natural diuretics that hydrate the human body because their flesh contains about 90% water. But the tough outer layer of the fruit (rind) also contains antioxidants which are beneficial to the skin. The water melon rind is rich in citrulline, an antioxidant that improves skin condition. Citrulline is also a pre-

119

cursor for the amino acid arginine which betters heart condition, immunity and blood circulation.

There's much more: Eating water melons revives libido in men, because the amino acid citrulline improves erection hardness in men and corrects erectile dysfunction. Mild diuretics such as water melons promote the release of sodium (salt) and water through the passing of urine from the body. There are artificial diuretics like water pills that cause forced elimination of urine from the body. Natural diuretics such as water melons also aid in elimination of water from the body and this is the reason eating water melons helps decrease high blood pressure.

Several workers in South Africa are documenting many plants used to manage skin diseases. In terms of bioprospecting for plants used to treat skin diseases as well as developing such plants into skin care products, South African research and development practitioners are continental leaders. This bioprospecting enterprise is driven by the motive to commercialize the production of biologically active natural products. Enormous investment into research and innovation of natural products has led to the production of many natural products for skin care and therapy in South Africa.

This is in contrast to other African countries that have neither greatly invested into bioprospecting nor moved closer to manufacturing. This way, many African countries still heavily rely on South Africa for skin care and health products containing plant materials such as tea, grape, cocoa, *Marula* and *Aloe*. Several of these natural products are incorporated into skin cosmetics, especially because of their antioxidant and sunscreen activities; few are made into anti-inflammatory and anti-microbial drugs for skin diseases.

Strangely though, plant products from Africa provide the active chemical compounds from which European and Indian companies now manufacture many drugs for skin and other diseases. Again, this mirrors the lack of African investment into innovation, value-addition and manufacturing of natural products. Natural skin products could be a huge money spinner for many African countries. Despite its great economic and health potential, many African countries (except South Africa) have not started production and value-addition of skin care natural products. This is regrettable.

Conspicuously, the Chinese, too, are missing in much of the R&D for natural products used for skin care and dermatological therapy. Chinese publications on skin products are much fewer than those on HIV/AIDS. This essentially means that Chinese interest and investments are more geared towards the discovery of novel treatments for AIDS than skin care products. Europeans on the other hand are clearly interested in natural products that work as sunscreens.

Though marred by the lack of equipment, the scientific community in Africa is documenting plants that are utilized in the management of skin diseases, especially during HIV infection. At the University of Namibia, this author is leading efforts to document and evaluate these plants for antimicrobial activities. Increased financial support would brighten the prospects of this important laboratory research effort, which is yet to advance to the next frontier of R&D. There are few projects aimed at processing African natural products to enhance value-addition. Unfortunately, many of these projects seem to concentrate on buying raw plant materials for export to European countries like Germany, where the plants are converted into drugs. The Devil's claw is a good case in point.

In East Africa, scientists in Ethiopia and Kenya are evaluating plants for their antimicrobial and anti-cancer actions on the human skin. In Asia, poor countries like India - perhaps due to the high burden of skin diseases emanating from below par sanitation - have buoyed investments into bioprospecting and biotechnological processing of natural products to manufacture cosmetics and drugs for skin diseases. India now supplies many African countries with drugs.

Conclusion and Recommendation

Three biological processes are associated with skin diseases: oxidation, inflammation, and microbial infection. In many different parts of the world, people use similar and different plants to manage various skin conditions and diseases. This chapter extensively describes plant species that are part of the natural pharmacopoeias for skin diseases in Africa, Asia and elsewhere. Natural products, especially those containing phenolics, act as powerful antioxidants that neutralise and destroy oxidation-causing free radicals. Excessive exposure of the skin to UV radiation from the sun also contributes to inflammatory skin diseases, the most common conditions in dermatology. Natural anti-inflammatory substances present in many plants ameliorate inflammatory diseases of the skin.

Natural products with beneficial and protective effects on the skin are usually rich in the following antioxidants: alpha-tocopherol, beta-carotene, genistein, silibin, myconoside, betacyanins, mesembryanthin, chlorophylls, hyperforin, procyanidins and catechins. Various natural products are rich in the following anti-inflammatory agents that prevent skin diseases: quercetin, curcumin, and alpha-bisabolol. Many extracts of plants have antimicrobial activity. Some plants with anti-HIV activity are also active against skin pathogens. Plants that contain crinane alkaloids confer broad-spectrum antibacterial action.

Plants have been greatly exploited and commercialized into products for skin care and health. Whereas many plant extracts are included in skin cosmetics, few are made into drugs for treating inflammatory disorders and microbial infections. In this respect, the potential to converting natural products into drugs for skin diseases is still largely unexploited. Authorities in Africa, both in the public and private sectors, should put more investments into the value-addition of natural products that promote skin health.

References

Abbasi, A.M., Khan, M.A., Ahmad, M., Zafar, M., Jahan, S., & Sultana, S. (2010). Ethnopharmacological application of medicinal plants to cure skin diseases and in folk cosmetics among the tribal communities of North-West Frontier Province, Pakistan. *Journal of Ethnopharmacology, 128*(2), 322-335.

Abe, R., & Ohtani, K. (2013). An ethnobotanical study of medicinal plants and traditional therapies on Batan Island, the Philippines. *Journal of Ethnopharmacology, 145*(2), 554-565.

Afolayan, A.J., Grierson, D.S., & Mbeng, W.O. (2014). Ethnobotanical survey of medicinal plants used in the management of skin disorders among the Xhosa communities of the Amathole District, Eastern Cape, South Africa. *Journal of Ethnopharmacology, 153*(1), 220-232.

Al-Gammal, S.Y. (1998). *Elecampane* and Job's disease. *Bulletin of the Indian Institute of History of Medicine (Hyderabad), 28*(1), 7-11.

AlGhamdi, K.M., AlHomoudi, F.A., & Khurram, H. (2013). Skin care: Historical and contemporary views. *Saudi Pharmaceutical Journal, 22*, 171-178.

Apone, F., Tito, A., Carola, A., Arciello, S., Tortora, A., Filippini, L., ... & Colucci, G. (2010). A mixture of peptides and sugars derived from plant cell walls increases plant defense responses to stress and attenuates ageing-associated molecular changes in cultured skin cells. *Journal of Biotechnology, 145*(4), 367-376.

Au, D.T., Wu, J., Jiang, Z., Chen, H., Lu, G., & Zhao, Z. (2008). Ethnobotanical study of medicinal plants used by Hakka in Guangdong, China. *Journal of Ethnopharmacology, 117*(1), 41-50.

Bhat, P., Hegde, G.R., Hegde, G., & Mulgund, G.S. (2014). Ethnomedicinal plants to cure skin diseases—An account of the traditional knowledge in the coastal parts of Central Western Ghats, Karnataka, India. *Journal of Ethnopharmacology, 151*(1), 493-502.

Chaudhari, P.M., Kawade, P.V., & Funne, S.M. (2011). Cosmeceuticals—a review. *Int. J. Pharm. Technol, 3*, 774-798.

Cheesman, L., Nair, J.J., & van Staden, J. (2012). Antibacterial activity of crinane alkaloids from *Boophone disticha* (Amaryllidaceae). *Journal of Ethnopharmacology, 140*(2), 405-408.

Chiller, K., Selkin, B.A., & Murakawa, G.J. (2001, December). Skin microflora and bacterial infections of the skin. In *Journal of Investigative Dermatology Symposium Proceedings* (Vol. 6, No. 3, pp. 170-174). Nature Publishing Group.

Choi, K.S., Kundu, J.K., Chun, K.S., Na, H.K., & Surh, Y.J. (2014). Rutin inhibits UVB radiation-induced expression of COX-2 and iNOS in hairless mouse skin: p38 MAP kinase and JNK as potential targets. *Archives of Biochemistry and Biophysics, 559*, 38-45.

De Spiegeleer, B., Boonen, J., Malysheva, S.V., Mavungu, J.D.D., De Saeger, S., Roche, N., ... & Veryser, L. (2013). Skin penetration enhancing properties of the plant N-alkylamide spilanthol. *Journal of Ethnopharmacology*, *148*(1), 117-125.

Deters, A.M., Meyer, U., & Stintzing, F.C. (2012). Time-dependent bioactivity of preparations from cactus pear (*Opuntia ficus indica*) and ice plant (*Mesembryanthemum crystallinum*) on human skin fibroblasts and keratinocytes. *Journal of Ethnopharmacology*, *142*(2), 438-444.

Ding, H., Chin, Y.W., Kinghorn, A.D., & D'Ambrosio, S.M. (2007, October). Chemopreventive characteristics of avocado fruit. In *Seminars in cancer biology* (Vol. 17, No. 5, pp. 386-394). Academic Press.

Dold, A.P., & Cocks, M.L. (2002). The trade in medicinal plants in the Eastern Cape Province, South Africa. *South African Journal of Science*, *98*(11 & 12), p-589.

Duraipandiyan, V., & Ignacimuthu, S. (2011). Antifungal activity of traditional medicinal plants from Tamil Nadu, India. *Asian Pacific Journal of Tropical Biomedicine*, *1*(2), S204-S215.

Gechev, T.S., Hille, J., Woerdenbag, H.J., Benina, M., Mehterov, N., Toneva, V., ... & Mueller-Roeber, B. (2014). Natural products from resurrection plants: Potential for medical applications. *Biotechnology Advances*.

Govindasamy, C., & Arulpriya, M. (2013). Antimicrobial activity of *Acanthus ilicifolius*: Skin infection pathogens. *Asian Pacific Journal of Tropical Disease*, *3*(3), 180-183.

Grace, O.M., Simmonds, M.S.J., Smith, G.F., & Van Wyk, A.E. (2008). Therapeutic uses of *Aloe* L. (Asphodelaceae) in Southern Africa. *Journal of Ethnopharmacology*, *119*(3), 604-614.

Haag, S.F., Tscherch, K., Arndt, S., Kleemann, A., Gersonde, I., Lademann, J., ... & Meinke, M.C. (2014). Enhancement of skin radical scavenging activity and *stratum corneum* lipids after the application of a hyperforin-rich cream. *European Journal of Pharmaceutics and Biopharmaceutics*, *86*(2), 227-233.

Halawany, H.S., 2012. A review of miswak (*Salvadora persica*) and its effect on various aspects of oral health. *The Saudi Dental Journal*, 24, 63–69.

Jeon, Y.J., Kim, B.H., Kim, S., Oh, I., Lee, S., Shin, J., & Kim, T.Y. (2013). Rhododendrin ameliorates skin inflammation through inhibition of NF-κB, MAPK, and PI3K/Akt signaling. *European Journal of Pharmacology*, *714*(1), 7-14.

Jong, M.C., Ermuth, U., & Augustin, M. (2013). Plant-based ointments versus usual care in the management of chronic skin diseases: A comparative analysis on outcome and safety. *Complementary Therapies in Medicine*, *21*(5), 453-459.

Katiyar, S.K. (2005). Silymarin and skin cancer prevention: anti-inflammatory, antioxidant and immunomodulatory effects. *International Journal of Oncology, 26*(1), 169-176.

Kaur, C.D., & Saraf, S. (2010). *In vitro* sun protection factor determination of herbal oils used in cosmetics. *Pharmacognosy Research, 2*(1), 22.

Kawagishi, H., Fukumoto, Y., Hatakeyama, M., He, P., Arimoto, H., Matsuzawa, T., ... & Sugiyama, K. (2001). Liver injury suppressing compounds from avocado (*Persea americana*). *Journal of Agricultural and Food Chemistry, 49*(5), 2215-2221.

Lall, N., & Kishore, N. (2014). Are plants used for skin care in South Africa fully explored? *Journal of Ehnopharmacology, 153*(1), 61-84.

Lephart, E.D., Sommerfeldt, J.M., & Andrus, M.B. (2014). Resveratrol: influences on gene expression in human skin. *Journal of Functional Foods, 10*, 377-384.

Leteane, M.M., Ngwenya, B.N., Muzila, M., Namushe, A., Mwinga, J., Musonda, R., ... & Andrae-Marobela, K. (2012). Old plants newly discovered: *Cassia sieberiana* DC and *Cassia abbreviata* Oliv. Oliv. root extracts inhibit in vitro HIV-1c replication in peripheral blood mononuclear cells (PBMCs) by different modes of action. *Journal of Ethnopharmacology, 141*(1), 48-56.

Lu, Q.Y., Arteaga, J.R., Zhang, Q., Huerta, S., Go, V.L.W., & Heber, D. (2005). Inhibition of prostate cancer cell growth by an avocado extract: role of lipid-soluble bioactive substances. *The Journal of Nutritional Biochemistry, 16*(1), 23-30.

Mabona, U., & Van Vuuren, S.F. (2013). Southern African medicinal plants used to treat skin diseases. *South African Journal of Botany, 87*, 175-193.

Mabona, U., Viljoen, A., Shikanga, E., Marston, A., & Van Vuuren, S. (2013). Antimicrobial activity of southern African medicinal plants with dermatological relevance: From an ethnopharmacological screening approach, to combination studies and the isolation of a bioactive compound. *Journal of Ethnopharmacology, 148*(1), 45-55.

Maroyi, A. (2014). Alternative medicines for HIV/AIDS in resource-poor settings: Insight from traditional medicines use in Sub-Saharan Africa. *Tropical Journal of Pharmaceutical Research, 13*(9), 1527-1536.

Martínez, G.J., & Barboza, G.E. (2010). Natural pharmacopoeia used in traditional Toba medicine for the treatment of parasitosis and skin disorders (Central Chaco, Argentina). *Journal of Ethnopharmacology, 132*(1), 86-100.

Mugisha, M.K., Asiimwe, S., Namutebi, A., Borg-Karlson, A.K., & Kakudidi, E.K. (2014). Ethnobotanical study of indigenous knowledge on medicinal and nutritious plants used to manage opportunistic infections associated with HIV/AIDS in western Uganda. *Journal of Ethnopharmacology, 155*, 194–202.

Nagata, J.M., Jew, A.R., Kimeu, J.M., Salmen, C.R., Bukusi, E.A., & Cohen, C.R. (2011). Medical pluralism on Mfangano Island: use of medicinal plants among persons living with HIV/AIDS in Suba District, Kenya. *Journal of Ethnopharmacology, 135*(2), 501-509.

Nair, J.J., & van Staden, J. (2014). Traditional usage, phytochemistry and pharmacology of the South African medicinal plant *Boophone disticha* (Lf) Herb. (Amaryllidaceae). *Journal of Ethnopharmacology, 151*(1), 12-26.

Ncube, B., Ndhlala, A.R., Okem, A., & van Staden, J. (2013). *Hypoxis* (Hypoxidaceae) in African traditional medicine. *Journal of Ethnopharmacology, 150*(3), 818-827.

Nicolaou, A. (2013). Eicosanoids in skin inflammation. *Prostaglandins, Leukotrienes and Essential Fatty Acids, 88*(1), 131-138.

Njoroge, G.N., & Bussmann, R.W. (2007). Ethnotherapeautic management of skin diseases among the Kikuyus of Central Kenya. *Journal of Ethnopharmacology, 111*(2), 303-307.

Ochwang'i, D.O., Kimwele, C.N., Oduma, J.A., Gathumbi, P.K., Mbaria, J.M., & Kiama, S.G. (2014). Medicinal plants used in treatment and management of cancer in Kakamega County, Kenya. *Journal of Ethnopharmacology, 151*(3), 1040-1055.

Okatch, H., Ngwenya, B., Raletamo, K.M., & Andrae-Marobela, K. (2012). Determination of potentially toxic heavy metals in traditionally used medicinal plants for HIV/AIDS opportunistic infections in Ngamiland District in Northern Botswana. *Analytica Chimica Acta, 730*, 42-48.

Okhuarobo, A., Ehizogie Falodun, J., Erharuyi, O., Imieje, V., Falodun, A., & Langer, P. (2014). Harnessing the medicinal properties of *Andrographis paniculata* for diseases and beyond: A review of its phytochemistry and pharmacology. *Asian Pacific Journal of Tropical Disease, 4*(3), 213-222.

Omoruyi, B.E., Bradley, G., & Afolayan, A.J. (2012). Antioxidant and phytochemical properties of *Carpobrotus edulis* (L.) bolus leaf used for the management of common infections in HIV/AIDS patients in Eastern Cape Province. *BMC Complementary and Alternative Medicine, 12*(1), 215.

Onifade, A.A., Jewell, A.P., Ajadi, T.A., Rahamon, S.K., & Ogunrin, O. O. (2013). Effectiveness of a herbal remedy in six HIV patients in Nigeria. *Journal of Herbal Medicine, 3*(3), 99-103.

Palamthodi, S., & Lele, S.S. (2014). Nutraceutical applications of gourd family vegetables: *Benincasa hispida, Lagenaria siceraria* and *Momordica charantia. Biomedicine and Preventive Nutrition, 4*(1), 15-21.

Patel, J.J., Acharya, S.R., & Acharya, N.S. (2014). *Clerodendrum serratum* (L.) Moon.–A review on traditional uses, phytochemistry and pharmacological activities. *Journal of Ethnopharmacology, 154*(2), 268-285.

Pei, S.J. (2001). Ethnobotanical approaches of traditional medicine studies: Some experiences from Asia. *Pharm. Biol., 39*, 74–79.

Pesewu, G.A., Cutler, R.R., & Humber, D.P. (2008). Antibacterial activity of plants used in traditional medicines of Ghana with particular reference to MRSA. *Journal of Ethnopharmacology, 116*(1), 102-111.

Policepatel, S.S., & Manikrao, V.G. (2013). Ethnomedicinal plants used in the treatment of skin diseases in Hyderabad Karnataka region, Karnataka, India. *Asian Pacific Journal of Tropical Biomedicine, 3*(11), 882-886.

Potdar, D., Hirwani, R.R., & Dhulap, S. (2012). Phyto-chemical and pharmacological applications of *Berberis aristata. Fitoterapia, 83*(5), 817-830.

Rajagopal, S., Kumar, R.A., Deevi, D.S., Satyanarayana, C., & Rajagopalan, R. (2003). Andrographolide, a potential cancer therapeutic agent isolated from *Andrographis paniculata. Journal of Experimental Therapeutics and Oncology, 3*(3), 147-158.

Ramos-e-Silva, M., Lima, C.M.O., Schechtman, R.C., Trope, B.M., & Carneiro, S. (2012). Systemic mycoses in immunodepressed patients (AIDS). *Clinics in Dermatology, 30*(6), 616-627.

Rodrigues, F., Palmeira-de-Oliveira, A., das Neves, J., Sarmento, B., Amaral, M. H., & Oliveira, M.B. (2013). *Medicago* spp. extracts as promising ingredients for skin care products. *Industrial Crops and Products, 49*, 634-644.

Rood, B. (2013). *Nature's own pharmacy*. Pretoria, South Africa: Protea Book House.

Saini, S., Kaur, H., Verma, B., Ripudaman, S.K., & Singh, K. (2009). *Kigelia africana* (Lam.) Benth:-An overview. *Nat. Prod. Rad., 8*(2), 190-197.

Seca, A.M., Grigore, A., Pinto, D.C., & Silva, A. (2014). The genus *Inula* and their metabolites: From ethnopharmacological to medicinal uses. *Journal of Ethnopharmacology, 154*(2), 286-310.

Shikov, A.N., Pozharitskaya, O.N., Makarov, V.G., Wagner, H., Verpoorte, R., & Heinrich, M. (2014). Medicinal Plants of the Russian Pharmacopoeia; their history and applications. *Journal of Ethnopharmacology, 154*, 481-536.

Tadeg, H., Mohammed, E., Asres, K., & Gebre-Mariam, T. (2005). Antimicrobial activities of some selected traditional Ethiopian medicinal plants used in the treatment of skin disorders. *Journal of Ethnopharmacology, 100*(1), 168-175.

Teshome, K., Gebre-Mariam, T., Asres, K., Perry, F., & Engidawork, E. (2008). Toxicity studies on dermal application of plant extract of *Plumbago zeylanica* used in Ethiopian traditional medicine. *Journal of Ethnopharmacology, 117*(2), 236-248.

Tsai, M.H., Lin, Z.C., Liang, C.J., Yen, F.L., Chiang, Y.C., & Lee, C.W. (2014). Eupafolin inhibits PGE2 production and COX2 expression in LPS-stimulated human dermal fibroblasts by blocking JNK/AP-1 and Nox2/p47 *phox* pathway. *Toxicology and Applied Pharmacology*, *279*(2), 240-251.

Van Damme, P., Van Den Eynden, V., & Vernemmen, P. (1922). Plant uses by the Topnaar of the Kuiseb Valley, Namib Desert. *Afrika Focus*, *8*, 223-252.

Wang, W., Bostic, T.R., & Gu, L. (2010). Antioxidant capacities, procyanidins and pigments in avocados of different strains and cultivars. *Food Chemistry*, *122*(4), 1193-1198.

Yu, H., Pardoll, D., & Jove, R. (2009). STATs in cancer inflammation and immunity: a leading role for STAT3. *Nature Reviews Cancer*, *9*(11), 798-809.

Ziegler, A., Jonason, A.S., Leffellt, D.J., Simon, J.A., Sharma, H.W., Kimmelman, J., ... & Brash, D.E. (1994). Sunburn and p53 in the onset of skin cancer. *Nature*, *372*(6508), 773-776.

Table 3.1: Plants used for treatment of skin diseases in Amathole, South Africa

Scientific name, Xhosa name	Plant parts, preparation	Skin diseases
Acacia karroo, Umnga	Bark, lotion	Ringworm, clean and soften facial skin
Agapanthus africanus, Isicakathi	Rhizome, decoction	Scabies and boils
Alepidea amatymbica, Iqwili	Rhizome, lotion	Perfume skin
Aloe ferox, Umhlaba	Leaves, sap squeezed from plant	Eczema, irritations, burns, wounds, insect bites, ring-worm, boils, pimples
Asclepias concolor, Itshongwe	Leaves, paste	pimples
Asparagus africanus, Umathunga	Leaves, infusion	Eczema, wounds
Capparis tomentosa, Intsihlo	Roots, infusion	Sore throat
Curtisia dentata, Uzintlwa	Bark, infusion of powder	Eczema
Dianthus thunbergii, Ungcane	Leaves, infusion	Bath to remove bad body odour
Digitaria eriantha, Injica	Leaves, decoction	Pimples
Dysphania ambrosioides, Imboya	Leaves, decoction	Pimples, eczema, itching
Emex australis, Inkunzane	Leaves, decoction	Prevent hair loss
Euphorbia bupleurifolia, Intsema	Leaves latex	Pimples, wounds, rashes
Harpephyllum caffrum, Umgwenye	Bark, decoction	Eczema, pimples, wounds
Hermannia geniculata, mpepho	Leaves, paste	Boils
Hypoxis argentea, Inongwe	Corm	ringworm, eczema, pimples
Lippia javanica, Inzinziniba	Leaves, infusion	Boils, scabies, wounds
Phytolacca americana, Umsobosobo	Leaves, paste	Boils
Rhus lucida, Intlokoshane	Bark, infusion	Scabies
Schotia afra, Umquqoba	Bark, decoction	Skin ulcers

(Adapted from Afolayan et al., 2014)

Table 3.2: Plant remedies used for skin diseases and skin care in Southern Africa

Scientific name	Medicinal uses	Chemical compounds
Aloe ferox (bitter aloe or Cape aloe); *Aloe aculeate*; *Aloe greatheadii*; *Aloe vera*	Sap is topically applied to treat wounds, dermatitis, acne, skin cancers, burns, and psoriasis; leaf extract is used to clear skin blemishes; sap treats eczema, skin cancer and burns; multi-purpose skin care functions and sunscreen	Chromones, anthraquinones, anthrones, anthrone-C-glycosides and other phenolic compounds
Aspalathus linearis (Rooibos tea)	Extracts from leaves lessen ageing and eczema; wash face in water solution made from tea to maintain good skin health	Rich in antioxidants; contains aspalathin, aspalalinin; flavo-noids like aspalathin, isoorientin, nothofagin, querce-tin and isoquercitrin
Calodendrum capense (Cape Chestnut tree)	Bark is an ingredient of skin oint-ment; oil extracted from seeds is included into soap; oil protects skin from UV; extracts treats psoriasis,	Oil is rich in antioxidants and fatty acids

	eczema, skin cracking and sagging	
Citrullus lanatus (water melon)	Full of antioxidant activity; used to treat enlarged liver, jaundice, kidney and blood pressure; oil from seeds is made into soap and face masks for delicate skin; flesh of fruits is part of sun lotions and cosmetics	Rich in vitamins A, B and C, arginine, carotenoids, lycopenes, carbohydrate, sodium, magnesium, potassium and water;
Diospyros lycioides (Monkey plum)	Bark/root decoctions are used for dysentery; bark and root decoctions are used for skin inflammation	Unknown
Diospyros mespiliformis (African ebony)	Leaf decoctions are used for whooping cough, fever, malaria, leprosy and dermatomycoses; extracts from leaves are used to alleviate skin infections and heal wounds	Unknown
Elaeis guineensis (oil palm)	Juice from leaves promotes wound healing; oils included in skin lotions and soap to treat skin infections	Major fatty acids are linoleic, palmitic, linolenic acids with trace amounts of oleic, stearic, arachidic, myristic, lauric, palmitoleic and margaric acids
Eriocephalus africanus (Cape snowbush or Rosemary)	Increases blood flow to the skin, hence restores a youthful glow; also promotes hair growth; oil is used in aromatherapy, cosmetics and perfume; leaf infusion treats inflammation and other dermal complications	Unknown
Eriocephalus punctulatus (Cape chamomile)	Commercial Cape chamomile oil, due to its pleasant odour, is used as a fragrance in skin care cosmetics and toiletries	2-Methylbutyl isobutyrate, 2-methylpropyl isobutyrate, p-cymene, α-pinene, 2-methylbutyl isovalerate and 3-methylbutyl isobutyrate
Eucalyptus camaldulensis	Leaves are used for colds and influenza, the oil is used as an antiseptic; bark infusion remedies pimples	Unknown
Ficus natalensis (Natal fig)	Leaves are used as poultices for wounds and boils	Unknown
Olea europaea (Olive tree)	Extracts from leaves and bark are applied topically to treat skin damage, such as contact dermatitis, atopic dermatitis, eczema including severe hand and foot eczema, psoriasis, thermal and radiation burns, other types of skin inflammation and ageing; used since ancient times as skin and hair conditioner	Olive oil contains fatty acids, triglycerides, tocopherols, squalene, carotenoids, sterols, polyphenols, chlorophylls, β-sitosterol, tocopherol; the main compound is Oleuropein (a complex phenol)
Pelargonium graveolens (Rose-scented pelargonium)	All plant parts, due to presence of geranium oil, are used for cleansing over-oily skin, and treating dermatitis, acne and eczema	Contains essential oils, phenolics and flavonoids
Sansevieria hyacinthoides (Devil's tongue, snake tongue)	Leaf decoctions are used topically for burns, wounds and swellings	Unknown
Schinziophyton rautanenii (known as Mungongo tree in Zambia and manketti in many other African countries	Oil is useful for skin protection and hydration, reduces inflammation, promotes cellular repair and tissue generation; supplements skin with	Seed oil has fatty acids, linoleic, oleic, palmitic, linolenic, and erucic acids, and lesser quantities of myristic and myristoleoic

	antioxidants; may play an important role in the reduction of photo-damage and photo-ageing due to free-radical oxidative stress	acids; also rich in vitamin E;
Sclerocarya birrea (Marula)	Oil is massaged into skin or used as body lotion for face, feet and hands; marula oil protects against dry and cracking skin; a shampoo for dry, damaged and fragile hair; oil improves skin hydration and smoothness and reduces skin redness	Marula oil contains oleic, linoleic and palmitic acid; has oxidative stability even during deep frying due to its fatty acid and tocopherol; contains monounsaturated fatty acids which make the oil very stable
Sideroxylon inerme (White milkwood)	Due to its antioxidant activity, it helps keep healthy skin; used for skin lightening; reduces melanin content by 37%	Contains the compound epigallocatechin gallate- the same active ingredient found in tea; exhibits great antioxidant and anti-tyrosinase actions
Sutherlandia frutescens (Cancer bush)	Leaf decoctions are used for washing wounds; also treats chicken pox, rheumatoid arthritis, dysentery and inflammation	Cycloartane-type triterpene glycosides
Withania somnifera (Winter cherry)	Leaves are used to heal open, septic and inflamed wounds; leaf decoction, infusion or tincture are applied for inflammation, haemorrhoids, rheumatism	Unknown
Ximenia americana (False sandalwood)	Traditionally used to treat skin problems, leprotic ulcers, mouth ulcers, haemorrhoids, abdominal pains, dysentery and venereal diseases; oil from the seed is used as an emollient, conditioner, skin softener and hair oil as well as included as an ingredient in lipsticks and lubricants; ximenynic acid (Ximenoil) improves blood circulation which help to keep skin young	Contains oleic, hexacos-17-enoic (ximenic), linoleic, linolenic and stearic acids; oil consists of very long chain fatty acids with up to 40 carbon atoms
Ziziphus mucronata (Buffalo thorn)	Extracts of plant parts heal boils, sores and swellings; decoctions of roots and bark treat respiratory infections, snake bites, dirrhoea and dysentery	Unknown

(Adapted from Lall & Kishore, 2014)

Table 3.3: Plants used to treat skin diseases in Southern Africa

Plant names	Plant parts	Mode of application	Skin condition treated
Acacia erioloba, Acacia mellifera	Wood ash; roots	Topical; poultice	Heals wounds, burns
Adansonia digitata (Baobab)	Leaves	Topical	Heals wounds
Bauhinia petersiana	Leaves	Extract applied topically	Heals wounds
Capparis tomentosa	Roots	Paste applied topically	Heals wounds
Cissampelos capensis	Rhizomes, roots	Paste applied topically	Treat sores and ulcers

131

	and leaves		
Combretum molle	Fresh or dry leaves	Applied topically as a dressing	Heals wounds
Cotyledon orbiculata	Leaf and leaf juice	Juice applied topically	removes corns and warts
Diospyros mespiliformis	Roots and leaves	Decoction	Heals wounds
Euclea divinorum	Roots and leaves	Applied topically on fresh bleeding wounds	Heals wounds
Glycyrrhiza glabra (liquorice root)	Roots, rhizomes	Topical	Treats skin inflammation
Harpagophytum procumbens (Devil's claw)	Roots	Ointment applied to skin	Treats sores, ulcers, boils
Hypericum perforatum (St. John's Wort)	Aerial parts	Topical application	Heals wounds
Ipomoea crassipes	Ground plant parts	Paste applied topically	Treat sores
Jatropha curcas, Jatropha zeyheri	Rhizome; sap	topical	Heals wounds, burns, boils
Kigelia africana (sausage tree)	Fruit	Decoction applied topically	Treats skin inflammation
Nymphaea caerulea	Leaves and stems	Poultice	Skin rashes
Opuntia vulgaris	Whole plant	Juice applied topically	Removes skin growths
Osmitopsis asteriscoides	Leaves	Applied topically	Treats cuts
Plantago afra	Leaves	Ointment	Relieves itching
Ricinus communis (castor bean)	Leaf, burnt-pulverized seeds and bark	Applied as poultice	Treats sores and boils
Sarcostemma viminale	Whole plant	Latex applied to skin	Treats skin lesions
Securidaca longepedunculata	Leaves or bark	Ointment	Heals wounds
Solanum capense; Solanum incanum	Crushed berries	Applied topically	Removes skin growths; treats furuncles and ringworm infections
Spermacoce natalensis (Insul-ansala)	Roots	Applied topically	Treats febrile skin rash
Terminalia sericea	Root sap or bark	topical	Heals wounds; leprosy
Trichilia emetica	Leaves or fruits	Poultice topically applied to skin	Eczema
Ximenia caffra	Roots	Applied topically	Treats septic sores
Ziziphus mucronata	Leaves, roots, bark	Decoction applied topically	Treats sores and boils

(Adapted from Mabona & Van Vuuren, 2013)

Table 3.4: Plants used to heal microbial infections of the skin in Southern Africa

Plant names	Plant parts	Mode of application and disease condition treated
Aristea ecklonii	Whole plant	Applied topically to treat shingles
Artemisia afra	Leaves	Decoction applied on acne and boils

Athrixia phylicoides (Bushman's tea)	Whole plant	Plant infusion applied on boils
Capparis tomentosa	Roots	Paste applied topically to treat leprosy
Chironia baccifera (Christmas berry)	Whole plant	Applied topically to treat leprosy, boils and acne
Combretum kraussii + Terminalia sericea	Roots	Mixed and applied topically to heal skin sores, ulcers, boils
Dichrostachys cinerea (Sickle bush)	Bark	Applied topically to treat abscesses
Elephantorrhiza elephantina + Pentanisia prunelloides	Tubers	Applied externally to heal eczema
Ficus natalensis, Ficus sur	Bark, leaves	Hot compress placed onto boils
Gunnera perpensa + Cassine transvaalensis	Rhizomes, bark	Taken orally to treat psoriasis
Lannea edulis	Bark	Applied topically to treat boils and abscesses
Momordica foetida + Pittosporum viridiflorum + Vernonia natalensis	Roots or leaves	Decoctions/ treating boils
Ochna serrulata	Roots	Decoction applied topically to treat gangrene infections
Senna italica	Roots	Applied topically to treat furuncles
Stephania abyssinica (Umbamba)	Powdered roots	Decoction applied topically to treat boils
Turbina oblongata (Ubhoqo)	Leaves	Applied topically to treat abscesses
Vernonia adoensis	Flowers	Applied topically to treat scabies
Withania somnifera (Poison gooseberry or winter cherry)	Leaves and berries	Ointment applied to treat abscesses

(Adapted from Mabona & Van Vuuren, 2013)

Table 3.5: Pharmacopoeia of plants used to treat skin diseases in Namibia

Scientific name of plant	Local name of plant	Skin diseases treated
Abrus precatorius	Isunde (L)	Boils
Acacia hockii; A. erioloba; A. erubescens; A. nigrescens	Mukotokoto (L)	Herpes zoster
Acanthosicyos naudinianus	Muputwi (Ru)	Body sores, fungal infection of skin
Albizia anthelmintica	Muhengutji (Ru)	Herpes zoster
Amaranthus thunbergii	Mboga (Ru)	Eczema
Annona senegalensis; Annona stenophylla	Malolo (L)	Herpes zoster, skin infections
Asparagus nelsii	Okawekamuthithi (O)	Eczema
Bauhinia petersiana	Muhusi (Ru)	Skin infections/sores
Capparis erythrocarpos; Capparis tomentosa	Ntulwantulwa (L)	Skin rashes; herpes zoster
Clerodendrum ternatum	Oshanyu (O)	Eczema
Combretum zeyheri	Mukenge (Ru)	Fungal infections of skin
Corchorus tridens	Okalyaoipute (O)	Wounds, boils
Diospyros mespiliformis	Unyandi (Ru)	General skin infections
Euclea divinorum	Mpumutwi (Ru)	Skin rashes
Ficus burkei	Mutata (Ru)	Skin rashes, eczema
Garcinia buchananii; Garcinia livingstonei	Mukononga (L)	Herpes zoster, Herpes simplex, skin rashes
Guibourtia coleosperma	Usivi (Ru)	General infections of the skin

Helinus integrifolius	Murore/ Murora (Ru)	Skin rash
Kigelia africana	Mupolota (L)	Herpes simplex
Kigelia africana	Uvhunguvhungu (Ru)	Boils, eczema, psoriasis, leprosy, syphilis, skin cancer, herpes simplex
Lannea stuhlmannii; Lannea zastrowiana	Rungomba (L)	Herpes zoster, Herpes simplex, skin infections
Lannea zastrowina	Mundowere (Ru)	Skin rashes, Herpes zoster
Ozoroa longipes	Mululira (Ru)	Skin rashes
Parinari curatellifolia	Mubula (L)	Skin rashes, herpes zoster, herpes simplex
Peltophorum africanum	Muparara (Ru)	General infections of the skin
Rhus quartiniana	Sikulikuli (Ru)	Skin rashes
Schrebera alata	Mulutuluha (L)	Skin rashes
Senna italic	Okatundangu (O)	Abscess
Solanum incanum	Nonduduwa (Ru)	Skin infections
Vigna dinteri	Omuyimbo (O)	Herpes simplex
Xylopia tomentosa	Munyambinyambi (Ru)	Fungal infections of the skin

Data collected by author; L = Lozi, O = Oshiwambo, Ru = Rukwangali

Table 3.6: Natural pharmacopoeia for skin cancer in Kenya

Scientific name of plant	Local name of plant
Abrus precatorius	Ndirakalu
Aeschynomene abyssinica	Olunyili
Albizia coriaria	Omubeli
Albizia gummifera	skin cancer Musenzeri/ Mukhonzuli
Bidens pilosa	Igwisi
Bridelia micrantha	Shikangania/ kamulondangombe/ shi kanyanga
Croton macrostachyus	Musutsu
Cyphostemma adenocaule	Mukoyegoye
Cyphostemma serpens	Lithunzune/ Maombola
Ekebergia capensis	Eshiruma
Gardenia volkensii	Eshiuna
Harungana madagascariensis	Musila/ Munamusayi
Hippocratea africana	Shikhalikhanga
Ipomoea cairica	Ndirande/Lilande
Justicia betonica	Shikuduli
Kigelia africana	Omurabe/Morabe
Macadamia tetraphylla	Muyundi
Mangifera indica	Liembe
Microglossa pyrifolia	Ingwe/Ingoyi/ Enguu
Oxygonum sinuatum	Rakaro
Pavetta abyssinica	Ombura
Persea americana	Kwa matsai
Phyllanthus fischeri	Lusarisari
Prunus africana	Mwilitsa/ Ishakulu/ Mwilitsa
Rhus vulgaris	Sungula
Sesbania sesban	Omukhule/ Olukhulila mbusi/ Lohori
Sida cordifolia	Lusatsa
Sida rhombifolia	Omukusa

Solanecio mannii	Livokho
Solanum aculeastrum	Indalandalua
Spathodea campanulata	Muthulio/Nandi
Spermacoce prince	Vikudhuli
Syzygium guineense	Musiema
Trichilia emetic	Munyama/irojo/ Musinzi
Urtica massaica	Elaila
Waltheria indica	Olundu lukhasi
Zanthoxylum gilletii	Shihumba/ Shikuma
Zanthoxylum rubescens	Shikhuma/ Shigulutsu/ Shughoma

(Adapted from Ochwang'i et al., 2014)

Table 3.7: Natural pharmacopoeia for skin diseases in Argentina

Plant species	Plant parts/preparation	Skin diseases treated
Allium cepa	Cataphylls/milled/poultice	Warts
Aspidosperma quebrachoblanco	Bark/infusion or decoction/wash	Boils, abscesses, rash, scabies
Capparis tweediana	Branches or twigs/infusion or decoction/wash	Eruptive diseases such as chickenpox and measles
Croton bonplandianus	Sap/unprepared/external use	Warts
Cucurbitella asperata	Root/infusion or decoction/wash	Boils and abscesses
Hippeastrum parodii	Bulb/unprepared/frictions and massages	Pimples, acnes, warts
Lanopila bicolor	Spores/unprepared/external use	Boils
Nicotiana glauca	Leaves/unprepared/poultice	Boils and abscesses; eruptive diseases like chickenpox and measles
Polygonum hispidum	Whole plant/infusion or decoction /wash	Eruptive diseases such as chickenpox and measles
Prosopis kuntzei	Leaves/ incision	Warts
Schinopsis balansae	Sap/infusion or decoction/wash	Mycosis, warts
Schinus fasciculata	Thorn/Incision of warts with two thorns	Warts
Usnea subflorida	Whole plant/unprepared; used as a pad inside shoes	Feet mycosis
Xanthium spinosum	Thorn/incision of warts	Warts
Zephyranthes carinata	Bulb/unprepared/frictions and massages	Eruptive diseases (chickenpox, measles), mycosis, dandruff

(Adapted from (Martínez & Barboza, 2010)

4

Natural Products in the Management of Sexually Transmitted Infections

Introduction

Change towards healthy lifestyles has rekindled a new anticipation and belief in the power of natural products to prevent and treat human diseases. Even so, in the management of sexually transmitted infections (STIs), the efficacy of natural products is often misunderstood by patients, medical doctors and the general public. Cultivated bananas (*Musa* spp.), lemons (*Citrus limon*) and paw-paw (*Carica papaya*) are good examples. Few people would agree that these common fruit plants may be used to treat gonorrhoea and syphilis; yet this is the case in many African countries like Zambia.

Natural products may not be a silver-bullet solution to the problem of STIs. However, because natural remedies are making a swift comeback, there are sentiments that phytotherapy, such as the use of bananas, lemons and paw-paw to treat STIs no longer belongs to the Dark Ages. Use of plants now presents a bright spot in our quest for knowable treatments for emerging as well as old diseases like STIs. Natural products, especially African plants, may cause a quantum leap in the discovery of novel medications that will rein in stubborn and drug-resistant STIs.

This chapter showcases natural products used in the management of STIs, common illnesses associated with AIDS. The chapter starts with a background review of the epidemiological synergy between HIV and other STIs. Then it details the global burden of STIs, aetiology, symptoms and management of STIs. As a case study, the chapter documents plants for treating STIs in Zambia. After the review of natural remedies for the management of general STIs, specific plants for the treatment of *Neisseria gonorrhoeae*, syphilis, warts, genital herpes, chancroid, *Candida albicans* and *Gardnerella vaginalis* are explained. Plants, fungi and algal species for the management of *Trichomonas vaginalis* are also given.

Epidemiological Synergy between HIV and Other STIs

Many studies have corroborated the association between HIV/AIDS and other STIs. As early as the 1990s, studies had already shown that there is an epidimiological synergy between HIV infection and conventional STIs (Wasserheit, 1992; Laga, Manoka, Kivuvu, Malele, Tuliza, & Nzila, 1993; Fleming & Wasserheit, 1999). According to Cohen (1998), the view that STIs enhance HIV transmission was no longer a hypothesis but a fact. Giordani, Vieira, Weizenmann, Rosemberg, Souza and Bonorino et al. (2011), citing several authorities, maintained that *Trichomonas vaginalis*, a parasite in the human urogenital tract that causes trichomoniasis characterized by vaginitis in women and urethritis in men, facilitates HIV-1 acquisition.

Galvin and Cohen (2004) also note that sexually transmitted diseases (STDs) that cause ulcers or inflammation greatly increase the efficiency of HIV transmission by enhancing both the infectiousness of and the susceptibility to HIV infection. In Africa, genital herpes has played a more important role than any other STI in driving HIV infection (Abu-Raddad, Magaret, Celum, Wald, Longini Jr., Self, & Corey, 2008). Globally, these authors find that remarkable increases in the incidence of STDs are associated with rapid increases in the spread of HIV in many areas. Similarly, HIV/AIDS is also related to the rapid spread and aggressive presentation of STDs like chancroid, gonorrhoea, syphilis and Kaposi's sarcoma. Treatment failure of chancroid, when the use of synthetic antibiotics becomes futile, is common in HIV-positive individuals. For this reason, targeted STD detection and treatment have a central role to play in HIV/AIDS prevention (Galvin & Cohen, 2004).

There exists a strong correlation between HIV infection and the occurrence of STIs. Because of HIV/AIDS, traditional STIs ride on the back of poor body immunity. Studies show that untreated STIs are important cofactors in the transmission of HIV. Van Vuuren and Naidoo (2010) argue that as HIV infection spreads, immunity is compromised and this leads to an upsurge of opportunistic infections including STIs. It is now well established that HIV/AIDS significantly escalates the risk and severity of traditional STIs. Stated differently, STDs may be regarded as opportunistic infections that are part of the AIDS-complex.

Global Burden of STIs

STIs are a global concern and enigma. According to the World Health Organization (WHO), the global burden of curable STIs (syphilis, gonorrhoea, chlamydia and trichomoniasis) was 448 million in 2005 and 499 million in 2008 (WHO, 2013). Data from WHO show that in 2008, the cases of chlamydia, gonorrhoea, syphilis and trichomoniasis were 105.7, 106.1, 10.6, and 270.4 million, respectively. The incidence of gonorrhoea increased by 21% from 2005 to 2008 (WHO, 2013).

STIs are spread primarily through person-to-person sexual contact. Nearly a million people acquire an STI, including HIV, every day (Chinsembu, 2009). Estimates suggest that the annual occurrence of STIs, including HIV, accounts for the loss of more than 51 million years of healthy life among men, women and children worldwide (Chinsembu, 2009). In developing countries, STIs account for 17% of economic losses caused by ill-health (Mayaud & Mabey, 2004). It is estimated that 80-90% of the global burden of STIs occurs in the developing world where there is limited or no access to diagnostics (Chinsembu, 2009).

In Southern Africa, transmission rates are reaching epidemic proportions where infections are currently one of the highest in the world. A study undertaken by Johnson (2008) found that 26% of all deaths which happened during the year 2000 were a consequence of STI infections. Chinsembu (2009) found that adolescents are the age group at greatest risk for nearly all STIs. Adolescents are often at a higher risk for acquiring STIs because they are unable to conceptualize actions and their consequences. STIs are more prevalent among adolescent women than men, thus two thirds of newly infected adolescents aged 15-19 years are female. For reasons of biology, gender and cultural norms, adolescent females are also more susceptible than males to STIs. Biologically, adolescent women face increased anatomical and physiological susceptibility to infection due to increased cervical ectopy.

Aetiology and Symptoms of STIs

STIs pose a serious health threat not only during the duration of the infection but also have long-range complications including infertility or congenital defects like conjunctivitis and blindness. In males, STIs may occur in the glands of the penis, in the upper urethra, prostrate and epididymis. In females the urethra and cervix are vulnerable to infection and the infection may ascend into the intra-abdominal organs.

There are more than 30 different sexually transmissible bacteria, viruses and parasites but only 19 of these are listed as the main causative agents of STIs. Bacterial pathogens include *Neisseria gonorrhoeae* (causes gonorrhoea or gonococcal infection), *Chlamydia trachomatis* (causes chlamydial infections), *Treponema pallidum* (causes syphilis), *Haemophilus ducreyi* (causes chancroid), *Lymphogranuloma venereum*, and *Klebsiella granulomatis* (previously known as *Calymmatobacterium granulomatis*, causes granuloma inguinale or donovanosis).

Haemophilus ducreyi is a fastidious gram-negative bacillus and is the aetiological agent of chancroid, a sexually transmitted genital ulcer disease. Nawrocki, Bedell and Humphreys (2013) revealed that chancroid facilitates the acquisition and transmission of HIV-1. Like other STIs, chancroid interacts with HIV via genital ulcers and thus increasing the infectiousness of HIV-positive individuals as well as the susceptibility of HIV-negative persons. Sethi, Singh, Samanta, and Sharma (2012) opine that the bacterium *Mycoplasma genitalium* is also an emerging sexually transmitted organism associated with non-gonococcal urethritis in men and several inflammatory reproductive tract syndromes (cervicitis, pelvic inflammatory disease and infertility) in women.

Viral STIs are mainly due to HIV (causes AIDS), herpes simplex virus type 2 (HSV-2, causes genital herpes), Papilloma viruses (cause genital warts and certain subtypes lead to cervical cancer in women), hepatitis B virus (causes hepatitis and chronic cases may lead to cancer of the liver), human herpes virus type 8 (HHV-8) causes Kaposi's sarcoma, Cytomegalovirus (causes inflammation in a number of organs including the brain, the eye and the bowel), and *Molluscum contagiosum* (pox virus) which triggers water warts. Parasitic organisms include *Trichomonas vaginalis* (causes vaginal trichomoniasis), and *Candida albicans* which causes genital candidiasis/thrush and vulvovaginitis in women and inflammation of the glans penis and foreskin (balano-posthitis) in men, and *Phthirus pubis* (pubic lice). Infections caused by *Ureaplasma urealyticum* cause urethritis, which may impair male fertility (Ochsendorf, 2008). *Oligella ureolytica* commonly infects the urinary tract and cervix.

Neisseria gonorrhoeae causes symptomatic infections of the cervix, urinary tract, mouth or rectum (Murray & Pizzorno, 1999). Untreated gonorrhoea and chlamydia cause life threatening conditions such as pelvic inflammation leading to chronic pelvic disease as well as infertility, ectopic pregnancy, neonatal ophthalmia and disseminated gonococcal infections. *Candida albicans* normally infects the skin and mucous membranes of the vagina (causes vaginitis characterzed by a foul smell) and head of the penis to invoke a condition known as balanitis (Murray & Pizzorno, 1999). *Gardnerella vaginalis* infects the female genital tract as a result of a disruption in the normal vaginal microflora. Its infections lead to endometritis, pelvic inflammatory disease and vaginal cellulites.

Then there is *Trichomonas vaginalis*, a common STI protozoan pathogen (protist) that causes profuse vaginal discharge in women and non-specific urethritis in men (Lewis, 2005). Scopel, dos Santos, Frasson, Abraham, Tasca, Henriques, and Macedo (2013) quoted WHO figures which put the global number of new trichomoniasis cases at about 174 million per year, the leading non-viral STI in the world. Trichomoniasis is associated with vaginitis, cervicitis, urethritis, prostatitis, epididymitis, cervical cancer, infertility and pelvic inflammatory disease. Metronidazole and tinidazole are the standard treatments for trichomoniasis (Moo-Puc, Robledo, & Freile-Pelegrin, 2008). Currently, 5-nitroimidazole drugs are the treatment of choice for trichomonosis, but the emergence of resistance has limited the effectiveness of this therapy (Scopel et al., 2013), opening new possibilities for the use of plant remedies.

Management of STIs

The three key steps in the management of STI patients are: making the correct diagnosis; prescribing the correct and effective treatment; and equipping the patient with information to promote safer sex and personal prophylaxis through counseling, contact tracing and condom promotion (Matondo, Chinsembu, & Kapembwa, 1998). Traditionally, management of STIs is based on laboratory diagnosis and prescription of treatment tailored to the etiological diagnosis. This has been the benchmark of medical practice for ages. Recently, there has been an urgent need for improved diagnostics of STIs in HIV endemic areas because studies in Sub-Saharan Africa have shown that STIs are important cofactors in the transmission of HIV infection.

However, due to non-availability of laboratory equipment in poor settings, coupled with the time-lag in waiting for laboratory results, patients are managed by covering for the common causes of the particular STD. This approach, known as syndromic STI management, is where the diagnosis is based on a combination of symptoms and signs which the patient presents (Matondo, Chinsembu, & Kapembwa, 1998; Johnson, Dorrington, Bradshaw, & Coetzee, 2011). Under syndromic management, all STI patients are treated according to the symptoms rather than deferring treatment until the results of laboratory tests are available. Other than the obvious incentive of receiving immediate treatment, this strategy is well suited for poor-resource settings as it avoids problems that may ensue from limited laboratory facilities, coordination of patient receipt of test results, the high cost of laboratory tests, and the limited sensitivity of certain tests (Johnson et al., 2011). That said, there are advantages and disadvantages of both etiological and syndromic management.

Regardless of the approach, the management of STIs is often based on these core principles: confidentiality; correct diagnosis; correct drug, dosage and route of drug administration; counseling; compliance; contact tracing; condom promotion; and clinical follow-up (Matondo, Chinsembu, & Kapembwa, 1998). Although effective STI patient management is the cornerstone of STI control, management of STIs remains one of the greatest challenges in healthcare delivery especially in developing countries. Several factors have compounded the problem of STI management: stigma, societal attitudes towards sex, inadequate resources, high levels of drug resistance, lack of diagnostic facilities and lack of trained health workers (Matondo, Chinsembu, & Kapembwa, 1998).

   Chinsembu (2009) discussed several challenges that hamper the treatment of STIs in public healthcare settings. For example, due to inadequate user-friendly health services, many STIs remain undetected and untreated. This is especially worrisome because many STIs are asymptomatic. Few countries have screening systems for STIs other than HIV. In resource-limited areas, STI clinics lack initiatives for diagnostics and treatment that take on board age- and gender-specific considerations and peculiarities. The issues of concern for treating and preventing STIs are similar to those for HIV/AIDS. But the focus of international discussions around STIs remain on three themes: access to treatment; increasing healthcare personnel to treat and test for STIs to reduce the risk of complications from untreated infections; and continued commitment by countries to finance treatment and prevention programmes sponsored by WHO.

   In the early days of the HIV epidemic when antiretroviral treatment was unaffordable, treatment of STIs received a lot of attention because of its impact on AIDS. Recently, the focus has shifted so much onto HIV/AIDS treatment that public attention for STIs has lost momentum and funding. Lack of surveillance is sweeping the STI problem under the carpet. Due to the plethora of challenges faced by public health facilities, a large proportion of the population in developing countries depends on herbal remedies for treating and managing STIs.

   Due to several challenges, for example stigma, lack of confidentiality and inadequate user-friendly facilities, many patients fail to seek therapy from official public health authorities. Corollary, the majority of STI patients in African countries elect to seek help from traditional healers (Peltzer, Mngqundaniso, & Petros, 2006). Traditional beliefs, cultural barriers and low socio-economic status are some of the reasons why the traditional healer is usually the first line of care for STI patients.

   Nevertheless, many persons with STIs find it difficult to present themselves to the public health authorities. In cultural societies, it is even more difficult to undress and allow someone else to inspect your private parts. For most persons with STIs, the reluctance to disclose information related to their genitalia is further reason why they initially seek help from traditional healers (Kamatenesi-Mugisha, Oryem-Origa, Odyek, & Makawiti, 2008). It is, therefore, not surprising that among all the diseases treated by traditional healers, symptoms related to STIs are one of the most frequently encountered (Peltzer et al., 2006). Patients suffering from STIs usually come to the clinic only after the use of traditional medicine has failed. This is the sad reality in most African settings where STIs are a silent epidemic, under-reported and swept under the carpet.

Dodet (2014) explains several barriers that limit the development of vaccines against STIs. She argues that critical scientific information is missing and this makes the feasibility and the likelihood of success of vaccines against genital herpes, chlamydia, gonorrhoea and trichomonas uncertain. According to Dodet (2014), the immunity induced by natural infection is absent or imperfect which seriously limits the capacity to define the types of immune responses that an effective vaccine must induce. Reliable animal models are unavailable and a number of crucial clinical questions are still unanswered about the goal of these vaccines and definition of endpoints for clinical trials. In the absence of a clear recognition of the need for vaccines against STIs, Dodet (2014) notes that there has been no motivation for public or private research and industry to invest into the development of vaccines against STIs.

Apart from the lack of vaccines against STIs, another major limitation in the management of STIs is the difficulty in the laboratory culturing of fastidious organisms responsible for STIs, such as *N. gonorrhoeae*, *O. urealytica*, *T. vaginalis*, *U. urealyticum*, *T. pallidum* and *H. ducreyi*. *Neisseria gonorrhoeae* remains the most commonly studied organism. Studies on *T. pallidum* (causative agent for syphilis) prove difficult as the pathogen cannot be cultured in bacteriological growth media. In spite of the difficulties associated with growing pathogens associated with STIs, there is a need to investigate the use of medicinal plants for the treatment of STIs, even if studies are only restricted to *N. gonorrhoeae*.

Management of STIs is a major challenge in many countries because of the emergency of drug resistant strains of STIs and HIV. Drug resistance has contributed to many unsuccessful cases of STI treatment, besides making STI treatment more expensive (Chinsembu, Matondo, & Banda, 1997). Indeed, the spread of resistance has crippled the efficacy of antibiotics thereby increasing treatment failure. According to Ison, Dillon and Tapsall (1998), *N. gonorrhoeae* is resistant to penicillin and tetracycline, antibiotics frequently used in developing countries. Strains of penicillinase-producing *N. gonorrhoeae* were first detected in 1976.

WHO recommends third-generation cephalosporins, fluoroquinolones and spectinomycin for the treatment of gonorrhoea. But *N. gonorrhoeae* has also developed resistance to quinolones. Ceftriaxones are useful against gonorrhoea yet remain expensive. There is also decreased susceptibility of *N. gononorrhoeae* to cephalosporins, the last class of effective antibiotics for the treatment of gonorrhoea. *Haemophilus ducreyi*, too, is resistant to sulphonamide, chloramphenicol, kanamycin and streptomycin.

Multiple drug resistance has made the treatment of STIs to become less effective and more complicated, opening new vistas in the use of natural products. In the developing counties of Africa, Asia and South America, many people rely on medicinal plants to manage STDs. It is amazing that some of these plant materials are impregnated with diverse and unique chemical compounds that can even overcome drug resistant strains of STIs.

The subsequent sections in this chapter detail plants and algal species that are harnessed in the management of general STIs, gonorrhoea, syphilis, warts, genital herpes, chancroid, fungal infections and trichomoniasis. Before that, plant species whose extracts are applied as ethnomedicines for STIs in Western Province and Chiawa, Zambia, are documented.

Case Study: Medicinal Plants for Managing STIs in Zambia

A little background about the socio-economic and health situation may help contextualize the use of plant remedies in the management of STIs within Western Province, Zambia. According to the Zambia Demographic Health Survey report, the Lozi people of Western Province are the least educated in Zambia with 9% of men and 22% of women aged 15-49 years having no formal education (Central Statistical Office Zambia and Macro International Inc., 2009). Only 34.4% have comprehensive knowledge of STIs including HIV.

Western Province is also the poorest in Zambia with 45.2% of households being in the lowest wealth quintile (Central Statistical Office Zambia and Macro International Inc., 2009). Annual unemployment rate is 29.2% among women and 26.8% among men. Most of these are absorbed in peasant agriculture, accounting for 67.9%. Only 31.3% of women have professional, technical, clerical, managerial and sales skills. About 99.5% of the people have no health insurance.

Teenage pregnancy and motherhood in Western Province is highest in Zambia at 35.6%. The province has the lowest age of sexual debut at 15.8 years for females and 15.7 years for males. About 53.9% of births are delivered at home; 5% being delivered by traditional birth attendants; the third highest in Zambia after Central and North-western provinces with 5.2% and 6.2%, respectively. Only a third of eligible pregnant women take intestinal parasite drugs and 19% had a urine sample test.

The Zambia Demographic Health Survey data show that the women of Western Province are the most promiscuous in Zambia, with 3.2% having more than two sexual partners and 28.1% having high risk sexual intercourse. Men in Western Province had the highest high risk intercourse in Zambia at 90.3%. About 3.1% of men reported an STI; 6.8% of women and 5.3% of men had syphilis (Central Statistical Office Zambia and Macro International Inc., 2009). In the siLozi language of western Zambia, STIs are commonly known as *matuku a sihule* or *butuku bwa sihule*; meaning 'diseases of prostitutes'.

According to the 2009 Zambia Demographic Health Survey, about 56.7% women and 74.9% of men never tested for HIV. Over 15.2% of adults aged

15-49 years and 7.7% of young people aged 15-24 years were HIV positive; but the Red Cross reported 30% adult HIV prevalence in Sesheke (IRIN, 2006). In 1992, quite early in the AIDS epidemic, sero-prevalence figures for HIV were 16% for blood donors and 41% for patients attending the clinic for STIs (Van Der Hoek, 1992). Over 25.7% of people do not access healthcare at clinics because drugs are not available.

Given the aforementioned socio-economic and health challenges, most of the Lozi people suffering from STIs use medicinal plants. Some of the plants used to manage STIs in Western Province, Zambia, are presented in Table 4.1. The botanical names, siLozi names, families, plant habits, plant parts used, treated STIs, and modes of plant remedy preparation and administration are shown. Ndubani and Höjer (1999) also documented 19 plants used by *n'ganga* (traditional healers) in the management of STIs in Chiawa, a rural community south-east of Lusaka, Zambia (Table 4.2).

Known as *matenda ye chihure* (literally meaning illnesses of prostitution), STIs in Chiawa are often diagnosed as three distinct syndromes: genital sores (*zvironda*), pus discharge (*kubunda ukono*) and swollen lymph nodes (*kazvimba mamota*) (Ndubani & Höjer, 1999). These STIs, obviously a result of sexual contact (*kutapukira*), are locally known as *songeya* (syphilis), *doroba* (gonorrhoea), and *bola-bola* (refers to swellings on the groins caused by *Lymphogranuloma inguinale* infection) (Ndubani & Höjer, 1999).

According to Ndubani and Höjer (1999), the term *doroba* connotes town, a reference to the perception that the source of gonorrhoea is in urban areas. *Bola-bola* is characterized by marked difficulties in walking, as the patient moves with legs far apart (*kutangasa makambo*). *Bola-bola* is a rewording for a ball, because the swellings in the groin resemble tennis balls. As the infection progresses, the swollen nodes burst, releasing pus.

Natural Products for Managing General STIs

A review of herbal medicines for STDs has been provided by Vermani and Garg (2002). The review analyses the scientific evidence and the rationalization of the use of these preparations in the prevention of transmission and treatment of STDs. Elsewhere, plant products are also candidates for novel therapies including topical microbicides against HSV-2 (Bourne, Bourne, Reising, & Stanberry, 1999). These papers provide firm support for the use of natural products both as traditional medicines as well as new therapies for preventing and managing STIs.

Van Vuuren (2008) plus Naidoo, Van Vuuren, Van Zyl and De Wet (2013) have shown that South African medicinal plants used for the treatment of STIs have antimicrobial activity. De Wet, Nzama and Van Vuuren (2012) as

145

well as De Wet and Ngubane (2014) recorded medicinal plants utilized in the treatment of STIs in Maputaland, Kwa-Zulu Natal, South Africa (Table 4.3). Semenya, Potgieter and Erasmus (2013a) documented plant species used to treat STIs in Limpopo Province, South Africa (Table 4.4).

Mabogo (1990) also reported the use of the following plants in the treatment of STIs among the Venda people of South Africa: *Adansonia digitata, Acacia karroo, Aloe chabaudii, Bolusanthus speciosus, Ekebergia capensis, Elephantorrhiza burkei, Grewia occidentalis, Osyris lanceolata, Pappea capensis, Peltophorum africanum, Pterocarpus angolensis* and *Ximenia caffra* (the large sour plum). Later, Nair, Mulaudzi, Chukwujekwu, van Heerden and van Staden (2013) found that water extracts of *X. caffra* leaves had good antibacterial activity; minimum inhibitory concentration (MIC) value of 0.049 mg/ml against *Staphylococcus aureus*. *Ximenia caffra* contains a novel antigonococcal agent, bisnorsesquiterpene vomifoliol, which has 63.1% activity against *N. gonorrhoeae* (Nair et al., 2013).

Essential oils from *Tarchonanthus camphoratus* and *Croton gratissimus* have extremely potent antimicrobial activity on STI pathogens. In an *in vitro* study on the activity of essential oils on microorganisms isolated from vaginal infections, *Cymbopogon* sp., *Melaleuca alternifolia, Leptospermum scoparium* and *Thymus vulgaris* were found to inhibit five vaginal pathogens (Van Vuuren & Naidoo, 2010). Tshikalange, Meyer, Lall, Munoz, Sancho, Van de Venter and Oosthuizen (2008) also documented the following plants used to manage syphilis, gonorrhea, herpes and HIV infections in Venda, Limpopo Province, South Africa: *Anredera cordifolia, Clerodendrum glabrum, Elaeodendron transvaalense, Polianthes tuberose, Rauvolfia caffra, Rotheca myricoides, Senna occidentalis, Senna petersiana and Zanthoxylum davyi.*

Mulaudzi, Ndhlala, Kulkarni, Finnie and van Staden (2011) studied the plant *Bolusanthus speciosus,* used commonly to treat STIs by the Venda people of South Africa. They found that *B. speciosus* is imbued with active compounds such as medicarpin, genistein, 6,60- dihydroxy-40-methoxy-2-arylbenzofuran (bolusanthin IV) and flavonoids. These compounds have significant antibacterial activity against *Bacillus subtilis, Escherichia coli* and *S. aureus*; thus justifying their ethnomedicinal usage for managing STIs.

Medicinal properties of South African *Aloe* species have been reviewed by Grace, Simmonds, Smith and Van Wyk (2008) and Amoo, Aremu and van Staden (2014). There are many reports that *Aloe ferox* is used to treat STIs. In the Eastern Cape, *A. ferox* is widely utilized in the traditional management gonorrhoea and syphilis. Since whole-leaf exudates of *Aloe* species have antimicrobial action and increase wound closure (Jia, Zhao, & Jia, 2008), they are often used as remedies for syphilitic wounds. *Aloe* species have various antimicrobial active compounds (Chen, Van Wyk, Vermaak, & Viljoen, 2012).

Kambizi, Sultana and Afolayan (2004) isolated and characterized aloe-emodin, aloin A and chrysophanol from *A. ferox*; these compounds are active against various bacterial strains. In their results, aloin A showed the lowest MIC against *S. aureus* (MIC = 62.5 mg/ml); aloe-emodin, an anti-cancer agent, was most effective against *E. coli* (MIC = 62.5 mg/ml); while chrysophanol was more active against *Staphylococcus epidermidis* (MIC = 31.25 mg/ml). The antibacterial properties of the aforementioned active compounds justify their use in the management of STIs caused by bacteria.

Semenya, Potgieter, Tshisikhawe, Shava and Maroyi (2012), in addition to Nair, Aremu and van Staden (2012) say that *Terminalia phanerophlebia*, also known as *amaNgwe ampofu* in the Zulu tribe, is a remedy for wounds, gynaecological conditions and STIs. These authors state that the *T. phanerophlebia* plant contains cholestane triterpenoids β-sitostenone and stigmast-4-ene-3,6-dione together with the commercial anti-inflammatory agent β-sitosterol as the active principles. Plants in the genus *Terminalia* have many antimicrobial properties including anti-HIV functions.

In Botswana, Okatch, Ngwenya, Raletamo and Andrae-Marobela (2012) documented seven plants whose root extracts are traditional remedies for STIs. The scientific (and Tswana) names of the plants are: *Dichrostachys cinerea* (*Moselesele*), *Maerua angolensis* (*Moretete/Moreketi*), *Mimusops zeyheri* (*Mmupudu*), *Albizia anthelminthica* (*Monoga*), *Plumbago zeylanica* (*Masigomabe*), *Clerodendrum ternatum* (*Legonyana*), and *Maytenus senegalensis* (*Mothono*). Other plants that are harvested and applied in the management of general STIs in Botswana are: *Senna abbreviata* (*Monepenepe*), *Diospyros lycioides* (*Letlhajwa*) and *Pavetta harborii* (*Legonyana*) (Leteane, Ngwenya, Muzila, Namushe, Mwinga, & Musonda et al., 2012).

STIs in Kenya are also managed using the following plants: *Harungana madagascariensis*, *Justicia betonica* (contains alkaloids like jusbetonin, 10H-quindoline; triterpenes, lignans), *Spathodea campanulata*, *Tabernaemontana stapfiana*, and *Vernonia lasiopus* (Ochwang'i, Kimwele, Oduma, Gathumbi, Mbaria, & Kiama, 2014). Several species in the genus *Vernonia* including *adoensis*, *aemulans*, *ambigua*, *amygdalina*, *colorata*, *guineensis* and *kotschyana*, are used in many African countries to treat gonorrhoea (Toyang & Verpoorte, 2013). Other Kenyan plants for treating STIs are *Carissa edulis* (gonorrhoea, syphilis), *Euphorbia cuneate* (gonorrhoea), *Rhamnus perinoides* (gonorrhoea), *Teclea simplicifolia* (gonorrhoea), *Harisonia abyssinica* (general STDs), *Withania somnifera* (gonorrhoea), *Clerodendrum myricoides* (gonorrhoea, syphilis) (Muthee, Gakuya, Mbaria, Kareru, Mulei, & Njonge, 2011).

In Bangladesh, a couple of plants are remedies for genitourinary tract and STIs characterized by painful urination: *Achyranthes aspera*, *Amaranthus spinosus*, *Crinum asiaticum*, *Hemidesmus indicus*, *Holarrhena pubescens*, *Ichnocarpus frutescens*, *Scoparia dulcis*, *Sida acuta*, *Tragia involucrate*, and *Vernonia cinerea* (Fahim Kadir,

Shahdaat Bin Sayeed, Islam Setu, Mostafa, & Mia, 2014). A 50:50 mixture of the dried bark of *Mangifera indica* and a dried root extract of *Carica papaya*, known by the name DAS-77®, is produced by Doynik Ventures in Ogun State, and marketed as a remedy for STIs in Nigeria (Awodele, Akindele, Aniete, & Adeyemi, 2013). Owing to the presence of antibacterial bioflavonoids, the leaf extract of *Ormocarpum trichocarpum*, known as *isiThibane* in isiZulu, South Africa, is also utilized in the treatment of STIs (Chukwujekwu, Amoo, & van Staden, 2013).

Extracts of the stem bark of *Sclerocarya birrea*, commonly known as *Marula*, are widely used in many parts of Southern Africa for the treatment of STIs (Sarkar, Chaudhary, Sharma, Yadav, Nema, & Sekhoacha et al., 2014). Chemicals in *Marula* function as anti-biofilm agents that repress quorum-sensing mediated virulence, thus limiting the pathogenicity of bacteria that cause STIs. In Zimbabwe, Maroyi (2011) revealed that STI syndromes are managed using extracts from the following plants: *Annona stenophylla*, *Brachystegia boehmii*, *Ozoroa insigns*, *Peltophorum africanum* and *Pouzolzia hypoleuca*. *Peltophorum africanum* has high amounts of alkaloids, saponins, cardiac glycosides and flavonoids.

Talwar, Dar, Rai, Reddy, Mitra and Kulkarni et al. (2008) formulated a polyherbal cream known as *Basant*. These authors stated that the *Basant* cream consists of diferuloylmethane (curcumin), purified extracts of *Emblica officinalis* (*Amla*), purified saponins from *Sapindus mukorossi*, *Aloe vera* and rose water along with pharmaceutically approved excipients and preservatives. *Basant* inhibits the growth of WHO strains and clinical isolates of *Neisseria gonorrhoeae*, including those resistant to penicillin, tetracycline, nalidixic acid and ciprofloxacin. Apart from inhibiting HIV-1, the *Basant* cream also works against *Candida* isolates that cause vulvovaginal candidiasis, including three isolates resistant to azole drugs and amphotericin B (Talwar et al., 2008).

Van Vuuren and Naidoo (2010) studied the antimicrobial actions of 25 plants used traditionally in Southern Africa to treat a host of STIs. Some of these plants are presented in Table 4.5. Evaluation of antimicrobial activity is based on the plant extracts having susceptibility to pathogens with MIC values below 8 mg/ml. Noteworthy activity is observed for plant extracts and oils having susceptibility to pathogens with MIC values of ≤ 1.0 mg/ml and ≤ 2.0 mg/ml, respectively (Van Vuuren & Naidoo, 2010).

Gonorrhoea

Naidoo and co-workers reported that leaf extracts of *Ximenia caffra* possess anti-gonnococcal activity. These scientists found that some plant species have noteworthy antimicrobial efficacies against one or more pathogens associated with STIs. Fyhrquist, Laakso, Garcia Marco, Julkunen-Tiitto and Hiltunen

(2014) described that hot decoctions of *Terminalia sericea* and *Terminalia kaiserana* are used for the management of gonorrhoea. *Terminalia* species possess ellagitannins, chemical ingredients active against multi-antibiotic resistant *N. gonorrhoeae*.

According to Semenya, Potgieter and Erasmus (2013b), tubers of *Hypoxis hemerocallidea*, a species listed as declining, are used by traditional healers from the Waterberg District, to treat gonorrhoea and HIV/AIDS. *Hypoxis hemerocallidea* extracts are sold in pharmacies, health shops and supermarkets in South Africa to help manage HIV/AIDS. These products are marketed under the names Moducare® (immune booster), Hypo-Plus® (energy booster and food supplement) and capsules consisting of the whole *H. hemerocallidea* herb.

In particular, Mulaudzi et al. (2011) affirm that the petroleum ether extracts of *X. caffra* leaves and roots, *Ekebergia capensis* leaves and *Bolusanthus speciosus* stems show good activity (greater than 70%) against *N. gonorrhoeae*. Despite being weakly mutagenic (Mulaudzi, Ndhlala, Kulkarni, Finnie, & Staden, 2013), extracts of *E. capensis* leaves showed the best inhibition level at 96%. The ethanol extracts of *B. speciosus* bark and *Osyris lanceolata* roots showed good inhibition points, 72% and 87%, respectively.

Semenya et al. (2012) submit that *Catharanthus roseus* is prescribed for the treatment of gonorrhoea. Although *C. roseus* contains poisonous alkaloids, the majority of Bapedi traditional healers still administer it orally to treat gonorrhoea. Its local name *lepolomo le le pinki la drop* alludes to the fact that currently the Bapedi people use it only for gonorrhoea and not in the treatment of other ailments. Gonorrhoea is also treated by the use of *Alternanthera pungens* and *Caesalpinia decapetala* extracts. Individual extracts of *Elaeis guineensis*, *Harpagophytum procumbens* (Devil's claw), *Pelargonium sidoides* and *Senecio serratuloides* are orally taken to alleviate gonorrhoea.

Using the disc diffusion method, Chomnawang, Trinapakul and Gritsanapan (2009) discovered that 19 out of 22 Thai plant extracts inhibit the growth of *N. gonorrhoeae*. The extracts of *Plumbago indica*, *Coscinium fenestratum*, *Alpinia conchigera* and *Caesalpinia sappan* have strong inhibitory action. *Coscinium fenestratum* is used in Thai traditional medicine for gonorrhoea treatment; it has broad-spectrum antimicrobial activity. Preparations of *Gomphrena globosa* (leaf), *Suregada multiflorum*, *Chromolaena odorata*, *G. globosa* (root and stem), *Ageratum conyzoides*, *Andrographis paniculata* and *Senna siamea* had moderate anti-gonococcal activity. The extracts of *Phyllanthus amarus*, *Plumeria obtusa*, *Amaranthus spinosus*, *Bixa orellana*, *Ardisia colorata*, *Artocarpus lacucha*, *Smilax corbularia*, *Garcinia mangostana* and *C. papaya* showed low anti-gonococcal activity with mean inhibition zone diameters of less than 9.3 mm.

Because results of disc diffusion techniques are not always reproducible and reliable, plants which gave high antigonococcal activities by disc diffusion method, namely *P. indica*, *C. fenestratum*, *A. conchigera* and *C. sappan*, were selected for further testing by determining their MIC values. The results revealed that the extract of *C. fenestratum* produced the strongest anti-gonococcal activity against *N. gonorrhoeae* ATCC 49226, with MIC value of 47.39 µg/ml whereas *C. sappan*, *P. indica* and *A. conchigera* gave MIC values of 130.21, 253.57 and 513.41 µg/ml, respectively (Chomnawang et al., 2009).

The researchers further examined the effects of *C. fenestratum* extracts against *N. gonorrhoeae* clinical isolates. Chomnawang and colleagues found MIC values varied between 19.51 and 112.14 µg/ml. These results confirm that the *C. fenestratum* stem crude extracts have anti-gonococcal activity. The anti-gonococcal active compound in *C. fenestratum* is berberine whose MIC values are 13.51 and 17.66 µg/ml against *N. gonorrhoeae* ATCC 49226 and a clinical isolate, respectively.

The MIC values for berberine isolated from *C. fenestratum* are higher than those for anti-gonococcal active compounds from other plants. For example, *Hymeneae palustris* in the Family Fabaceae contains the active compounds hydnocarpin-D, 5'-methoxyhydnocarpin-D, and palstatin whose MIC values against *N. gonorrhoeae* are 0.5, 0.625, and 1 µg/ml, respectively (Pettit, Meng, Stevenson, Doubek, Knight, & Cichacz, et al., 2003). Against *N. gonorrhoeae*, luteolin- another active compound from *H. palustris* - has MIC value of 16–32 µg/ml.

Mollik, Hossan, Paul, Taufiq-Ur-Rahman, Jahan and Rahmatullah (2010) working in rural Bangladesh found that gonorrhoea was treated by the use of thirteen medicinal plants: *Celosia cristata*, *B. orellana*, *Jatropha curcas*, *Drynaria quercifolia*, *Arachis hypogaea*, *Senna alata*, *Uraria picta*, *Sterculia foetida*, *Amomum aromaticum*, *Ruellia tuberosa*, *A. vera*, *Citrus aurantifolia*, and *Euphorbia hirta*. *Celosia cristata* has well-known antimicrobial functions; reason the plant is applied in the management of gonorrhoea as well as genital wounds and herpes. *Bixa orellana*, a plant with natural pigments employed as food colour additives and lipsticks, also has broad-spectrum antibacterial activity thus is used to alleviate gonorrhoea. A shrub native to Mexico, *S. alata* is known to have antimicrobial activity even at very low concentrations, mostly due to the presence of flavonoids.

Extracts from two Cameroonian medicinal plants *Bersama engleriana*, which has 80% inhibitory activity against HIV reverse transcriptase and the bark of *Vitellaria paradoxa*, are effective against ten *N. gonorrhoeae* strains, with MIC values closer or lower than for gentamycin, below 100 µg/ml on most strains (Mbaveng, Kuete, Mapunya, Beng, Nkengfack, Meyer, & Lall, 2011). Telefo, Lienou, Yemele, Lemfack, Mouokeu and Goka et al. (2011) indicated that water extracts of *Ficus sycomorus* roots or leaves and *Cissus quadrangularis* stems are taken orally to treat gonorrhoea in Cameroon.

In several African countries, De Villiers, Van Vuuren, Van Zyl and Van Wyk (2010), citing several studies, reported that infection with *N. gonorrhoeae* is treated with various plants belonging to the genus *Cussonia*. It has been reported that gonorrhoea is treated with *Cussonia holstii* and *Cussonia spicata* in Tanzania. In culture, *N. gonorrhoeae* is sensitive to extracts of *Cussonia* species. The anti-gonorrhoeal activity of the species tested had MIC values between 0.02 and 0.7 mg/ml. The methanolic extract of *Cussonia nicholsonii* (methanol extract) had the most noteworthy activity with a MIC value of 0.02 mg/ml (De Villiers et al., 2010). In addition, methanolic extracts of *Schefflera umbellifera* and *Seemannaralia gerrardii* had notable activity against *N. gonorrhoeae*.

Maroyi (2011), working in Zimbabwe, found that people use *Albizia antunesiana*, *Senna abbreviata*, *Elephantorrhiza goetzei* and *Lannea edulis* as natural remedies for gonorrhoea. These four plants are known to have antimicrobial properties. Extracts of *A. antunesiana* are also useful in treating *bola-bola* (groin swellings caused by *L. inguinale*) and gonorrhoea in Chiawa, Zambia. *Senna abbreviata*, whose bark infusion is taken orally, has antibacterial properties perhaps because of the high amounts of tannins and flavonoids. It is also used to treat STIs in the Blouberg area of Limpopo Province in South Africa.

Juice squeezed from the leaves of *Asclepias curassavica* is administered orally as a remedy for gonorrhoea in India (Duraipandiyan & Ignacimuthu, 2011). *Oxygonum sinuatum*, *Rhus vulgaris*, *Senna didymobotrya* and *Solanum aculeastrum* are plant remedies for gonorrhoea in Kenya (Ochwang'i, Kimwele, Oduma, Gathumbi, Mbaria, & Kiama, 2014). Endowed with active compounds such as friedelin (a triterpenoid with antibacterial action), epifriedelinol, beta-amyrin, beta-sitosterol and naringin, the plant *Drynaria quercifolia* is active against *N. gonorrhoeae* (Mithraja, Irudayaraj, Kiruba, & Jeeva, 2012). Other plants exploited in the treatment of gonorrhoea are *Achyranthes aspera*, *Hibiscus rosa-sinensis and Ricinus communis* (De Boer & Cotingting, 2014) and *Fibraurea tinctoria* (Galappathie, Palombo, Yeo, Ley, Tu, Malherbe, & Mahon, 2014). Van Vuuren and Naidoo (2010) found high antimicrobial activity against *N. gonorrhoeae* from *Hypericum aethiopicum* root extracts (0.25 mg/ml).

Syphilis

Semenya et al. (2012) documented that *Aristea ecklonii*, *Elephantorrhiza elephantine* and *Kigelia africana* are individually used to manage syphilis. Unfortunately, *K. africana* is known to be cytotoxic. In the Indian Ocean island of Madagascar, people utilize *Acalypha andringitrensis* and *Acalypha radula* as remedies for syphilis (Seebaluck, Gurib-Fakim, & Mahomoodally, 2014).

In Nigeria, *Acalypha fimbriata* is applied in the management of syphilis. Ethanolic leaf extracts of *A. fimbriata* contain saponins, tannins, flavonoids and glycosides. In general, plant species from the genus *Acalypha* contain principle bioactive phytochemicals such as tannins, flavonoids, phenolics, saponins, alkaloids, terpenoids, coumarins, anthocyanins and anthraquinones which undoubtedly justify their antimicrobial and healing properties for STIs.

Cissus quadrangularis stem extracts are a remedy for syphilis in Cameroon (Telefo et al., 2011). A water decoction of *Cussonia arborea* root is applied topically to heal syphilitic sores in Zambia (Ndubani & Höjer, 1999). Infusions of *Cussonia zimmermannii* leaves (De Villiers et al., 2010), whole plant preparations of *Aristea ecklonii*, and a paste prepared from the rhizomes, roots and leaves of *Cissampelos capensis* (Mabona, Viljoen, Shikanga, Marston, & Van Vuuren, 2013) are applied topically to treat syphilis. *Aristea ecklonii* is known to have noteworthy antibacterial and 100% antifungal activities.

The dietary spice *Solanum melongena*, commonly known as *Aubergine*, is applied as a natural remedy for syphilis and gonorrhoea in Cameroon (Tekwu, Askun, Kuete, Nkengfack, Nyasse, Etoa, & Beng, 2012). In Uganda, the plants *Zehneria scabra* and *M. senegalensis* are exploited as remedies for syphilis (Mugisha, Asiimwe, Namutebi, Borg-Karlson, & Kakudidi, 2014). *Ficus sur* and *Peltophorum africanum* are collected in Zimbabwe to alleviate syphilis (Maroyi, 2011). The following plants are used to treat syphilis in Bangladesh: *Siegesbeckia orientalis, Borassus flabellifer, Brassica campestris, Basella alba, Mimusops elengi, Nigella sativa, Clerodendrum indicum, Colocasia esculenta* and *Argyreia speciosa* (Mollik et al., 2010).

Genital Warts

Fathi and Tsoukas (2014) explained that podophyllotoxin, a purified extract from members of the genus *Podophyllum*, binds to cellular microtubules to induce wart necrosis by inhibiting mitosis. Fathi and Tsoukas (2014) also mention polyphenon E, approved for use against external genital and peri-anal warts in the United States of America in 2006. The active ingredient in polyphenon E is a green tea extract, thought to contain antioxidant, antiviral and anti-tumour sinecatechins. Likewise, extracts of *Anacardium occidentale* and *Viscum capense* are topically smeared to shrink genital warts (Lall & Kishore, 2014). *Acalypha fimbriata* is also used in the management of warts in Nigeria.

Genital Herpes

Some of the anti-herpes drugs like ganciclovir and foscarnet produce toxic side-effects. In addition, the emergence of virus strains resistant to commonly used anti-herpesvirus drugs is a growing problem, particularly in immunocompromised patients. Corollary, many patients with genital herpes still use herbal preparations to manage the disease. Xiong, Luo, Hou, Xiao and Yang (2011) pointed out that a number of anthraquinones and anthrones isolated from plants and lichens exhibit virucidal activity against enveloped viruses including HSV-2, the causative agent of genital herpes. These authors showed that emodin (3-methyl-1,6,8-trihydroxyanthraquinone), extracted and purified from *Rheum tanguticum*, prevents HSV-2 attachment and penetration; thus has anti-herpesvirus activity *in vitro* and *in vivo*. Therefore, emodin is believed to be a promising agent in the clinical therapy of HSV infection, comparable to the standard anti-HSV drug acyclovir.

Rheum tanguticum is a member of the rhubarb group of plants that belong to the genus *Rheum* in the family Polygonaceae. It is one of the oldest and best-known traditional Chinese medicines. Ye, Han, Chen, Zheng and Guo (2007) explained that rhubarb contains pharmaceutically relevant compounds such as sennosides, anthraquinones, stilbenes, glucose gallates, naphthalenes and cate-chins. Since genital herpes has played a more important role than any other STI in driving HIV prevalence in Africa (Abu-Raddad et al., 2008), use of *R. tanguticum* to control HSV-2 infection may concurrently reduce the spread of HIV in African populations.

Many studies including the one by Koch, Reichling, Schneele and Schnitzler (2008) have named essential oils of various plants as anti-herpes agents. The use of tea tree oil- the essential oil of *Melaleuca alternifolia* - for the treatment of recurrent herpes labialis is one such example. Camomile oil also finds therapeutic application as a virucidal agent for topical treatment of herpes genitalis (Koch et al., 2008). *Vernonia amygdalina* is harvested for use as a treatment for genital herpes in Tanzania (Toyang & Verpoorte, 2013). Extracts of *Boehmeria nivea* and *Polygonum cuspidatum* are harnessed as remedies for hepatitis B virus while those for *Carissa edulis* and *Phyllanthus urinaria* are applied against HSV-2 infections (Mukhtar, Arshad, Ahmad, Pomerantz, Wigdahl, & Parveen, 2008).

Chancroid

Nawrocki et al. (2013) bemoaned that chancroid is endemic in regions of Africa and Asia, but because these areas are bereft of accurate diagnostic tests for *H. ducreyi*, the actual prevalence of chancroid is unknown. Nawrocki and co-workers warn that strains of *H. ducreyi* have now acquired plasmid mediated mechanisms of resistance to several classes of antibiotics (azithromycin, ceftri-axone ciprofloxacin and erythromycin). The rise of antibiotic resistance and the prevalence of chancroid in resource-poor environments have opened new vistas in the development of alternative treatment options mainly based on natural products.

One of the natural products that thwarts the growth of *H. ducreyi* is resveratrol (3,5,4'-trihydroxystilbene), a polyphenolic phytoalexin produced by some flowering plants in response to unfavourable environmental conditions such as fungal infection or injury (Trela & Waterhouse, 1996). A proven anti-HIV agent, resveratrol is also commonly found in food and drink products such as peanuts, grapes and red wine. In their experiments, Nawrocki et al. (2013) showed that resveratrol has bacteriostatic and bactericidal actions against *H. ducreyi*. At par with this experimental evidence, resveratrol (and red wine?) may be used as a topical microbicide to prevent chancroid especially in women.

Candida albicans

Van Vuuren and Naidoo (2010) showed that leaf extracts of *Psidium guajava* have notable action against *C. albicans* (0.75 mg/ml). Galappathie, Palombo, Yeo, Ley, Tu and Malherbe et al. (2014) found that *Pyrenaria* sp. have significant activity against *C. albicans* with minimum fungicidal concentration of 50 µg/ml; hence these plants are used to treat vaginomycosis. Noteworthy susceptibility of *C. albicans* was noted with aqueous extracts of *Syzygium cordatum*, MIC value of 0.1 mg/ml. According to Van Vuuren and Naidoo (2010), the aqueous extracts of *Bowiea volubilis* leaf material (0.5 mg/ml), *Euclea natalensis* (0.5 mg/ml), *Catharanthus roseus* (0.5 mg/ml) and *S. cordatum* (0.1 mg/ml) demonstrated noteworthy activity against *C. albicans*.

Trichomonas vaginalis and Gardnerella vaginalis

Trichomonas vaginalis showed antimicrobial susceptibility to eighteen plant extracts studied by Van Vuuren and Naidoo (2010), with the most noteworthy activity observed for *Tarchonanthus camphoratus* leaf material (0.5 mg/ml). *Hypoxis latifolia* produced noteworthy activity against *T. vaginalis* at 0.75 mg/ml. *Schefflera umbellifera* and *Seemannaralia gerrardii* have noteworthy activities against *T. vaginalis* (De Villiers et al., 2010).

Marine fungi also possess anti-*Trichomonas* activity. *Hypocrea lixii* and *Penicillium citrinum* have significant growth-inhibitory activity (up to 100%) against *T. vaginalis* ATCC 30236 and fresh clinical isolates, including a metronidazole-resistant isolate. Minimum inhibitory concentration values of *H. lixii* and *P. citrinum* samples for all isolates tested, including the metronidazole-resistant isolate, were 2.5 mg/ml (Scopel et al., 2013).

Lycorine, an alkaloid from plants belonging to the Amaryllidaceae family, arrests the cell cycle of *T. vaginalis* (Giordani et al., 2011). Moo-Puc et al. (2008) evaluated the efficacy of seaweeds on *T. vaginalis* trophozoites. Their results indicated that 44% of the seaweeds studied had high to moderate anti-*T. vaginalis* activity. *Lobophora variegata* and *Udotea conglutinata* showed the highest anti-*T. vaginalis* activity with IC_{50} values of 1.39 and 1.66 µg/ml, respectively. Extracts of these two algae also had low selectivity index (SI), defined as the ratio of cytotoxicity to biological activity, according to the formulae $SI = CC_{50}$ MDCK cells/IC_{50} *T. vaginalis*.

Van Vuuren and Naidoo (2010) also found that extracts of the five plants *Polygala fruticosa* (0.2 mg/ml), *Hypericum aethiopicum* root extract (0.2 mg/ml), *Tarchonanthus camphoratus* (0.7 mg/ml), *Croton gratissimus* (1.0 mg/ml) and *Psidium guajava* (1.0 mg/ml) displayed noteworthy activities against *Gardnerella vaginalis*. *Polygala fruticosa* and the root extract of *H. aethiopicum* exhibit highest antimicrobial activity towards *G. vaginalis* at 0.2 mg/ml (Van Vuuren & Naidoo, 2010).

A Closer Look at Natural Products for STIs

The transmission and epidemiology of HIV/AIDS and other STIs are intertwined; they spread synergistically and in tandem. Owing to poor immunity, persons infected with HIV can very easily be infected with other STIs. In such HIV/AIDS individuals, presentation of traditional STIs is usually aggressive and severe. In short, HIV/AIDS does not only spur the transmission of classical and curable STIs (chancroid, gonorrhoea syphilis and trachomoniasis) but also magnifies their presentation, making them very difficult to treat and manage. Coupled with the emergence of drug resistance, STIs are always an eminent threat and real menace during HIV infection as most cases are not amenable to therapy.

In every society, STIs are difficult to diagnose and treat because of the fact that patients are reluctant to come to the fore, mainly because STIs are perceived as diseases for promiscuous individuals, commercial sex workers and casual prostitutes. STIs are a silent epidemic. Since most patients do not want to seek treatment at hospitals and public health clinics, they usually seek the services of traditional healers who dispense natural products. Others administer self-medications of a simple nature, for example root concoctions of common plants such as bananas, paw-paw, lemon and mangoes.

The chapter has documented more than 200 different plants for the treatment and management of STIs. These plants have proven antimicrobial efficacy against *H. ducreyi*, *N. gonorrhoeae*, *T. pallidum*, *T. vaginalis*, HSV-2 and *C. albicans*. Most of the plants are found in several African countries such as Botswana, Cameroon, Kenya, Madagascar, Namibia, Nigeria, South Africa, Uganda, Zimbabwe and Zambia. A few ethnomedicinal plants used in the management of STIs are from other developing countries outside Africa, for example Bangladesh and India, but almost none are from developed countries.

This perhaps alludes to STIs being a public health problem of resource-poor communities in developing countries.

Except for marine algae and fungal species utilized in the treatment of *T. vaginalis* infection, all the natural products reviewed in this chapter are strictly plant species. All this said, most of the African studies on natural products used in the management of STIs are conducted in South Africa. This mirrors the strong South African research capability in the emerging fields of bio-prospecting and drug discovery.

Unfortunately, compared to natural products for skin diseases, there is a conspicuous failure towards commercialization of traditional plant products used in the management of STIs. One of the few commercial herbal remedies for STIs is DAS-77®, a phytotherapy for STIs produced by Doynik Ventures in Ogun State, Nigeria. Therefore, there is an urgent need for African countries to add value and commercialize natural products used in the management of STIs. This is critical given the high burden of STIs in Africa.

With the rising incidence of resistance to antibiotics and other drugs used to treat STIs, many patients are turning to natural products for the management of stubborn STIs. For instance, there are several plant products that are able to treat antibiotic-resistant gonorrhoea. For socio-economic reasons, the use of natural products still remains cheaper and discrete as many patients secretly seek treatment from traditional healers, mainly at night. Finally, natural products embody a new promise in the development of novel drugs for treating STIs.

Conclusions and Recommendations

This chapter presents over 200 different natural products (including 120 entries of plants in the tables) that are utilized in the management of STDs such as chancroid, gonorrhoea, syphilis, genital warts, genital herpes, trichomoniasis and vaginal thrush. Many of the plants are used as ethnomedicines, hence have not been tested for antimicrobial activity. *Neisseria gonorrhoeae* accounts for the lion's share of ethnomedicinal plants that have been subjected to antimicrobial testing against STIs. Since *N. gonorrhoeae* is relatively easy to culture, fresh cultures are available for antimicrobial testing.

Although *C. albicans* and *G. vaginalis* are also easy to culture and their laboratory strains are available, it is surprising that many medicinal plant extracts have not been tested against this fungus and bacterium, respectively. Few plant species have been tested for activity against viral and protozoan STIs, mainly because viruses and protozoan parasites are difficult to grow and maintain in the laboratory. Working on viruses may also require laboratories to increase their safety level, a major constraint in most African laboratories conducting research on natural products. Starting with ethnobotanical inventories of plants used to manage STIs in Western Province and the small south-eastern town of Chiawa in Zambia, the chapter also details medicinal plants utilized in the treatment of STIs in Kwa-Zulu Natal and Limpopo provinces in South Africa. A few plants from other African countries including Botswana, Cameroon, Kenya, Namibia, Nigeria, Uganda and Zimbabwe are also documented. Common plants like *Aloe ferox, Sclerocarya birrea, Terminalia sp., Ximenia caffra, Hypoxis hemerocallidea* and *Kigelia africana* are being used to manage various STDs. The available evidence of the plants' antimicrobial properties and active chemical compounds justifies the use of ethnomedicinal plants as natural medicines for STDs. However, more efforts are needed to commercialise current natural products as well as to discover novel active ingredients that may be developed into newer drugs to combat drug resistant STIs.

References

Abu-Raddad, L.J., Magaret, A.S., Celum, C., Wald, A., Longini Jr., I.M., Self, S.G., Corey, L., (2008). Genital herpes has played a more important role than any other sexually transmitted infection in driving HIV prevalence in Africa. *PLoS One*, 3, e2230.

Amoo, S.O., Aremu, A.O., & van Staden, J. (2014). Unraveling the medicinal potential of South African *Aloe* species. *Journal of Ethnopharmacology*, *153*(1), 19-41.

Awodele, O., Akindele, A.J., Aniete, J., & Adeyemi, O.O. (2013). Preliminary antimicrobial evaluation of DAS-77®—A polyherbal medicine. *Journal of Herbal Medicine*, *3*(2), 52-56.

Bourne, K.Z., Bourne, N., Reising, S.F., & Stanberry, L.R. (1999). Plant products as topical microbicide candidates: assessment of in vitro and in vivo activity against herpes simplex virus type-2. *Antiviral Research*, *42(3)*, 219-226.

Central Statistical Office (CSO) [Zambia] and Macro International Inc. (2009). *Zambia Demographic and Health Survey 2007*. Calverton, Maryland, USA: CSO and Macro International Inc.

Chen, W., Van Wyk, B.E., Vermaak, I., & Viljoen, A.M. (2012). Cape aloes—A review of the phytochemistry, pharmacology and commercialisation of *Aloe ferox*. *Phytochemistry Letters*, *5*(1), 1-12.

Chinsembu, K.C. (2009). Sexually transmitted infections in adolescents. *The Open Infectious Diseases Journal*, 3, 107-117.

Chinsembu, K.C., Matondo, P. & Banda, S.S. (1997). *Sexually transmitted diseases: A training manual for health workers*. Published by Ministry of Health/USAID/AIDSCAP, Lusaka, Zambia.

Chomnawang, M.T., Trinapakul, C., & Gritsanapan, W. (2009). *In vitro* antigonococcal activity of *Coscinium fenestratum* stem extract. *Journal of Ethnopharmacology*, *122*(3), 445-449.

Chukwujekwu, J.C., Amoo, S.O., & van Staden, J. (2013). Antimicrobial, antioxidant, mutagenic and antimutagenic activities of *Distephanus angulifolius* and *Ormocarpum trichocarpum*. *Journal of Ethnopharmacology*, *148*(3), 975-979.

Cohen, M. S. (1998). Sexually transmitted diseases enhance HIV transmission: no longer a hypothesis. *The Lancet*, *351*, S5-S7.

De Boer, H.J., & Cotingting, C. (2014). Medicinal plants for women's healthcare in southeast Asia: A meta-analysis of their traditional use, chemical constituents, and pharmacology. *Journal of Ethnopharmacology*, *151*(2), 747-767.

De Villiers, B.J., Van Vuuren, S.F., Van Zyl, R.L., & Van Wyk, B.E. (2010). Antimicrobial and antimalarial activity of *Cussonia* species (Araliaceae). *Journal of Ethnopharmacology*, *129*(2), 189-196.

De Wet, H., & Ngubane, S.C. (2014). Traditional herbal remedies used by women in a rural community in northern Maputaland (South Africa) for the treatment of gynaecology and obstetric complaints. *South African Journal of Botany*, *94*, 129-139.

De Wet, H., Nzama, V.N., & Van Vuuren, S.F. (2012). Medicinal plants used for the treatment of sexually transmitted infections by lay people in northern Maputaland, KwaZulu–Natal Province, South Africa. *South African Journal of Botany*, *78*, 12-20.

Dodet, B. (2014). Current barriers, challenges and opportunities for the development of effective STI vaccines: Point of view of vaccine producers, biotech companies and funding agencies. *Vaccine*, *32*(14), 1624-1629.

Duraipandiyan, V., & Ignacimuthu, S. (2011). Antifungal activity of traditional medicinal plants from Tamil Nadu, India. *Asian Pacific Journal of Tropical Biomedicine*, *1*(2), S204-S215.

Fahim Kadir, M., Shahdaat Bin Sayeed, M., Islam Setu, N., Mostafa, A., & Mia, M.M.K. (2014). Ethnopharmacological survey of medicinal plants used by traditional health practitioners in Thanchi, Bandarban Hill Tracts, Bangladesh. *Journal of Ethnopharmacology*, *155*, 495-508.

Fathi, R., & Tsoukas, M.M. (2014). Genital warts and other HPV infections: Established and novel therapies. *Clinics in Dermatology*, *32*(2), 299-306.

Fleming, D.T., & Wasserheit, J.N. (1999). From epidemiological synergy to public health policy and practice: The contribution of other sexually transmitted diseases to sexual transmission of HIV infection. *Sexually Transmitted Infections*, *75*(1), 3-17.

Fyhrquist, P., Laakso, I., Garcia Marco, S., Julkunen-Tiitto, R., & Hiltunen, R. (2014). Antimycobacterial activity of ellagitannin and ellagic acid derivate rich crude extracts and fractions of five selected species of *Terminalia* used for treatment of infectious diseases in African traditional medicine. *South African Journal of Botany*, *90*, 1-16.

Galappathie, S., Palombo, E.A., Yeo, T.C., Ley, D.L.S., Tu, C.L., Malherbe, F.M., & Mahon, P.J. (2014). Comparative antimicrobial activity of South East Asian plants used in Bornean folkloric medicine. *Journal of Herbal Medicine*, *4*(2), 96-105.

Galvin, S.R., & Cohen, M.S. (2004). The role of sexually transmitted diseases in HIV transmission. *Nature Reviews Microbiology*, *2*(1), 33-42.

Giordani, R.B., Vieira, P.D.B., Weizenmann, M., Rosemberg, D.B., Souza, A.P., Bonorino, C., ... & Tasca, T. (2011). Lycorine induces cell death in the amitochondriate parasite, *Trichomonas vaginalis*, via an alternative non-apoptotic death pathway. *Phytochemistry*, *72*(7), 645-650.

Grace, O.M., Simmonds, M.S.J., Smith, G.F., & Van Wyk, A.E. (2008). Therapeutic uses of *Aloe* L. (Asphodelaceae) in Southern Africa. *Journal of Ethnopharmacology*, *119*(3), 604-614.

IRIN (2006). Namibia: Curbing HIV/AIDS along a transport corridor. IRIN News.

Ison, C.A., Dillon, J.A.R., & Tapsall, J.W. (1998). The epidemiology of global antibiotic resistance among *Neisseria gonorrhoeae* and *Haemophilus ducreyi*. *The Lancet*, 351, s8-s11.

Jia, Y., Zhao, G., & Jia, J. (2008). Preliminary evaluation: The effects of *Aloe ferox* Miller and *Aloe arborescens* Miller on wound healing. *Journal of Ethnopharmacology*, *120*(2), 181-189.

Johnson, L.F., Dorrington, R.E., Bradshaw, D., & Coetzee, D.J. (2011). The effect of syndromic management interventions on the prevalence of sexually transmitted infections in South Africa. *Sexual and Reproductive Healthcare*, *2*(1), 13-20.

Johnson, L.F. (2008). The interaction between HIV and other sexually transmitted infections in South Africa: A model-based evaluation. Doctoral thesis, University of Cape Town, Cape Town, South Africa.

Kamatenesi-Mugisha, M., Oryem-Origa, Odyek, O., & Makawiti, D.W. (2008). Medicinal plants used in the treatment of fungal and bacterial infections in and around Queen Elizabeth Biosphere Reserve, western Uganda. *African Journal of Ecology*, 46, 90–97.

Kambizi, L., Sultana, N., & Afolayan, A.J. (2004). Bioactive compounds isolated from *Aloe ferox*: A plant traditionally used for the treatment of sexually transmitted infections in the Eastern Cape, South Africa. *Pharmaceutical Biology*, 42, 636–639.

Koch, C., Reichling, J., Schneele, J., & Schnitzler, P. (2008). Inhibitory effect of essential oils against herpes simplex virus type 2. *Phytomedicine*, *15*(1), 71-78.

Laga, M., Manoka, A., Kivuvu, M., Malele, B., Tuliza, M., Nzila, N., ... & Piot, P. (1993). Non-ulcerative sexually transmitted diseases as risk factors for HIV-1 transmission in women: Results from a cohort study. *AIDS*, *7*(1), 95-102.

Lall, N., & Kishore, N. (2014). Are plants used for skin care in South Africa fully explored?. *Journal of Ethnopharmacology*, *153*(1), 61-84.

Leteane, M.M., Ngwenya, B.N., Muzila, M., Namushe, A., Mwinga, J., Musonda, R., ... & Andrae-Marobela, K. (2012). Old plants newly discovered: *Cassia sieberiana* DC and *Cassia abbreviata* Oliv. Oliv. root extracts inhibit in vitro HIV-1c replication in peripheral blood mononuclear cells (PBMCs) by different modes of action. *Journal of Ethnopharmacology*, *141*(1), 48-56.

Lewis, D.A. (2005). Trichomoniasis. *Medicine*, 33, 66–67.

Mabona, U., Viljoen, A., Shikanga, E., Marston, A., & Van Vuuren, S. (2013). Antimicrobial activity of southern African medicinal plants with dermatological relevance: From an ethnopharmacological screening approach, to combination studies and the isolation of a bioactive compound. *Journal of Ethnopharmacology*, *148*(1), 45-55.

Mabogo, D.E.N. (1990). *The ethnobotany of the Vhavenda*. MSc. Thesis. University of Pretoria, South Africa.

Maroyi, A. (2011). An ethnobotanical survey of medicinal plants used by the people in Nhema communal area, Zimbabwe. *Journal of Ethnopharmacology*, *136*(2), 347-354.

Matondo, P., Chinsembu, K.C., & Kapembwa, M.S. (1998). *Sexually transmitted disease syndromes: A text and atlas*. Lusaka, Zambia: Xpress Yourself.

Mayaud, P., & Mabey, D. (2004). Approaches to the control of sexually transmitted infections in developing countries: old problems and modern challenges. *Sexually Transmitted Infections*, 80, 174-82.

Mbaveng, A.T., Kuete, V., Mapunya, B.M., Beng, V.P., Nkengfack, A.E., Meyer, J.J.M., & Lall, N. (2011). Evaluation of four Cameroonian medicinal plants for anticancer, antigonorrheal and antireverse transcriptase activities. *Environmental Toxicology and Pharmacology*, *32*(2), 162-167.

Mithraja, M.J., Irudayaraj, V., Kiruba, S., & Jeeva, S. (2012). Antibacterial efficacy of *Drynaria quercifolia* (L.) J. Smith (Polypodiaceae) against clinically isolated urinary tract pathogens. *Asian Pacific Journal of Tropical Biomedicine*, *2*(1), S131-S135.

Mollik, M.A.H., Hossan, M.S., Paul, A.K., Taufiq-Ur-Rahman, M., Jahan, R., & Rahmatullah, M. (2010). A comparative analysis of medicinal plants used by folk medicinal healers in three districts of Bangladesh and inquiry as to mode of selection of medicinal plants. *Ethnobotany Research and Applications*, *8*, 195-218.

Moo-Puc, R., Robledo, D., & Freile-Pelegrin, Y. (2008). Evaluation of selected tropical seaweeds for *in vitro* anti-trichomonal activity. *Journal of Ethnopharmacology*, *120*(1), 92-97.

Mugisha, M.K., Asiimwe, S., Namutebi, A., Borg-Karlson, A.K., & Kakudidi, E.K. (2014). Ethnobotanical study of indigenous knowledge on medicinal and nutritious plants used to manage opportunistic infections associated with HIV/AIDS in western Uganda. *Journal of Ethnopharmacology*, 155, 194–202.

Mukhtar, M., Arshad, M., Ahmad, M., Pomerantz, R.J., Wigdahl, B., & Parveen, Z. (2008). Antiviral potentials of medicinal plants. *Virus Research*, *131*(2), 111-120.

Mulaudzi, R.B., Ndhlala, A.R., Kulkarni, M.G., Finnie, J.F., & van Staden, J. (2011). Antimicrobial properties and phenolic contents of medicinal plants used by the Venda people for conditions related to venereal diseases. *Journal of Ethnopharmacology, 135*(2), 330-337.

Mulaudzi, R.B., Ndhlala, A.R., Kulkarni, M.G., Finnie, J.F., & Staden, J. V. (2013). Anti-inflammatory and mutagenic evaluation of medicinal plants used by Venda people against venereal and related diseases. *Journal of Ethnopharmacology, 146*(1), 173-179.

Murray, M.T., & Pizzorno, J.E. (1999). *Textbook of Natural Medicine*. Churchill Living, China.

Muthee, J.K., Gakuya, D.W., Mbaria, J.M., Kareru, P.G., Mulei, C.M., & Njonge, F.K. (2011). Ethnobotanical study of anthelmintic and other medicinal plants traditionally used in Loitoktok district of Kenya. *Journal of Ethnopharmacology, 135*(1), 15–21.

Naidoo, D., Van Vuuren, S.F., Van Zyl, R.L., & De Wet, H. (2013). Plants traditionally used individually and in combination to treat sexually transmitted infections in northern Maputaland, South Africa: Antimicrobial activity and cytotoxicity. *Journal of Ethnopharmacology, 149*(3), 656-667.

Nair, J.J., Aremu, A.O., & van Staden, J. (2012). Anti-inflammatory effects of *Terminalia phanerophlebia* (Combretaceae) and identification of the active constituent principles. *South African Journal of Botany, 81*, 79-80.

Nair, J.J., Mulaudzi, R.B., Chukwujekwu, J.C., Van Heerden, F.R., & van Staden, J. (2013). Antigonococcal activity of *Ximenia caffra* Sond. (Olacaceae) and identification of the active principle. *South African Journal of Botany, 86*, 111-115.

Nawrocki, E.M., Bedell, H.W., & Humphreys, T.L. (2013). Resveratrol is cidal to both classes of *Haemophilus ducreyi*. *International Journal of Antimicrobial agents, 41*(5), 477-479.

Ndubani, P., & Höjer, B. (1999). Traditional healers and the treatment of sexually transmitted illnesses in rural Zambia. *Journal of Ethnopharmacology, 67*(1), 15-25.

Ochsendorf, F.R. (2008). Sexually transmitted infections: Impact on male fertility. *Andrologia*, 40, 72–75.

Ochwang'i, D.O., Kimwele, C.N., Oduma, J.A., Gathumbi, P.K., Mbaria, J.M., & Kiama, S.G. (2014). Medicinal plants used in treatment and management of cancer in Kakamega County, Kenya. *Journal of Ethnopharmacology, 151*(3), 1040-1055.

Okatch, H., Ngwenya, B., Raletamo, K.M., & Andrae-Marobela, K. (2012). Determination of potentially toxic heavy metals in traditionally used medicinal plants for HIV/AIDS opportunistic infections in Ngamiland District in Northern Botswana. *Analytica Chimica Acta, 730*, 42-48.

Peltzer, K., Mngqundaniso, N., & Petros, G., (2006). HIV/AIDS/TB knowledge, beliefs and practices of traditional healers in KwaZulu-Natal, South Africa. *AIDS Care*, 18, 608–613.

Pettit, G.R., Meng, Y., Stevenson, C.A., Doubek, D.L., Knight, J.C., Cichacz, Z., Pettit, R.K., Chapuis, J.C., Schmidt, J.M. (2003). Isolation and structure of palstatin from the Amazon tree *Hymeneae palustris*. *Journal of Natural Products*, 66, 259–262.

Sarkar, R., Chaudhary, S. K., Sharma, A., Yadav, K.K., Nema, N.K., Sekhoacha, M., ... & Sen, T. (2014). Anti-biofilm activity of Marula–A study with the standardized bark extract. *Journal of Ethnopharmacology*, *154*(1), 170-175.

Scopel, M., dos Santos, O., Frasson, A.P., Abraham, W.R., Tasca, T., Henriques, A.T., & Macedo, A.J. (2013). Anti-*Trichomonas vaginalis* activity of marine-associated fungi from the South Brazilian Coast. *Experimental Parasitology*, *133*(2), 211-216.

Seebaluck, R., Gurib-Fakim, A., & Mahomoodally, F. (2014). Medicinal plants from the genus *Acalypha* (Euphorbiaceae)–A review of their ethnopharmacology and phytochemistry. *Journal of Ethnopharmacology* (in press).

Semenya, S.S., Potgieter, M.J., & Erasmus, L.J.C. (2013a). Indigenous plant species used by Bapedi healers to treat sexually transmitted infections: Their distribution, harvesting, conservation and threats. *South African Journal of Botany*, *87*, 66-75.

Semenya, S.S., Potgieter, M.J., & Erasmus, L.J.C. (2013b). Bapedi phytomedicine and their use in the treatment of sexually transmitted infections in Limpopo Province, South Africa. *African Journal of Pharmacy and Pharmacology*, *7*(6), 250-262.

Semenya, S., Potgieter, M., Tshisikhawe, M., Shava, S., & Maroyi, A. (2012). Medicinal utilization of exotic plants by Bapedi traditional healers to treat human ailments in Limpopo province, South Africa. *Journal of Ethnopharmacology*, *144*(3), 646-655.

Sethi, S., Singh, G., Samanta, P., & Sharma, M. (2012). *Mycoplasma genitalium*: An emerging sexually transmitted pathogen. *The Indian Journal of Medical Research*, *136*(6), 942.

Talwar, G.P., Dar, S.A., Rai, M.K., Reddy, K.V.R., Mitra, D., Kulkarni, S. V., ... & Verma, J.K. (2008). A novel polyherbal microbicide with inhibitory effect on bacterial, fungal and viral genital pathogens. *International Journal of Antimicrobial Agents*, *32*(2), 180-185.

Tekwu, E.M., Askun, T., Kuete, V., Nkengfack, A.E., Nyasse, B., Etoa, F. X., & Beng, V.P. (2012). Antibacterial activity of selected Cameroonian dietary spices ethno-medically used against strains of *Mycobacterium tuberculosis*. *Journal of Ethnopharmacology*, *142*(2), 374-382.

Telefo, P.B., Lienou, L.L., Yemele, M.D., Lemfack, M.C., Mouokeu, C., Goka, C.S., ... & Moundipa, F.P. (2011). Ethnopharmacological survey of plants used for the treatment of female infertility in Baham, Cameroon. *Journal of Ethnopharmacology, 136*(1), 178-187.

Toyang, N.J., & Verpoorte, R. (2013). A review of the medicinal potentials of plants of the genus *Vernonia* (Asteraceae). *Journal of Ethnopharmacology, 146*(3), 681-723.

Trela, B.C., & Waterhouse, A.L. (1996). Resveratrol: isomeric molar absorptivities and stability. *J. Agric. Food Chem.*, 5, 1253–1257.

Tshikalange, T.E., Meyer, J.J.M., Lall, N., Munoz, E., Sancho, R., Van de Venter, M., & Oosthuizen, V. (2008). *In vitro* anti-HIV-1 properties of ethnobotanically selected South African plants used in the treatment of sexually transmitted diseases. *Journal of Ehnopharmacology, 119*(3), 478-481.

Van Der Hoek, W. (1992). AIDS in Zambian district. *Nederlands Tijdschrift Voor Geneeskunde*, 136(49), 2432-2435.

Van Vuuren, S.F. (2008). Antimicrobial activity of South African medicinal plants. *Journal of Ethnopharmacology, 119*(3), 462-472.

Van Vuuren, S.F., & Naidoo, D. (2010). An antimicrobial investigation of plants used traditionally in southern Africa to treat sexually transmitted infections. *Journal of Ethnopharmacology, 130*(3), 552-558.

Vermani, K., & Garg, S. (2002). Herbal medicines for sexually transmitted diseases and AIDS. *Journal of Ethnopharmacology, 80(1)*, 49-66.

Wasserheit, J.N. (1992). Epidemiological synergy: Interrelationships between human immunodeficiency virus infection and other sexually transmitted diseases. *Sexually Transmitted Diseases, 19*(2), 61-77.

WHO [World Health Organization] (2013). *Baseline report on global sexually transmitted infection surveillance 2012.* Geneva, Switzerland: WHO.

Xiong, H.R., Luo, J., Hou, W., Xiao, H., & Yang, Z.Q. (2011). The effect of emodin, an anthraquinone derivative extracted from the roots of *Rheum tanguticum*, against herpes simplex virus *in vitro* and *in vivo*. *Journal of Ethnopharmacology, 133*(2), 718-723.

Ye, M., Han, J., Chen, H., Zheng, J., Guo, D. (2007). Analysis of phenolic compounds in rhubarbs using liquid chromatography coupled with electrospray ionization mass spectrometry. *Journal of the American Society for Mass Spectrometry*, 18, 82–91.

Table 4.1 "Medicinal plants for managing STIs in Western Province, Zambia"

Botanical name	Lozi name	Family name	Habit	Parts used	STIs treated	Preparation and administration
Abrus precatorius	Mupitipiti	Fabaceae	Climber	Roots	Gonorrhoea, Chlamydia, syphilitic ulcers, genital herpes	Boiled and taken orally as an infusion; topical application to wounds
Acacia mellifera	Kakumbwe	Fabaceae	Shrub	Stem bark, roots	Syphilis	Boil in water and drink solution
Acacia nilotica	Mukotokoto	Fabaceae	Tree	Leaves, roots, stem bark	Gonorrhoea, Chlamydia symptoms in men	Pound, add warm water, and drink
Adansonia digitata	Mubuyu	Malvaceae	Tree	Stem bark, leaves, roots	General STIs	Boil in water, drink decoction
Afzelia quanzensis	Muwande	Fabaceae	Tree	Stem bark, roots	General STIs	Crush in water, oral
Albizia versicolor	Mububa	Fabaceae	Tree	Stem bark	Gonorrhoea, Chlamydia symptoms in men	Dry, boil and drink solution
Ampelocissus obtusata	Munsansa	Vitaceae	Climber	Roots	Syphilitic rashes, Genital herpes	Cold infusion used as a dressing to heal wounds
Baikiaea plurijuga	Mukusi	Fabaceae	Tree	Stem bark	Syphilis	Decoctions and infusions are taken orally
Boscia albitrunca	Kabombwa-mutemwa	Capparaceae	Tree	Roots	Syphilis, HIV/AIDS	Boil in water, drink while warm
Brachystegia spiciformis	Mutuya	Fabaceae	Tree	Stem bark	General STIs	Boil in water, drink solution while tepid
Burkea Africana	Musheshe	Fabaceae	Tree	Roots, stem bark	Gonorrhoea, HIV/AIDS	Dried plant parts are pounded into powder, boiled in water, sieved, and filtrated is introduced into urethra
Capparis tomentosa	Chiwezeze	Capparaceae	Climber	Roots	Syphilis rashes; HIV/AIDS	Boil roots boiled in water, mixed with tea, and drunk; drink tepid decoction; decoction of roots is used as a topical wash for rashes
Cissampelos	ltende	Menisperma-	Climber	Roots,	Syphilis,	Powdered dry roots

165

mucronata		ceae	er	leaves	Chancroid	are mixed with Vaseline and applied to sores; root decoction is drunk
Cleome gynandra	Namanga	Capparaceae	Shrub	Leaves	Chancroid	Boil, disinfect wounds
Clerodendrum myricoides	Mutume	Lamiaceae	Shrub	Stem bark, roots	General STI syndromes	Boil in water, drink decoction in small amounts using tea spoon
Clerodendrum uncinatum	Mubwanyo	Lamiaceae	Shrub	Roots	Gonorrhoea	Crush dry roots, mix in boiled water, drink
Colophospermum mopane	Mupane	Fabaceae	Tree	Stem bark	Syphilis	Macerate, boil in water, drink decoction; bark extract is applied to sores
Combretum apiculatum	Mukalanga	Combreta-ceae	Shrub	Leaves	General STI syndromes	Boil leaves in water, drink warm solution
Combretum hereroense	Mububu	Combreta-ceae	Shrub	Leaves	Gonorrhoea, Chlamydia symptoms in men	Crush leaves, suspend in water, drink cold infusion
Combretum imberbe	Muzwili	Combreta-ceae	Tree	Leaves	General STIs	Crush leaves, suspend in water, drink infusion
Combretum mossambicense	Silutombolwa	Combreta-ceae	Climb-er	Whole plant	Gonorrhoea, syphilis	Cut into small pieces, pound, put in water, drink cold infusion
Commiphora angolensis	Mubwabwa	Burseraceae	Tree	Stem bark	Gonorrhoea, Chlamydia symptoms in men	Pound dry material, mix with water, drink
Croton gratissimus	Mukena	Euphorbia-ceae	Tree	Leaves	Syphilis	Exudate from crushed leaves is applied to sores
Dichrostachys cinerea	Museleseke	Fabaceae	Shrub	Roots, stem bark, leaves	General STI syndromes especially syphilis	Crush plant materials, mix with water, drink filtrate; leaves are drunk as a tea; chew leaves and apply paste to syphilis sores; topical application of dried bark powder to sores or skin eruptions
Dioscorea hirtiflo-ra	Mantembe	Dioscoreace-ae	Climb-er	Leaves	Syphilitic sores, Chancroid	Grind fresh leaves and apply to sores
Diospyros lycioides	Mupichu	Ebenaceae	Shrub	Leaves	Gonorrhoea, syphilis	Leaves are soaked in cold water for 3 days, solution is drank
Entandrophragma	Mupamena	Meliaceae	Tree	Roots,	Gonorrhoea;	Roots are boiled in

caudatum				fruits	genital warts	water, solution is drunk; fruit peels are burnt, mixed with Vaseline, rubbed onto genital warts
Euclea divinorum	Musokola	Ebenaceae	Shrub	Stems, leaves	Syphilis, genital herpes	Boil and wash syphilitic ulcers
Euphorbia benthamii	Kabomba	Euphorbiaceae	Shrub	Leaves	Gonorrhoea, Chlamydia symptoms in men	Boil a handful of leaves in pot of water. Take one cup of decoction three times a day
Ficus natalensis	Mutaba	Moraceae	Tree	Leaves	Genital warts	Pound leaves, rub into warts
Helinus integrifolius	Mulalawa	Rhamnaceae	Climber	Roots	Gonorrhoea, syphilis, HIV/AIDS	Macerate, soak in cold water, drink infusion
Indigofera ormocarpoides	Kungandofu	Leguminosae	Shrub	Leaves	Syphilis	Fresh leaves are boiled in boiled and solution is drunk
Ipomoea verbascoidea	Litalala	Convolvulaceae	Climber	Roots	Gonorrhoea	Roots are boiled and the solution is drank
Kigelia africana	Muzungula	Bignoniaceae	Tree	Fruit	Syphilis	Exudate is used as a dressing for wounds; boil in water, drink decoction
Lannea stuhlmannii	Musamba	Anacardiaceae	Tree	Roots	Gonorrhoea, syphilis	Crushed fresh roots are soaked in warm water, drink solution
Momordica balsamina	Lombwalombwa	Cucurbitaceae	Climber	Whole plant	Gonorrhoea, syphilis, HIV/AIDS	Boil, decoction is taken with porridge
Peltophorum africanum	Munyele	Fabaceae	Tree	Stem bark, roots	General STIs	Boil cut plant materials in water. Drink decoction
Plumbago zeylanica	Sikalutenta	Plumbaginaceae	Shrub	Leaves	Generally treats all STI symptoms	Macerate leaves into paste which is applied to sores and rashes; crush dried leaves, mix with water or honey solution and drink
Sansevieria kirkii	Lukushe	Asparagaceae	Climber	Roots	Most STIs	Boil fresh roots with water and drink solution while tepid
Sclerocarya caffra	Mulula	Anacardiaceae	Tree	Stem bark, leaves	Gonorrhoea, HIV/AIDS	Pound plant materials, boil in water, drink concoction
Securidaca longepedunculata	Muiinda	Polygalaceae	Shrub	Stem bark,	Syphilis, gonorrhoea	Dry materials, crush, mix with

				roots		water, sieve, drink filtrate
Senna abbreviata	Mululwe	Fabaceae	Tree	Stem bark, roots	Gonorrhoea, HIV/AIDS	Macerate in water, drink
Senna occidentalis	Changu	Fabaceae	Shrub	Roots	Gonorrhoea	Boiled, orally taken as a tea
Solanum panduri-forme	Ntulwantul-wa	Solanaceae	Shrub		HIV/AIDS	Cut, macerate in warm water, drink solution
Strychnos coccu-loides	Muhuluhulu	Loganiaceae	Tree	Roots	Gonorrhoea	Crush in water and drink solution
Strychnos innocua	Muzimbiko-lo, Muteme	Loganiaceae	Tree	Roots	Gonorrhoea, Chlamydia symptoms in men	Root decoction is taken orally
Strychnos potato-rum	Mu-lombelombe	Loganiaceae	Tree	Roots	Syphilis	Boiled and taken orally
Terminalia sericea	Muhonono	Combreta-ceae	Tree	Roots, leaves	Gonorrhoea, syphilis	Macerate materials together, boil in water, drink decoc-tion
Trichilia emetica	Musikili	Meliaceae	Tree	Stem bark, leaves	Gonorrhoea, syphilis	Soak crushed bark and leaves in water, drink small amounts of solution; boil in water, decoction is drunk; powdered dry roots applied to wounds
Ximenia america-na	Mutente	Olacaceae	Tree	Stem bark	Bacterial vaginosis, gonorrhoea	Apply powder to vagina; dissolve stem powder in water and drink
Ximenia caffra	Mulutulua	Olacaceae	Shrub	Roots	General STI conditions	Cut roots into very small pieces, mix with water, boil, and drink solution
Ziziphus mucro-nata	Mukalu	Rhamnaceae	Tree	Stem bark	Gonorrhoea, syphilis, Chlamydia symptoms in men	Boil in water for half an hour, drink solution; wash urethra; powder is applied to wounds

Table 4.2: Medicinal plants for managing STIs among the Kore-kore people of Chiawa District, Zambia

Scientific name	Kore-kore name of plant	STI treated	Plant parts
Albizia antunesiana	Muriranyenze	Bola-bola, gonorrhoea	Roots, leaves
Azanza garckeana	Munego	Gonorrhoea	Roots, stem bark
Commiphora mossambicensis	Muchabobo	Bola-bola	Roots
Croton megalobotrys	Muchape	Bola-bola, gonorrhoea, syphilis	Roots, stem bark
Cussonia arborea	Mufenje	Syphilis	Roots, stem bark
Diplorynchus condylocarpon	Mutowha	Gonorrhoea	Roots
Fic sur	Mukuyu	Bola-bola, gonorrhoea, syphilis	Roots
Kigelia africana	Muveve	Gonorrhoea	Roots, stem bark
Ormocarpum trichocarpum	Mupotanzou	Bola-bola, syphilis	Roots, leaves
Rauvolfia caffra	Mukashu	Syphilis	Roots
Senna abbreviata	Muveneka	Bola-bola, gonorrhoea	Roots, stem bark
Solanum incanum; Solanum delagoense	Muhnundurwa	Bola-bola, gonorrhoea, syphilis	Roots
Strychnos spinosa; Strychnos cocculoides	Mutamba	Bola-bola, gonorrhoea, syphilis	Fruits, roots
Ximenia caffra	Mtswanza	Gonorrhoea	Roots

Adapted from Ndubani and Höjer (1999)

Table 4.3: Medicinal plants for managing STIs in Maputaland, KwaZulu-Natal Province, South Africa

Scientific name of plants	Vernacular name of plants	STI treated
Adenia gummifera	Impindamshaya	Gonorrhoea, HIV/AIDS
Albizia adianthifolia	Igowane	Gonnorhoeae, syphilis
Bidens pilosa	Uqandolo	Syphilis
Bridelia cathartica	-	General STIs
Carica papaya	Upopo	Candida, gonnorheae
Clematis brachiata	Ufufuno	Syphilis
Combretum molle	Umbondo	Gonorrhoea, syphilis
Erianthemum dregei	Iphakama	Gonorrhoea
Euphorbia hypericifolia	Umaphipha	Gonnorhoeae
Hypoxis hemerocallidea	Inkomfe	HIV/AIDS
Ipomoea batatas	Ubhatata	Gonorrhoea
Kigelia africana	Umvongothi	Syphilis, gonorrhoea
Mimusops caffra	Amasethole	Gonorrhoea
Musa acuminata	Ubhanana	Sores on genitals
Pyrenacantha kaurabassana	Inzema	Genital warts, herpes
Ranunculus multifidus	Uxhaphozi	Syphilis, genital warts, gonorrhoea
Sclerocarya birrea	Umganu	Candida, gonorrhoea
Senecio serratuloides		Syphilis
Syzygium cordatum	Umdoni	Gonorrhoea
Tabernaemontana elegans	Umkhadlu	Gonorrhoea
Terminalia sericea	Imkhonono	General STIs
Trichilia dregeana	Umkhuhlu	Gonorrhoea, syphilis

Data from De Wet and Ngubane (2014), Naidoo et al. (2013), and De Wet et al. (2012)

Table 4.4: Medicinal plants for managing STIs in Limpopo Province, South Africa

Scientific name of plant	Bapedi name of plant	STI treated
Aloe marlothii	Kgopha-ya-go-ema	Gonorrhoea
Cotyledon orbiculata	Tsebe-ya-kolobe	Gonorrhoea
Eucomis pallidiflora	Mathuba-difala	Chlamydia
Gethyllis namaquensis	Naka-tsa-tholo	Chlamydia
Helichrysum caespititium	Bokgatha	Gonorrhoea
Hypoxis hemerocallidea	Titikwane	Gonorrhoea, HIV/AIDS
Hypoxis obtusa	Monna-maledu	Chlamydia
Ipomoea obscura	Kgomodimaswi	Gonorrhoea
Jatropha zeyheri	Unknown	Gonorrhoea
Myrothamnus flabellifolius	Boka	HIV/AIDS
Peltophorum africanum	Mosehla	HIV/AIDS
Protea caffra	Unknown	Chlamydia
Sclerocarya birrea	Morula	HIV/AIDS
Senna italica	Mankgane	Gonorrhoea
Zanthoxylum capense	Senokomaropa	HIV/AIDS
Ziziphus mucronata	Mokgalo	Gonorrhoea, Chlamydia

Adapted from Semenya et al. (2013)

Table 4.5: Medicinal plants for managing STIs in Southern Africa

Scientific name of plant	Zulu name of plant	STIs treated
Carpobrotus edulis	Ikhambi-lamabulawo, umgongozi	Herpes simplex virus, *Candida albicans*
Senna occidentalis	Isinyembane, umnwanda-nyoka	Gonorrhoea, syphilitic sores, swollen testicles
Cissus quadrangulis	Isinwazi	Gonorrhoea
Croton gratissimus	Ihubeshane-elikhulu, ilabele, ilethi, intumbanhlosi, umhluka, umhuluga	Sores associated with STIs
Euclea natalensis	Ichitamuzi, idungamuzi, inkunzane, emnyama, isinzimane, umzimane	Syphilis,
Polygala fruticosa	Ithethe	Gonorrhoea
Strelitzia reginae	Isagudu, isigude	Enemas for inflamed glands associated with STIs
Terminalia sericea	Amangwe, umkhonono	Syphilis, gonorrhoea, *Candida albicans*

Adapted from Van Vuuren and Naidoo (2010)

5 Natural Products for Oral Health

Introduction

Due to high costs, many people hardly buy and use commercial oral hygiene products. Toothpaste and toothbrushes are beyond the reach of the majority poor. Yet, with increasing incidences of oral diseases especially due to HIV/AIDS, many poor folks turn to the use of plant products to prevent and treat oral infections like dental caries and periodontal disease - the most common infectious diseases of humans.

The goal of this chapter is to elucidate natural products for oral health. To this end, the following themes are discoursed:

- Oral cavity as a hive of microbes and site for diseases
- Dental caries and periodontal disease in African human fossils
- Oral diseases during HIV infection
- Synthetic versus natural products in oral health
- Rhein and raisins
- Pomegranate, chamomile and honey
- Essential oils
- Green tea and probiotics
- Chewing sticks
- African pharmacopoeia
- Asian pharmacopoeia
- Brazilian and Mexican folk medicines

To start with, here is a case study of a common oral hygiene plant, *Diospyros mespiliformis*. Known as *Mchenja* in many parts of Zambia, *D. mespiliformis* extracts have now been incorporated into Toothache Master, one of several herbal medicinal formulations produced by a small enterprise in Kabwe, Zambia. It is worth noting that my reference to *Toothache Master* is not in any way a marketing promotion for the product. On the contrary, mention of *D. mespiliformis* and *Toothache Master* is a footnote in the trove of indigenous knowledge relating to the herbal pharmacopoeia for oral diseases.

Case Study: *Mchenja* in *Toothache Master*

It was Wednesday 12th November 2014. Flying on an Air Namibia aeroplane from Windhoek (Namibia) to Lusaka (Zambia), Kazhila Chinsembu was *enroute* to the small rural town of Zambezi to attend his mother's funeral, having succumbed to cancer of the stomach on 9th November 2014. The following day, while travelling on a Lusaka-Solwezi bus, passengers were greeted by a young entrepreneur of natural products, a representative from the Final Hope Natural Medicines Ltd., located in Kabwe, Central Province, Zambia.

With a small bag on his back, the young entrepreneur got onto the bus in Kabwe, formerly Broken Hill town. After a few minutes' drive, he started to advertise his merchandise to passengers. One of the products, *Toothache Master*, caught Chinsembu's attention. It was a fine brown blend of plant powder applied to heal toothache. According to instructions on the product label, a little powder is applied directly onto the aching tooth. Or, a quarter teaspoon of the *Toothache Master* powder is dissolved in 25 ml of tepid water and used as a mouthwash.

Upon arrival in Solwezi, while resting in the room at Mwaka Lodge, Chinsembu would turn himself into a guinea pig. The *Toothache Master* mouthwash was, indeed, what he had expected throughout the journey. It was made from a plant, or at least the principal plant, was *D. mespiliformis* or *Mchenja*. As a young boy, growing up in Chileng'a, Zambezi District, Chinsembu had gotten used to *Mchenja*. Many people in Zambezi use the plant, which grows by the beaches and in the plains of the Zambezi River, as a chewing stick and toothbrush. *Mchenja* whitens teeth and confers good breath.

Indeed, that night, as Chinsembu went to sleep, he was relieved that, finally, a local entrepreneurial initiative, albeit, rudimentary in terms of production capacity, was adding value to local medicinal flora. It was amazing to see that a local plant, *Mchenja*, was now increasingly being recognized as an agent for oral hygiene. That is how it should be.

Oral Cavity as a Hive of Microbes and Site for Diseases

The human oral cavity is heavily colonized by disease-causing microbes such as viruses, protozoa, fungi, Archaea and the true bacteria (Eubacteria). More than 500 different types of bacteria have been isolated from the mouth most of which are innocuous. Distribution and diversity of Archaea (e.g. *Methanobrevibacter oralis*, *Methanobrevibacter* spp., *Methanobacterium* spp., *Methanosarcina* spp., *Thermoplasmata* spp.) in oral diseases has been reviewed by Maeda, Hirai, Mineshiba, Yamamoto, Kokeguchi and Takashiba (2013).

Okumura (2011) stated that resistance to oral bacterial infections is provided by the oral mucosa membrane, which acts as a mechanical and physical barrier, and saliva which contains unique host defense peptides, also termed antimicrobial peptides. The mechanical shield of the oral epithelium consists of stratified keratinocytes which form a strengthened structure. Okumura (2011) enumerated several types of host defense peptides including defensins, cathelicidins, and histatins. Host defense peptides are mostly cationic, have amphipathic structures and provide non-specific, rapid defenses against invading pathogens.

Successful adherence of pathogenic microorganisms to host buccal cavity tissues is the first step in the initiation of oral pathologies. Oral microbes are responsible for two common diseases of humans: dental caries and the periodontal diseases. Dental caries and periodontal diseases are the most common infectious diseases affecting humans. Allaker and Douglas (2009) also affirm that plaque-related diseases are probably the most common bacterial diseases of humans.

Periodontitis involves inflammation around the tooth. It is a serious gum infection that damages the soft tissue and bone that supports the tooth. Periodontitis is associated with members of the indigenous oral microbiota including *Aggregatibacter actinomycetemcomitans, Eikenella corrodens, Fusobacterium nucleatum, Porphyromonas gingivalis, Prevotella intermedia, Tannerella forsythia, Enterococcus faecalis* and *Treponema denticola* (Amir Alireza, Afsaneh, Seied Hosein, Siamak, Afshin, & Zeinab et al., 2014). *Porphyromonas gingivalis, P. intermedia* and *A. actinomycetemcomitans* are regarded as the major pathogens in advancing periodontitis (Allaker & Douglas, 2009).

Gingivitis is a mild and reversible form of periodontal disease, but periodontitis causes permanent damage to tooth-supporting tissues and may lead to tooth loss (Bonifait, Marquis, Genovese, Epifano, & Grenier, 2012). While as many as 700 different bacterial species may be present in sub-gingival plaque samples, strong experimental evidence has emerged to implicate *P. gingivalis*, a gram-negative anaerobic bacterium often found in association with *T. forsythia* and *T. denticola*, as one of the key pathogens in periodontitis (Azelmat, Larente, & Grenier, 2014). *Methanobrevibacter oralis* is the dominant archaeal species in sub-gingival plaque (Maeda et al., 2013).

Dental caries is the medical term for tooth decay or cavities. It is a polymicrobial disease caused by specific bacteria that produce acid which destroys the tooth's enamel and the layer under it (dentin). Allaker and Douglas (2009) state that dental caries (dental decay) is a destructive condition of the dental hard tissues and that, if left unchecked, can progress to inflammation and death of vital pulp tissue, with eventual spread of infection to the periapical area of the tooth and beyond. The disease process involves acidogenic plaque bacteria, including *Streptococcus mutans*, *Streptococcus sobrinus* and *Lactobacillus* sp.

Similarly, in individuals who repeatedly ingest high levels of carbohydrates- more so those that drink beer, the frequency of acid production leads to erosion of the buffering capacity of saliva and sustained reductions in pH. In turn, this favours the growth of oral microbiota that grows well in acidic environments. Aciduric bacterial species, particularly *S. mutans* and lactobacilli continue to produce acid and thus exacerbate the damage to dental hard tissues. *Streptococcus mutans* and *S. sobrinus*, the main acidogenic components of dental biofilm, break down exogenous dietary carbohydrates to produce lactic acid, resulting in demineralization of tooth enamel (Bonifait et al., 2012).

Biofilm is a dense non-calcified mass composed of microorganisms, *Streptococcus mitis* and *Streptococcus sanguis* being the pioneers (Batista, Diógenes Alves Uchôa Lins, de Souza Coelho, do Nascimento Barbosa, Moura Belém, & Alves Celestino, 2014). It is a matrix rich in bacterial extracellular polysaccharides and salivary glycoproteins, firmly attached to the teeth and other hard surfaces of the oral cavity. The development of the oral biofilm is a major factor responsible for the emergence of various diseases including dental cavities, gingivitis and periodontitis (Barbieri, Tonial, Lopez, Sales Maia, Santos, & Ribas et al., 2014). As dental biofilm matures, colonization shifts towards facultative and anaerobic bacterial species leading to supra-gingival plaque accumulation and gingival inflammation which are the first clinical signs of periodontal disease (Bonifait et al., 2012).

While caries and periodontitis are bacterial diseases, Wade (2013) makes the case that they are not infectious diseases *sensu stricto* because they result from a complex interaction between the commensal microbiota, host susceptibility and environmental factors such as diet and smoking. Periodontitis, in particular, appears to result from an inappropriate inflammatory reaction to the normal microbiota, exacerbated by the presence of some disease-associated bacterial species. In consequence to pathogens that cause oral diseases, people should always engage in regular oral hygiene practices, especially brushing with toothpastes, or rinsing with mouthwashes. Brushing, a common physical method of biofilm removal is practically important but sometimes difficult to perform as it requires reasonable control, time, motivation and manual dexterity (Batista et al., 2014).

Dental Caries and Periodontal Disease in African Human Fossils

Dental caries and periodontal disease are evident in human fossils. Lacy (2014) has established that the cranium of Broken Hill man, found in 1921 at Broken Hill mines in Kabwe, Zambia (then Northern Rhodesia), exhibits dental caries on ten teeth, multiple periapical lesions, periodontal disease, severe anterior dental wear and hypercementosis. The diet of Broken Hill man is believed to have been rich in protein and similar to that of recent tropical hunter-gatherers. Although Broken Hill man is undated, he is assumed to have lived during the Middle Pleistocene Age, about 11,000 years Before Present. Now kept at the Natural History Museum in London - against the consent of the Zambian government - Broken Hill man is one of the fewest known archaic *Homo* fossils from Southern Africa.

Lacy (2014) diagnosed Broken Hill man and revealed dentoalveolar abnormalities, possibly attributable to ignorance to use toothpicks, excessive honey consumption and lead poisoning. It is argued that exposure to lead, ingested through diet, may have produced the extensive caries and periodontal disease. Lacy (2014) concludes that these oral pathological conditions had morbidity consequences for Broken Hill man. In retrospect, these findings point to Broken Hill man's apparent lack of indigenous knowledge about the use of medicinal plants for managing oral diseases. On the other hand, these findings may well attest the fact that dental caries and periodontal disease are the most common infections of humans, even during the days of Broken Hill man in the Middle Pleistocene Age.

Coincidentally, it is in Broken Hill town, now Kabwe, that *Toothache Master* - a natural product that treats dental caries and periodontal disease, was conceived by Final Hope Natural Medicines Ltd. Today, the inhabitants of Kabwe still suffer from many oral health pathologies as they are still heavily polluted by lead from the closed mine that operated for over 90 years till June 1994. Lead concentrations of up to 51,188 mg/kg dry weight have been observed in soils around Kabwe. In fact, due to lead, Kabwe is among the ten most heavily polluted towns in the world. The production of *Toothache Master* in Kabwe may be a reflection of the increasing know-how about natural products for oral health. This is unlike in the days of Broken Hill man and other early men.

Oral Diseases during HIV Infection

Oral hygiene is very important in HIV/AIDS. The oral microbiome and the immunobiology of periodontal disease and caries have been reviewed by Costalonga and Herzberg (2014). These authors argue that impairment of the gingival immune response leads to the pathology of periodontal tissue. Oral diseases are intimately linked to HIV/AIDS. During HIV infection, periodontal diseases are a sign of progression to AIDS. Depletion of CD4 cells is the hallmark of HIV infection. Initial immune suppression is indicated by CD4 levels below 500 and signals the first appearance of systemic and oral opportunistic infections. In HIV-infected subjects, increased progression and aggression of periodontitis is related to lower CD4 counts. High viral load, too, is associated with increased tooth loss. There are significant associations between a CD4 count of less than 200 with periodontitis and oral hairy leukoplakia in HIV-infected pregnant women.

It is not surprising that more than one third of people who are seropositive for HIV and approximately 90% of people with AIDS develop HIV associated oral lesions during the course of the disease. HIV can also enter the mouth via gingival crevicular fluid (Wade, 2013). Studies have shown that oral health and periodontal status closely reflect the immune status of an individual. HIV-infected patients have an increased risk of developing more aggressive periodontitis. Oxidative stress in the oral cavity also increases the risk of aggressive periodontitis (Avezov, Reznick, & Aizenbud, 2014). Oral cancer is among the commonest malignancies in HIV/AIDS, with 900,000 new global cases diagnosed annually (Lopes, de Angelis, Prudente, de Souza, Cardoso, & de Azambuja Ribeiro, 2012).

In HIV/AIDS persons, oral candidiasis is an opportunistic infection of the oral cavity caused by an overgrowth of *Candida* species, the most common being *Candida albicans* (Bonifait et al., 2012). The most prevalent forms of oral candidiasis are pseudomembranous candidiasis (also called thrush) and erythematous candidiasis, which includes denture stomatitis. The yeast *C. albicans* is frequently associated with infections in HIV-positive patients (Sardi, Almeida, & Giannini, 2011). Occurrence of opportunistic oropharyngeal candidiasis is a clinical alarm for the onset of AIDS (Alili, Türp, Kulik, & Waltimo, 2014). Put differently, there is strong synergy between oral candidiasis and AIDS.

The majority of oral candidiases are caused by the opportunistic pathogen *C. albicans*, followed by non-albicans *Candida species* such as *Candida glabrata*, *Candida krusei*, *Candida tropicalis*, *Candida dubliniensis* and Candida *guilliermondii*. Due to HIV/AIDS, increased prevalence of resistance against anti-*Candida* agents is now widely recognized in the global oral healthcare community. HIV-associated gingivitis and HIV-associated periodontitis do not respond well to conventional therapy and often progress very rapidly. HIV-associated periodontitis is characterized by rapid destruction of the periodontal supporting apparatus and severe soft tissue damage. Even worse, in some HIV-associated periodontitis cases, more than 90% of the attachment is destroyed in as little as 3 to 6 months, resulting in early tooth loss. In HIV infected adults, treatment failure of periodontal diseases and losses of teeth are warning bells for AIDS.

Published research before the introduction of highly active antiretroviral therapy (HAART) indicates a significantly greater prevalence of periodontitis in HIV-infected patients when compared to sero-negative individuals. However, antiretroviral therapy has markedly helped to de-escalate the proliferation of periodontal pathogens thus reducing the clinical manifestation of periodontitis. HAART provides a protector effect, keeping the pathogenic sub-gingival microbiota under control, even in previous cases of severe immunodeficiency. Indeed, the introduction of HAART has decreased the frequency of several oral diseases such as candidiasis, hairy leukoplakia and Kaposi's sarcoma.

Despite the importance of HAART in alleviating oral diseases, many have long believed that our indigenous plant species are impregnated with phytochemicals and chemical ingredients that inhibit the growth of oral pathogens. These plant extracts may be included into formulations of commercial toothpastes and mouthwashes or developed into novel drugs for oral pathogens. In retrospect, phytochemical and antimicrobial knowledge of our indigenous flora could play a crucial role in managing oral diseases brought on by HIV/AIDS. In addition, the rapid increase in antibiotic resistance and the side effects they cause has opened real possibilities in the application of natural plant extracts for oral diseases during HIV infection.

Synthetic versus Natural Products in Oral Health

Allaker and Douglas (2009) explained that upkeep of oral hygiene is often premised on the use of chemical agents. For instance, mouthrinses are often employed in the prevention and treatment of oral infections. Mouthrinses may contain fluorides, alcohols, detergents and other antimicrobial substances. Toothpastes also contain fluorides and other antimicrobials including triclosan and zinc citrate. Synthetic antimicrobials include povidone iodine products, flourides, phenol derivatives, chlorhexidine and cetyl pyridinium chloride. Antibiotics like ampicillin, erythromycin, penicillin, tetracycline and vancomycin are also widely used in dentistry to inhibit bacterial growth (Jang, Cha, Choi, & Cha, 2014).

However, the available evidence demonstrates that most antibiotics and synthetic oral hygiene products still have mixed clinical effects. For instance, synthetic substances have several adverse effects such as vomiting, diarrhoea and teeth staining (Alviano, Alviano, Diniz, Antoniolli, Alviano, Farias, et al., 2008). Oral microbes are also developing resistance to antibiotics and oral health products containing these synthetic chemicals. In the wake of these shortcomings, natural antibacterial substances are now attracting attention as useful antimicrobials to be incorporated into mouthrinses and toothpastes. Compounds possessing antimicrobial activities against oral pathogens may be isolated from edible plants and plants traditionally used as oral remedies (Rivero-Cruz, Zhu, Kinghorn, & Wu, 2008).

In this light, Allaker and Douglas (2009) noted that the increasing challenges of resistance to synthetic antimicrobials have opened new vistas in the search for alternative natural products. They assert that since plants are the source of more than 25% of prescription and over-the-counter preparations, the potential of natural agents for oral prophylaxis and treatment is vehemently important. They also emphasized that mainstream medicine is increasingly receptive to the use of antimicrobials derived from plant sources, as traditional antimicrobial agents become ineffective against both existing and emerging microbial diseases. As one would expect, the rise of herbal medicines has rekindled fresh interest in the prowess of plant extracts to control plaque and other oral diseases (Lobo, Fonteles, Marques, Jamacaru, Fonseca, de Carvalho et al., 2014).

For many years now, Listerine™ Essential Oils Rinse, which contains the natural active ingredients thymol, eucalyptol, methyl salicylate and menthol, has been in widespread use (Allaker & Douglas, 2009). Thymol is a natural monoterpene phenol derivative of cymene and an isomer of carvacrol (Nabavi, Marchese, Izadi, Curti, Daglia, & Nabavi, 2015). An antimicrobial, thymol is commonly used in dental preparations to inhibit foul-odour producing bacteria. Nabavi et al. (2015) mentioned studies where thymol deters the growth of bacteria known to be resistant to antibiotics such as penicillin. According to Allaker and Douglas (2009), eucalyptol is an antimicrobial agent while methyl salicylate and menthol act as cleaning agent and local anaesthetic, respectively. Even more important, thymol possesses various biological and pharmacological benefits attributable to its anti-mutagenic, anti-tumour, antioxidant, and anti-inflammatory functions.

One does not need to search very far to find natural products that inhibit the adhesion of periodontopathogenic bacteria. Common products like milk, honey, tea (*Camellia sinensis*), cranberries (*Vaccinium macrocarpon*), edible mushroom (*Lentinus edodes*), common coffee (*Coffea arabica*), barley coffee (*Hordeum vulgare*), grapes (*Vitis vinifera*), and alcohol-free red wine are some of the representative natural foods and beverages that inhibit adhesion of bacteria in the buccal cavity (Signoretto, Canepari, Stauder, Vezzulli, & Pruzzo, 2012). Extracts of miswak, tea tree oil, peppermint, green tea and *Manuka* honey have all been incorporated into synthetic oral hygiene products to enhance their antimicrobial efficacies.

In the same vein, Rivero-Cruz et al. (2008) assert that during the quest for potential anti-plaque agents from natural sources, several compounds of plant origin show plenty of growth inhibitory activity against oral pathogens, e.g. the naphthalene glucosides, diospyrosides A–D and some flavonoids including kaempferol, myricetin and rhamnocitrin. These authors argue that plant-derived antimicrobial compounds may serve as alternatives to the commonly used chemicals for dental plaque and oral disease control.

Delfan, Bahmani, Rafieian-Kopaei, Delfan and Saki (2014) conducted an ethnobotanical study of medicinal plants used to relieve toothache in Lorestan Province, Iran. Some of the plants used to treat toothache are *Daphne mucronata* (mazerion), *Vitis vinifera* (grape), and *Glycyrrhiza glabra* (liquorice). At the Department of Oral Medicine, School of Dentistry, Tehran University of Medical Sciences, Mansourian, Boojarpour, Ashnagar, Beitollahi and Shamshiri (2014) found that the plant extracts of *Syzygium aromaticum* or clove oil and *Punica granatum* (pomegranate) had good activity against oral *C. albicans*.

Remarkably, the antifungal action of *S. aromaticum* was better than that for nystatin, an antifungal drug first isolated from *Streptomyces noursei* in 1950 by Elizabeth Lee Hazen and co-workers. *S. aromaticum* contains high amounts of eugenol, a known antifungal agent. *Punica granatum* has definite anti-candida activity, but the magnitude of this activity is less than for nystatin or *S. aromaticum*. Against cariogenic and periodontopathogenic bacteria, clove oil and eugenol are effective natural antibacterial agents; both have synergistic effects with antibiotics ampicillin and gentamicin (Moon, Kim, & Cha, 2011).

Elsewhere, the leaf juice of *Phyllanthus reticulatus*, a shrub that grows in India, Bangladesh, China and the Malay Islands, heals bleeding gums (Kumar, Sharma, Kumar, Kumar, & Arya, 2014). *Phyllanthus reticulatus*, which contains tannins and phenolic compounds, increases the immune system's phagocytic activity and neutrophil adhesion. In view of its immune-stimulatory properties, *P. reticulatus* is also used in the management of HIV/AIDS in Tanzania.

As we have seen before, most plants used in the management of oral infections are infused with several useful antimicrobial phytochemicals such as simple phenols, phenolic acids, quinones, flavones, flavonoids, flavonols, tannins, coumarins, terpenoids, essential oils, alkaloids, lectins and antimicrobial peptides. The actions of flavonoids are classically attributed to their antioxidant properties. According to Petti and Scully (2009), polyphenols help prevent oral diseases via mechanisms like antioxidant activity and neutralization or modulation of human and microbial enzymes. They assert that regular and frequent dietary intake of polyphenols helps alleviate symptoms of oral cancer.

Shi, Hui, Zhang, Hong-Ying, Guang-Li and Ying et al. (2014) indicate that several alkaloids isolated from natural herbs exhibit anti-proliferation, antibacterial, antiviral and anti-metastatic effects on various types of oral cancers both *in vitro* and *in vivo*. The compounds 2',6'-dihydroxy-4'-geranyloxyacetophenone (1) and 2',6'-dihydroxy-4'-farnesyloxy-acetophenone (2) are oxyprenylated secondary metabolites extracted from plants belonging to the Rutaceae family. Bonifait et al. (2012) elucidated that compounds (1) and (2) are potential natural molecules for the prevention and treatment of common oral infections including dental caries, periodontal disease and candidiasis. The two compounds also inhibit proliferation of cancer cells.

Contrary to the common assumption that food has a negative impact on oral health, the common edible mushroom shiitake, *Lentinula edodes*, protects against dental caries. Shiitake mushroom contains several therapeutic benefits such as antioxidant and antimicrobial properties. Frequent mouth rinses with shiitake mushroom extracts may reduce the metabolic activity of dental bio-film. Shiitake mushroom also has antibiotic action which can be harnessed by incorporating its extracts into mouth washes and toothpastes.

Evolution of resistance by oral pathogens to single plant extracts has brought a new justification for poly-herbal oral therapies involving two or more plant combinations. In this vein, the growth of dental bacteria is inhibited by a poly-herbal tablet of the plants *Azadirachta indica*, *Mangifera indica*, *Hemidesmus indicus*, *Caryophyllus aromaticus*, *Cinnamomum zeylanicum*, *Quercus infectoria*, *Emblica officinalis*, *Terminalia belerica* and *Terminalia chebula*. Shosaikoto is another medicinal plant mixture used in China and Japan to treat oral infections.

Rhein and Raisins

Azelmat et al. (2014) studied the effects of rhein, a major anthraquinone found in rhubarb root, on the periodontopathogen *P. gingivalis*. Their data reveal that rhein has significant activity against the oral bacterium *P. gingivalis*, the gram-negative anaerobe most commonly associated with gum diseases. Using polymerase chain reaction assays, they found that rhein impairs the pathogenicity of *P. gingivalis* by reducing transcription of genes coding for important virulence factors. Rhein inhibits the activity of gingipains, enzymes that provide peptides and amino acids to aid the growth of *P. gingivalis*.

Rivero-Cruz et al. (2008) demonstrated the power of raisins in improving oral health. Raisins are dried grapes, the fruits of the plant *Vitis vinifera* (family Vitaceae). Experiments show that phytochemicals in raisins suppress growth of oral bacteria associated with dental diseases. Besides being a traditional and popular snack food, raisins contain polyphenols, antioxidants, flavonoids and iron that favour overall human health. Various phytochemicals found in raisins include triterpenes, fatty acids, flavonoids, amino acids, hydroxycinnamic acids and 5-hydroxymethyl-2-furaldehyde. Oleanolic acid, oleanolic aldehyde and 5-(hydroxymethyl)-2-furfural stall the growth of *P. gingivalis*, with minimum inhibitory concentration values ranging from 3.5 to 488 µg/ml (Rivero-Cruz et al., 2008). Besides its antibacterial benefits, oleanolic acid also plays valuable pharmacological functions due to its anti-inflammatory, anti-tumour and anti-HIV properties.

Pomegranate, Chamomile and Honey

Bailly (2009) believes that good old drugs from plants and microbes remain essential. In this light, Batista et al. (2014) conducted a randomized controlled clinical trial to evaluate the effectiveness of a mouthrinse with pomegranate (*P. granatum*) and chamomile (*Matricaria recutita*) plant extracts, against chlorhexidine 0.12% in gingiva bleeding condition. The mouthrinses with the herbal products were equally effective for this oral condition, producing antimicrobial and anti-inflammatory properties similar to that of chlorhexidine 0.12%.

According to Batista et al. (2014), *M. recutita* contains flavonoids and volatile oil rich in terpenoids such as alpha-bisabolol, azulene, matricine and chamazulene. These components provide the anti-inflammatory, antispasmodic and antibacterial activity of the chamomile. *Punica granatum* prevents and fights oral diseases due to its antioxidant, antiviral, antiparasitic, antifungal and anticancer properties. It has antibacterial action against *S. aureus* and *Salmonella typhi*. Its anti-inflammatory, healing and antiseptic activities are attributable to the large amounts of tannin in the fruit skin (Batista et al., 2014).

In their review of novel antimicrobial therapies for dental plaque-related diseases, Allaker and Douglas (2009) write that *Manuka* honey, derived from the flowers of the *Manuka* tree in New Zealand, is widely utilized in the treatment of cariogenic and periodontopathic bacteria. Along a similar trajectory, propolis is added to *Colgate Herbal Propolis* toothpaste manufactured by Colgate-Palmolive in Brazil and exported to many African countries including Namibia and Zambia. Propolis is a resinous product collected by honeybees from various plant sources. It is a substance used in defence of the beehive including embalming invaders which bees have killed but cannot transport out of the hive. A multifunctional material (bee glue) used by bees to make and maintain their hives, propolis contains flavonoids, phenolic acids and their esters.

In relation to the external environment, propolis lowers the concentration of bacteria and moulds in the hive. Antibacterial activity of Brazilian propolis against oral bacteria has been demonstrated in experiments. Consequently, propolis is an old remedy in modern medicine. Due to its pharmaceutical properties, it is incorporated into biocosmetics, food supplements and formulations of medicinal natural products. It has long been known as a relatively non-toxic natural remedy with antibiotic, antifungal and antiviral activities. Interestingly, propolis suppresses HIV-1 replication and increases immune responses in humans. The addition of propolis to the Colgate toothpaste is by no means a fluke as it is clearly aimed at utilizing its well established activities against periodontopathogenic microorganisms. *Herbal Colgate* toothpaste consisting of chamomile, eucalyptus, myrrh and sage is made by Colgative- Palmolive (China) Co. Ltd., Guangzhou, China.

Essential Oils

All over the world, traditional healers prescribe essential oils for a variety of diseases. In their status review vis-à-vis the medicinal properties of essential oils, Raut and Karuppayil (2014) refer to various pharmacological and biological activities such as anti-inflammatory, antibacterial, antifungal, anticancer, anti-mutagenic, antiviral and anti-protozoal properties associated with essential oils. They mention that essential oils are complex mixtures of low molecular weight compounds extracted from plants by steam distillation and various solvents.

Raut and Karuppayil (2014) state the characteristic aroma and biological properties of essential oils are founded in their two major constituents: terpenoids and phenylpropanoids. Emergence of drug resistant strains of oral pathogens, increasing cases of immune-compromised individuals due to HIV/AIDS, and several limitations of current regimens of pharmaceutical drugs have motivated people to use essential oils for oral health. Essential oils of medicinal importance distributed in selected plant families have been provided by Raut and Karuppayil (2014).

Thymus vulgaris essential oil exhibits extremely strong activity against 120 bacterial strains of *Staphylococcus*, *Enterococcus*, *Escherichia* and *Pseudomonas* isolated from patients with infections of the oral cavity (Nabavi et al., 2015). Through a multiplicity of evidence-based examples, Allaker and Douglas (2009) state that essential oils extracted from tea tree, eucalyptus, lavandula and rosmarinus (rosemary) are widely applied as inhibitory agents against cariogenic and periodontopathic bacteria. *Curcuma longa* essential oil prevents cytogenetic damage to oral sub-mucous cells (Raut & Karuppayil, 2014).

Leaning on experimental evidence from other studies, Sardi et al. (2011) found that the essential oils of *Achillea millefolium*, *Mikania glomerata* and *Stachys byzantina* all had strong activity against oral *C. albicans*. In addition, essential oils obtained from the leaves of *Coriandrum sativum* displayed antifungal activity against established biofilm and planktonic cells of *C. albicans* isolated from periodontal pockets. Allaker and Douglas (2009), working in the fields of oral microbiology and pathology in the United Kingdom, assert that tea tree oil confers strong broad-spectrum antibacterial action. Their studies show that tea tree oil contains about 100 chemical components, mostly monoterpenes, sesquiterpenes and associated alcohols. Of all these chemicals, terpinen-4-ol which acts through the disruption of microbial cell membranes has the greatest antimicrobial activity.

According to Allaker and Douglas (2009), essential oil mouthrinses effectively destroy oral pathogens through various mechanisms: disruption of the cell wall, inhibition of key enzymes, slowing down replication, reduction of endotoxin release and disaggregation of bacteria in the early plaque matrix. On the other hand, chlorhexidine acts through three mechanisms: it mediates loss of cellular contents through leakages in the cell wall, disrupts pellicle formation, and inhibits formation of the plaque matrix.

In terms of clinical efficacy against plaque and gingivitis, Allaker and Douglas (2009) note that essential oil inhibits supragingival plaque by up to 56% and gingivitis by up to 36%, while chlorhexidine decreases plaque by up to 61% and reduces gingivitis by up to 80%. Notwithstanding the superior clinical effects of chlorhexidine, the authors admit the superior personal appeal and acceptability of essential oils. In comparison to chlorhexidine, essential oil natural remedies offer four advantages: they do not cause teeth staining, do not alter taste perception, do not promote dental or supragingival calculus formation and their efficacy is not diminished in the presence of toothpaste.

Through a randomized double-blind controlled trial, Lobo et al. (2014) verified the use of essential oil from the plant *Lippia sidoides* in the treatment of dental caries in children. The plant is popularly known as *Alecrim-Pimenta* in north-eastern Brazil. Lobo and co-workers convincingly showed that toothpaste containing *L. sidoides* essential oil produced significant reductions in salivary *S. mutans* in children with dental caries. In the trial, *L. sidoides* essential oil toothpaste demonstrated a reduction of salivary *S. mutans* after 5 days of treatment. Most importantly, Lobo and collaborators discovered that significantly low colonies of *S. mutans* were maintained throughout the study and these numbers did not revert to baseline levels during subsequent analysis at 30, 60, 180 and 365 days post-treatment.

The toothpaste formulation of *L. sidoides* essential oil mainly has a gram-positive antibacterial spectrum in addition to a limited action against gram-negative bacteria. The two major constituents of *L. sidoides* oil are phenolic compounds: Thymol (50–59%) and carvacrol (7–16%). Current experimental data are unanimous about the remarkable broad-spectrum antimicrobial actions of essential oils extracted from *L. sidoides*. Indeed, carvacrol and thymol have shown broad-spectrum antimicrobial activities against yeasts and bacteria.

Green Tea and Probiotics

Experimental evidence appears to be decisive that green tea contains multi-purpose antimicrobial phytochemicals. It is, therefore, not surprising that Narotzki, Reznick, Aizenbud and Levy (2012) point to the beneficial role of green tea in oral health. Based on their review, green tea works against dental caries induced by bacteria. That is not all. Tea polyphenols possess antiviral properties and abolish bad breath (halitosis) through modification of odourant sulphur components. Narotzki et al. (2012) explain that green tea polyphenols diminish oral cavity oxidative stress and inflammation, especially caused by nicotine and acrolein, the two most harmful compounds in cigarette smoke. In Japan, there is a popular notion that green tea makes the mouth clean as well as an old tradition that those who drink copious amounts of green tea rarely get tooth decay (Signoretto et al., 2012).

Allaker and Douglas (2009) also indicated that data from animal and human trials support the use of green tea in the control of dental caries. They cited studies which show that flavonoids in green tea control plaque-related diseases and dental caries. Extracts of green tea destroy oral bacteria *S. mutans* and *S. sobrinus* through the inhibition of three factors: bacterial adherence, acid production, and glucosyl transferase activity, an enzyme involved in the formation of extracellular polysaccharides.

In relation to periodontitis, Allaker and Douglas (2009) opined that the inhibition of the periodontal pathogens *Porphyromonas* and *Prevotella* species has been demonstrated with extracts of green tea. They also quote studies where green tea extracts restrain cysteine proteinase, one of the key enzymes in the virulence of *P. gingivalis*. Experiments in diseased animals also show that extracts of green tea decrease periodontal pocket depths and proportions of black pigmented gram-negative bacteria.

In addition, Avezov et al. (2014) indicated that consumption of products with antioxidant activity promotes oral health. In this regard, green tea as an excellent source of the polyphenol and antioxidant epigallocatechin-3-gallate plays a beneficial role in alleviating oral oxidative stress and inflammation. In the main, green tea defends healthy oral cells from malignant transformation and induces local apoptosis in oral cancer cells. Consequently, there is a growing interest in the oral health benefits of green tea.

Not less important, probiotics like yoghurts also control the growth of microorganisms including cariogenic streptococci associated with oral diseases (Allaker & Douglas, 2009). Probiotics are defined as live microorganisms which, when administered in adequate amounts, confer a health benefit on the host. Again, Allaker and Douglas (2009) cite studies where probiotics such as *Lactobacillus rhamnosus* CG, *Lactobacillus casei*, *Lactobacillus reuteri* and *Bifidobacterium* have all demonstrated the capacity to change colonization of cariogenic bacteria and thus prevent dental caries. The oral administration of probiotics controls periodontal disease. For example, application of *L. reuteri* to subjects with moderate and severe gingivitis reduced plaque levels and gingival inflammation.

Tong, Ni and Ling (2014) describe the use of nisin, a natural antimicrobial peptide, first isolated from *Lactococcus lactis* by Mattick and Hirsch in 1947. Nisin is one of the oldest known and most widely studied lantibiotics, a class of peptide antibiotics. Tong and co-workers have elucidated the antibacterial efficacy of nisin against pathogenic bacteria related to dental caries. They have observed that nisin is a caries-preventive agent due to its inhibition of common cariogenic-relevant bacteria: *Streptococcus sanguinis*, *Streptococcus gordonii*, *S. mutans*, *S. sobrinus*, *Lactobacillus acidophilus*, *Lactobacillus fermenti*, *L. casei*, *Actinomyces viscosus* and *Actinomyces naeslundii*.

Chewing Sticks

In many African and Middle East countries, a number of plants are used as chewing sticks to maintain good oral health. Africans that use chewing sticks have fewer carious lessons than those that use toothbrushes (Oshomoh & Idu, 2012). In Saudi Arabia, *Arak* chewing sticks are used by Muslims for cleaning teeth during the whole day (Ibrahim, Alaraidh, Al-Homaidan, Mostafa, & EL-Gaaly, 2014). WHO supports the use of chewing sticks as an effective tool for oral hygiene.

Chewing sticks are made from many plant species: *Acacia arabica*, *Anogeissus leiocarpa*, *A. indica*, *Diospyros lycioides*, *Distemonanthus benthamianus*, *Fagara zanthoxyloides*, *Garcinia kola*, *Glyphea brevis*, *Massularia acuminata*, *Sorindeia warneckei*, *Terminalia glaucescens*, *Vernonia amygdalina* and *Vitex doniana* (Alili et al., 2014). Within an individual stick, the active antimicrobial ingredients may be heterogeneous. *Fagara zanthoxyloides*, a chewing stick in Nigeria, consists of antimicrobial alkaloids and the species *S. warneckei* inhibits the growth of the periodontal pathogens *P. gingivalis* and *Prevotella melaninogenica* (Allaker & Douglas, 2009). *Glyphea brevis* twigs are also utilized in Nigeria as antimicrobial chewing sticks for cleaning teeth (Oshomoh & Idu, 2012).

Globally, the most commonly used chewing stick is *Salvadora persica* (Aboul-Enein, 2014). It has many synonyms such as *Salvadora indica*, *Arak*, *Meswak*, *Peelu*, mustard tree, or natural toothbrush tree (Chaurasia, Patil, & Nagar, 2013). Natural chewing sticks made of *S. persica* may be considered to be the first toothbrush of mankind, having been used by ancient Babylonians, Greeks, Romans, Jews and Egyptians. The plant also serves as natural toothpaste with antibacterial, anti-caries and anti-periopathic disinfectants having anti-plaque and antifungal properties (Chaurasia et al., 2013). Aboul-Enein (2014) also reiterated that in addition to its mechanical properties on plaque removal, *S. persica* also possesses antibacterial and antifungal properties. As a chewing stick, *S. persica* is used by many people who cannot afford commercial western toothbrush and toothpaste in rural areas of developing countries.

Twigs of the *S. persica* tree have a selective inhibitory effect on the level of certain bacteria in saliva, particularly the oral streptococci (Allaker & Douglas, 2009). In Saudi Arabia, scientists found that *S. persica* extracts have high antioxidant activities mainly due to the presence of flavonoids and phenolics (Ibrahim et al., 2014). Non-enzymatic antioxidants like flavonoids and phenolics reduce oral pathogenesis by preventing the disintegration of macromolecules (lipids, proteins, nucleic acids) and cell membranes.

Aboul-Enein (2014) revealed evidence-based studies and clinical trials where the use of *S. persica* was an effective oral hygiene plant. Interestingly, WHO recommends and encourages the use of *S. persica* as a readily-available, low-cost, simple and effective plant tool to promote oral hygiene including diminishing foul breath, polishing teeth and strengthening gums. *Salvadora persica*, too, has strong anti-cariogenic properties. Alili et al. (2014) demonstrated that *S. persica* displays antifungal activity against all *Candida* species. This is credited to the plant's volatile oils and compounds.

Other several studies corroborate that *S. persica* contains many different natural chemical compounds essential for good oral and dental hygiene (Chaurasia et al., 2013): fluorides, silica, tannic acid, gallic acid, resins, alkaloids (salvadorine), sinigrin, sulfur, vitamin C, sodium bicarbonate, chlorides, calcium, benzyl isothoicyanate, salicylic acids, sterols, trimethylamine, saponins, flavonoids, β-sitosterol, manisic acid, salvadourea [1,3-bis-(3-methoxy-benzyl)-urea and sulfur containing mustard oil.

Studies cited by Chaurasia et al. (2013) indicate different biological actions of *S. persica*'s chemical ingredients. For example, silica acts as an abrasive material to remove stains on teeth. Denture bases treated with tannic acid show reduced counts of *C. albicans*. Salvadorine has bactericidal activity while essential oils confer characteristic aroma and antiseptic action. The sulfur compounds in *S. persica* have bactericidal properties and sodium bicarbonate is a mild abrasive and dentifrice.

Aboul-Enein (2014) quoted several studies where benzyl isothiocyanate, one of the active ingredients of *S. persica*, is the main bactericidal agent against oral pathogens that mediate periodontal disease. Benzyl isothiocyanate is mostly active against gram-negative bacteria. However, Amir Alireza et al. (2014) showed that *S. persica* extracts were effective against both gram-negative and gram-positive bacteria.

A number of commercial preparations worldwide include *S. persica* extracts: *Sarkan* toothpaste (UK), *QualiMeswak* toothpaste (Switzerland) *Epident* toothpaste (Egypt), *Siwak-F* toothpaste (Indonesia), *Dentacare Miswak Plus* (Saudi Arabia), *Fluoroswak* and *Miswak* (Pakistan).

African Pharmacopoeia

Medicinal plants such as *Conyza sumatrensis*, *Aeschynomene abyssinica*, *Sida rhombifolia* and *Triumfetta rhomboidea* are used to manage carcinoma of the gums in Kenya (Ochwang'i, Kimwele, Oduma, Gathumbi, Mbaria, & Kiama, 2014). Ocheng, Bwanga, Joloba, Borg-Karlson, Gustafsson and Obua (2014) studied the antibacterial activities of extracts from Ugandan medicinal plants used for oral care (Table 5.1). Pulp juice prepared from fresh roots of *Zanthoxylum chalybeum* and *Euclea latidens* show activities against bacteria associated with periodontal disease and dental caries. Antibacterial activities were also demonstrated for solvent extracts of *Helichrysum odoratissimum*, *Z. chalybeum*, *Lantana trifolia*, and *Cymbopogon nardus*.

The antimicrobial effects of South African plants commonly utilized as ethnomedicines for oral diseases were studied by More, Tshikalange, Lall, Botha, and Meyer (2008). The plants *Annona senegalensis*, *Englerophytum magalismontanum*, *Dicerocarym senecioides*, *Euclea divinorum*, *Euclea natalensis*, *Solanum panduriforme* and *Parinari curatellifolia* displayed minimum inhibitory concentration values ranging from 25.0 mg/ml to 0.8 mg/ml. All the plants had moderate cytotoxicity. *Annona senegalensis* and *E. natalensis* had excellent therapeutic indices greater than 20. Plus, *Diospyros lycioides* demonstrated growth inhibitory activity against the oral pathogens *S. mutans* and *P. gingivalis*.

In South Africa, a leaf decoction of *Dodonaea viscosa* (hopbush) is traditionally used for the treatment of oral thrush and as a mouthwash for toothaches and related problems. Crude extracts of *D. viscosa* were bactericidal to *S. mutans* and significantly reduced its biofilm formation thus demonstrating potency in ameliorating oral infections. *Euclea natalensis* suppressed the growth of *S. mutans* and inhibited *A. viscosus* and *C. albicans*.

Asian Pharmacopoeia

Rasingam, Jeeva and Kannan (2012) enumerated eleven plant tooth twigs used by the inhabitants of Andaman and Nicobar Island, India, to treat dental caries. Some of the plants are *Acacia nilotica*, *A. indica* (neem), *Ficus benghalensis*, *Jatropha curcas* and *Pongamia pinnata*. Neem is used as a chewing stick throughout the world. In Tamilnadu, India, fruit paste from *Solanum surattense* is applied to heal toothache while the young stems of *A. nilotica* are employed as toothbrush in addition to being a treatment for toothache (Munuswamy, Thirunavukkarasu, Rajamani, Elumalai, & Ernest, 2013). *Moringa oleifera* leaf extracts inhibit the growth of dental plaque bacteria.

Bixa Orellana, commonly known as *Annatto* or the lipstick tree, is also useful in alleviating cancer of the mouth. Ziech, Anestopoulos, Hanafi,

Voulgaridou, Franco and Georgakilas et al. (2012) reported that withaferin A, a steroid lactone derived from the roots and leaves of *Withania somnifera*, heals oral cancer. Twigs of *Jatropha* are utilized as toothbrush and cure gum problems in Nepal. *Pongamia pinnata* contains antimicrobial and antioxidant compounds like chalcones, flavones, furanoflavonoids, isoflavones and pyranoflavonoids.

In China, roots of *Scutellaria baicalensis*, known as the *Huang-Qin* plant, cause apoptosis of cancerous cells. A panel of 15 oral bacterial pathogens were inhibited by baicalein, a flavonoid originally isolated from the roots of *S. baicalensis* (Jang et al., 2014). Baicalein bestows numerous pharmacological benefits not least antiviral, antibacterial, antifungal, antioxidant, anti-cancer and anti-inflammatory activities.

Against oral bacteria, there is a synergistic effect between baicalein and antibiotics ampicillin or gentamicin. Indeed, a time-kill study showed that the growth of the tested bacteria was completely attenuated after 1–6 hours post-treatment with baicalein, regardless of whether baicalein was administered alone or with ampicillin or gentamicin (Jang et al., 2014). In the treatment of oral pathogens, these results are important because *S. baicalensis* extracts and pure baicalein (5,6,7-trihydroxyflavone) are not antagonist to antibiotics in addition to being effective antibacterial agents in their own right. This means that extracts of *S. baicalensis* may be administered together with antibiotics, without any pharmacological problems.

Scientists at the Matsumoto Dental University in Japan have shown that *Kampo* herbal medicines are useful in treating periodontal disease and drug-induced gingival overgrowth (Ara, Hattori, Imamura, & Wang, 2010). One of the *Kampo* medicine plants is *Shosaikoto*. Since *Shosaikoto* decreases lipopolysaccharide-induced prostaglandin production by gingival fibroblasts, it reduces inflammation of periodontal tissue.

Barbieri et al. (2014) refer to studies in South Korea where *Polygonum cuspidatum* (Polygonaceae) roots are traditionally used to maintain good oral health. Extracts of *P. cuspidatum* reduce the viability of *S. mutans* and *S. sobrinus* cells, inhibit sucrose dependent adherence, decrease synthesis of water-insoluble glucan formation and reduce glycolytic acid production and acid environment tolerance. The inhibitory effects of *P. cuspidatum* are linked to the presence of alkaloids, phenolics and terpenes/-sterols.

Fucoidan, a complex sulphated polysaccharide found in the cell walls of several edible brown algae including *Fucus vesiculosus*, is an important agent against oral bacteria (Lee, Jeong, Choi, Na, & Cha, 2013). Fucoidan inhibits bacterial cell wall synthesis. Apart from being a natural antibiotic, fucoidan also boosts the immune system by enhancing the action of natural killer cells and macrophages. Corollary to these findings, fucoidan may be a useful candidate in the treatment of cariogenic and periodontopathogenic bacteria.

Microcystis aeruginosa and *Phormidium corium* are effective against oral diseases in India (Madhumathi & Vijayakumar, 2014). The reason is because phytochemicals like alkaloids, phenolics and steroids are present in these two cyanobacterial species that inhibit the growth of oral *C. albicans* and *S. mutans*. Antimicrobial action of these two blue-green algae is also premised on their novel chemical active ingredients such as microginins and cyalobolide B, present in *M. aeruginosa* and *P. corium*, respectively. In antimicrobial assays, *P. corium* extracts show activity against HIV reverse transcriptase and *S. aureus*. But caution should be taken because extracts of *M. aeruginosa* are known to contain hepato- and neuro-toxins (commonly called microcystins); these toxins do kill even larvae of mosquitoes *Aedes aegyptii*.

Rhodomyrtus tomentosa is an evergreen shrub native to Southeast Asia. Its active chemical compound, rhodomyrtone, is isolated from leaves. Studies in Thailand show leaf extracts of *R. tomentosa* have antibacterial activity against oral microorganisms including *S. aureus* ATCC 25923, *S. mutans* (clinical isolate) and *C. albicans* ATCC 90028 with minimum inhibitory concentrations of 31.25, 15.62 and 1000 μg/ml, respectively (Limsuwan, Homlaead, Watcharakul, Chusri, Moosigapong, & Saising et al., 2014). Rhodomyrtone also displays antibacterial activity with minimum inhibitory concentrations of 0.78 μg/ml and 0.39 μg/ml against *S. aureus* ATCC 25923 and *S. mutans*, respectively. Leaf extracts of *R. tomentosa* and rhodomyrtone are useful in prophylaxis and therapy of oral infections.

In Malaysia, extracts of two local ethnomedicinal plants *Piper betle* and *Brucea javanica* inhibit the adherence of seven oral *Candida* species (Nordin, Wan Harun, & Abdul Razak, 2013). *Piper betle* extracts drastically reduce the adherence of *C. tropicalis*, *C. albicans* and *C. krusei* by 86.01%, 61.41% and 56.34%, respectively (Nordin et a., 2013). *Brucea javanica* exhibits similar inhibitory effects on *C. tropicalis* (89.86%), *Candida lusitaniae* (88.95%), *C. albicans* (79.74%), *C. glabrata* (76.85%) and *C. krusei* (67.61%).

Brazilian and Mexican Folk Medicines

In Brazilian folk medicine, extracts of the plants *Aristolochia cymbifera*, *Cocos nucifera*, *Caesalpinia pyramidalis* and *Ziziphus joazeiro* are popularly used to treat oral diseases (Alviano et al., 2008). Laboratory assays confirmed that *A. cymbifera* extract induced the highest bactericidal effect against oral bacteria, followed by *C. nucifera*, *Z. joazeiro* and *C. pyramidalis* extracts, respectively. *Caesalpinia ferrea* fruit extract inhibits *in vitro* growth of oral pathogens in planktonic and biofilm models justifying its traditional use in the management of oral infections (Sampaio, Pereira, Dias, Costa, Conde, & Buzalaf, 2009). The crude extract of *C. ferrea* contains tannins (major constituent), anthraquinones, alkaloids, depsides, depsidones, flavonoids, lactones, saponins, sugars, sesquiterpenes and triterpenes. These phytochemicals confer many oral health functions.

In ethnobotanical surveys of plants used to treat oral diseases, the following plants were frequently cited: *Aloe vera*, *Anacardium occidentale*, *Schinus terebinthifolius*, *Chenopodium ambrosioides* and *P. granatum* (Vieira, Amaral, Maciel, Nascimento, Libério, & Rodrigues, 2014). Determination of minimum inhibitory concentration demonstrated that *P. granatum*, *Psidium guajava* and *S. terebinthifolius* had similar activity to 0.12% chlorhexidine, the positive control. Surprisingly, *C. ambrosioides*, though widely used, did not display any antimicrobial activity in lab tests (Vieira et al., 2014).

In other studies conducted in Brazil, Barbieri et al. (2014) showed that preparations of *S. terebinthifolius* and *Croton urucurana* inhibit biofilms formed by *S. mutans* and *C. albicans* strains. Their results show biofilms of *C. albicans* were more efficiently inhibited by extracts of *S. terebinthifolius*. The anti-adherent potential of both plants on *in vitro* biofilms formed by *C. albicans* and *S. mutans* were confirmed, suggesting the importance of these extracts in the prevention of oral diseases mediated by oral biofilms.

Compounds produced by *S. terebinthifolius* exhibit antimicrobial, anti-inflammatory and anti-ulcer properties. Phenolic compounds, anthraquinones, terpenoids and alkaloids are believed to confer these pharmacological functions. The plant also contains the compounds apigenin, methyl gallate and gallic acid which inhibit adherence of biofilms. *Croton urucurana* has anti-inflammatory, anti-haemorrhagic and antifungal properties.

Other Brazilian herbal products with the potential to control oral biofilms were cited by Barbieri et al. (2014): extracts of peas (*Pisum sativum*), lectins from pitombeira (*Telisia esculenta*), and crude extracts from mulberry leaves (*Morus alba*). Having undergone pharmaceutical evaluations, these plant extracts are now added to mouthwashes, toothpastes and other oral hygiene products; in order to make the oral hygiene products more amenable to the prevention of oral biofilm formation.

Eugenia calycina (family Myrtaceae), an endemic plant species in Brazil, produces an essential oil with remarkable activity against anaerobic bacteria *Prevotella nigrescens* and *P. gingivalis* (Sousa, de Morais, Vieira, Napolitano, Guzman, & Moraes et al., 2015). At low minimum inhibitory concentrations, *E. calycina* essential oil has a higher selectivity against oral bacteria and lower toxicity towards HeLa cells. These findings illustrate that *E. calycina* is a promising plant for the management of oral pathogenic bacteria.

In Mexico, traditional healers and patients use many plants as medicines to treat oral diseases. Rosas-Piñón, Mejía, Díaz-Ruiz, Aguilar, Sánchez-Nieto and Rivero-Cruz (2012) obtained high inhibitory effects against oral pathogens *S. mutans* and *P. gingivalis* with ethanolic extracts of *Haematoxylon brasiletto*, *P.*

granatum, Iostephane heterophyla, Bursera simaruba, Cedrela odorata and *Rhus standleyi* (12.5–65.0 µg/ml) as well as water extracts of *H. brasiletto, P. granatum, I. hetero-phyla, Amphipterygium adstringens, Argemone mexicana, C. odorata, Eysenhardtia polystachya, Persea americana, Syzygium aromaticum, Cinnamomun zeylanicum, Cnidoscolus multilobus* and *R. standleyi* (10.5–78.0 µg/ml). These laboratory results no doubt mean the plants have antibacterial effects thus justifying their use in the traditional medicine for oral infections.

A Closer Look at Natural Products against Oral Infections

It is ironic to note that the most common infectious diseases of humans are oral diseases; not HIV/AIDS, not influenza, and not tuberculosis. Even fossil evidence reveals early humans like Broken Hill man, who lived in modern-day Zambia in the Middle Pleistocene Age more than 11,000 years before present, suffered a great deal from dental caries and periodontal diseases. Nowadays, the increasing incidence of dental caries and periodontitis is inextricably linked to dysfunctional immunity experienced during HIV/AIDS. Oral diseases are one of the clear manifestations of AIDS, a part of the AIDS complex that evolves when CD4 counts are as low as 200.

In developing countries, the numbers of oral health facilities and practitioners including dentists are very low, too inadequate to meet demand. There is less than one dentist for every 100,000 people in Africa; the least number of dentists is in Angola. The increasing incidence of oral diseases due to HIV/AIDS, coupled with the lack of oral health facilities and person-power, has created a natural demand for the use of plant products to treat oral diseases. But there is another reason for the shift to natural products. Resistance of pathogens to conventional drugs for oral therapy is increasing public interest towards natural products for oral health. Whilst natural products are not a replacement for oral antibiotics, fungicides or virucides, they provide more options from which to select new treatments for diseases of the oral cavity.

Even without bioprospecting, many common natural products alleviate oral infections. Milk, honey, green tea, cranberries, edible mushrooms, liquorice, alcohol-free red wine, grapes, raisins, essential oils, rhein, pomegranate, chamomile, and probiotics such as those in yoghurt have been shown to reduce symptoms of oral diseases. Green tea has polyphenol antioxidants like epigallocatechin-3-gallate which reduce oral oxidative stress, inflammation and malignancy. In addition, many antimicrobial substances are present in chewing sticks, the most common being miswak (*S. persica*).

The use of *Mchenja* (*D. mespiliformis*) as a chewing stick is even more significant because the plant has antipyretic, anti-inflammatory, antibacterial, antiparasitic, anti-HIV and antifungal properties. *Diospyros mespiliformis* is found in

191

many parts of Central, Southern, Eastern and West Africa where it is also used in the treatment of fever, whooping cough, wounds, malaria, pneumonia, syphilis, leprosy, dermatomycoses, helminths and facilitation of childbirth. The broad antimicrobial functions of *D. mespiliformis* are accredited to the presence of two active compounds, diosquinone and plumbagin. Diosquinone also displays anti-cancer activity while plumbagin is a known anti-HIV agent.

For the treatment of oral diseases, this chapter describes, albeit, in a non-exhaustive manner- close to 100 species of plants and blue-green algae (*M. aeruginosa* and *P. corium*). Chemical ingredients have also been isolated from fungal and bacterial species. In general, these species are impregnated with several useful antimicrobial phytochemicals that fight oral diseases: phenols, phenolic acids, quinones, flavones, flavonoids, flavonols, tannins, coumarins, terpenoids, essential oils, alkaloids, monoterpenes, sesquiterpenes, lectins, naphthalene glucosides, diospyrosides, kaempferol, myricetin, rhamnocitrin, eugenol, oleanolic acid, oleanolic aldehyde and antimicrobial peptides.

Specifically, many active chemical ingredients isolated from natural products ward off oral infections, for example: 2',6'-dihydroxy-4'-geranyloxyacetophenone, 2',6'-dihydroxy-4'-farnesyloxy-acetophenone, 5-(hydroxymethyl)-2-furfural, benzyl isothiocyanate, alpha-bisabolol, salvadourea [1,3-bis-(3-methoxy-benzyl)-urea, azulene, matricine and chamazulene. While many of these active chemical ingredients may be laced into drugs and other oral health products, use of their raw source plant materials is significantly justifiable, as is the case with *S. persica* chewing sticks which are recommended by WHO.

On the face of it, the use of natural products for oral health is quite prominent especially in resource-poor settings. But a closer scrutiny of the literature cited in this chapter shows that bioprospecting for and antimicrobial studies of natural products for oral health were mainly conducted in the following countries (in decreasing magnitude): India, South Africa, Brazil (where 8 million people do not have teeth), Japan, France, Egypt, Iran, Mexico, Kenya, Switzerland, Nigeria, Australia, Uganda and the United Kingdom. There is somewhat an emerging dichotomy when one looks at natural products for oral health in these countries. Work on basic research, mouthwashes and value-addition is synonymous with Brazil, European countries and Australia. Already Brazil and China are adding natural products to Colgate toothpaste. On the other hand, African and Asian countries mostly focus on the antimicrobial testing of natural products. Countries such as Iran and Egypt conduct substantial research on plants used as chewing sticks.

In Africa, research on natural products for treating oral diseases is far much less when compared to other natural remedies for AIDS-related diseases such as skin and sexually transmitted infections, tuberculosis, or diarrhoea. The reasons for this imbalance are not entirely clear, but one possibility is that because morbidity and mortality due to oral infections are usually inconspicuous, natural products for oral diseases have not received their fair share of research attention and funding. Against this backdrop, there is an urgent need to accelerate bioprospecting efforts, antimicrobial testing and isolation of active compounds from African plants and other natural products that may be used to manufacture new drugs and hygiene products for oral health.

To improve our understanding of the link between food and oral health, an international European Union (EU) sixth framework programme consortium project (NUTRIDENT, FOOD-CT-2006-36210) was commissioned with the overall aim of identifying beverage/food constituents that are able to reduce the risk of two major dental diseases, caries and gingivitis. This 2.2 million Euro project was implemented between 2006 and 2010. Despite this EU project, there is still a global paucity of data about the quality, safety and efficacy of herbal products used in oral health. Therefore, given the possible adverse interactions between natural product formulations and conventional drugs, caution should be exercised when using herbal medicines. Natural products can destroy oral health as much as they can help restore its bright future.

Conclusions and Recommendations

The mouth is a hive of activity for microorganisms and protozoal parasites. Many of these microbes become increasingly pathogenic in the course of HIV infection. Therefore, oral infections are becoming poignant and serious opportunistic diseases associated with AIDS. Oral diseases should therefore be part and parcel of current HIV/AIDS research and interventions. Despite this recognition, clinical management of oral diseases still faces many challenges that necessitate the use of natural agents including food products, beverages, and ethnomedicinal plants.

This chapter has reviewed common natural products employed in oral health: rhein, raisins, pomegranate, chamomile, honey, essential oils, green tea, probiotics, and chewing sticks made from plants like *D. mespiliformis* and *S. persica*. More importantly, the chapter has provided a relatively small sample of plants (especially from African, Asian, Brazilian/Mexican pharmacopoeias) whose antimicrobial properties against oral pathogens have been elucidated through laboratory experimentation and human trials. Some active chemical principles have been isolated from medicinal plants used against oral pathogens.

With respect to natural products for oral health, there is an urgent need to increase research efforts aimed at identifying more natural products that possess antimicrobial efficacy targeting oral pathogens. More studies should also focus on toxicological safety of natural products in addition to isolation and characterisation of active chemical compounds. These endeavours may lead to value-addition and commercialization of natural products that may be used to manufacture novel products and drugs for the treatment of oral infections associated with HIV/AIDS.

References

Aboul-Enein, B.H. (2014). The miswak (*Salvadora persica* L.) chewing stick: Cultural implications in oral health promotion. *The Saudi Journal for Dental Research, 5*(1), 9-13.

Alili, N., Türp, J.C., Kulik, E.M., & Waltimo, T. (2014). Volatile compounds of *Salvadora persica* inhibit the growth of oral *Candida* species. *Archives of Oral Biology, 59*(5), 441-447.

Allaker, R.P., & Douglas, C.W. (2009). Novel anti-microbial therapies for dental plaque-related diseases. *International Journal of Antimicrobial Agents, 33*(1), 8-13.

Alviano, W.S., Alviano, D.S., Diniz, C.G., Antoniolli, A.R., Alviano, C.S., Farias, L.M., ... & Bolognese, A.M. (2008). *In vitro* antioxidant potential of medicinal plant extracts and their activities against oral bacteria based on Brazilian folk medicine. *Archives of Oral Biology, 53*(6), 545-552.

Amir Alireza, R.G., Afsaneh, R., Seied Hosein, M.S., Siamak, Y., Afshin, K., Zeinab, K., ... & Amir Reza, R. (2014). Inhibitory activity of *Salvadora persica* extracts against oral bacterial strains associated with periodontitis: An *in-vitro* study. *Journal of Oral Biology and Craniofacial Research (in press)*.

Ara, T., Hattori, T., Imamura, Y., & Wang, P.L. (2010). Development of novel therapy for oral diseases using *Kampo* medicines. *Journal of Oral Biosciences, 52*(2), 100-106.

Avezov, K., Reznick, A.Z., & Aizenbud, D. (2014). Oxidative stress in the oral cavity: Sources and pathological outcomes. *Respiratory Physiology and Neurobiology (in press)*.

Azelmat, J., Larente, J.F., & Grenier, D. (2014). The anthraquinone rhein exhibits synergistic antibacterial activity in association with metronidazole or natural compounds and attenuates virulence gene expression in *Porphyromonas gingivalis. Archives of Oral Biology (in press)*.

Bailly, C. (2009). Ready for a comeback of natural products in oncology. *Biochemical Pharmacology, 77*(9), 1447-1457.

Barbieri, D.S., Tonial, F., Lopez, P.V., Sales Maia, B.H., Santos, G.D., Ribas, M.O., ... & Vicente, V.A. (2014). Antiadherent activity of *Schinus terebinthifolius* and *Croton urucurana* extracts on in vitro biofilm formation of *Candida albicans* and *Streptococcus mutans. Archives of Oral Biology (in press)*.

Batista, A.L.A., Diógenes Alves Uchôa Lins, R., de Souza Coelho, R., do Nascimento Barbosa, D., Moura Belém, N., & Alves Celestino, F.J. (2014). Clinical efficacy analysis of the mouthrinsing with pomegranate and chamomile plant extracts in the gingival bleeding reduction. *Complementary Therapies in Clinical Practice, 20*(1), 93-98.

Bonifait, L., Marquis, A., Genovese, S., Epifano, F., & Grenier, D. (2012). Synthesis and antimicrobial activity of geranyloxy-and farnesyloxy-acetophenone derivatives against oral pathogens. *Fitoterapia, 83*(6), 996-999.

Chaurasia, A., Patil, R., & Nagar, A. (2013). Miswak in oral cavity–An update. *Journal of Oral Biology and Craniofacial Research, 3*(2), 98-101.

Costalonga, M., & Herzberg, M. C. (2014). The oral microbiome and the immunobiology of periodontal disease and caries. *Immunology Letters (in press)*.

Delfan, B., Bahmani, M., Rafieian-Kopaei, M., Delfan, M., & Saki, K. (2014). A review study on ethnobotanical study of medicinal plants used in relief of toothache in Lorestan Province, Iran. *Asian Pacific Journal of Tropical Disease, 4*, S879-S884.

Ibrahim, M.M., Alaraidh, I.A., Al-Homaidan, A.A., Mostafa, E.M., & EL-Gaaly, G.A. (2014). Assessment of antioxidant activities in roots of *Miswak Salvadora persica*) plants grown at two different locations in Saudi Arabia. *Saudi Journal of Biological Sciences (in press)*.

Jang, E.J., Cha, S.M., Choi, S.M., & Cha, J.D. (2014). Combination effects of baicalein with antibiotics against oral pathogens. *Archives of Oral Biology, 59*(11), 1233-1241.

Kumar, S., Sharma, S., Kumar, D., Kumar, K., & Arya, R. (2014). Immunostimulant activity of *Phyllanthus reticulatus* Poir: A useful plant for infectious tropical diseases. *Asian Pacific Journal of Tropical Disease, 4*, S491-S495.

Lacy, S.A. (2014). The oral pathological conditions of the Broken Hill (Kabwe) 1 cranium. *International Journal of Paleopathology, 7*, 57-63.

Lee, K.Y., Jeong, M.R., Choi, S.M., Na, S.S., & Cha, J.D. (2013). Synergistic effect of fucoidan with antibiotics against oral pathogenic bacteria. *Archives of Oral Biology, 58*(5), 482-492.

Limsuwan, S., Homlaead, S., Watcharakul, S., Chusri, S., Moosigapong, K., Saising, J., & Voravuthikunchai, S.P. (2014). Inhibition of microbial adhesion to plastic surface and human buccal epithelial cells by *Rhodomyrtus tomentosa* leaf extract. *Archives of Oral Biology, 59*(12), 1256-1265.

Lobo, P.L.D., Fonteles, C.S.R., Marques, L.A.R.V., Jamacaru, F.V.F., Fonseca, S.G.D.C., de Carvalho, C.B.M., & de Moraes, M.E.A. (2014). The efficacy of three formulations of *Lippia sidoides* Cham. essential oil in the reduction of salivary *Streptococcus mutans* in children with caries: A randomized, double-blind, controlled study. *Phytomedicine, 21*(8), 1043-1047.

Lopes, C.F.B., de Angelis, B.B., Prudente, H.M., de Souza, B.V.G., Cardoso, S.V., & de Azambuja Ribeiro, R.I.M. (2012). Concomitant consumption of marijuana, alcohol and tobacco in oral squamous cell carcinoma development and progression: recent advances and challenges. *Archives of Oral Biology, 57*(8), 1026-1033.

Madhumathi, V., & Vijayakumar, S. (2014). Identification of novel cyano-bacterial compounds for oral disease through in vitro and *insilico* approach. *Biomedicine and Aging Pathology (in press)*.

Maeda, H., Hirai, K., Mineshiba, J., Yamamoto, T., Kokeguchi, S., & Takashiba, S. (2013). Medical microbiological approach to Archaea in oral infectious diseases. *Japanese Dental Science Review, 49*(2), 72-78.

Mansourian, A., Boojarpour, N., Ashnagar, S., Beitollahi, J.M., & Shamshiri, A.R. (2014). The comparative study of antifungal activity of *Syzygium aromaticum*, *Punica granatum* and nystatin on *Candida albicans:* An *in vitro* study. *Journal de Mycologie Médicale/Journal of Medical Mycology, 24*(4), e163-e168.

Moon, S.E., Kim, H.Y., & Cha, J.D. (2011). Synergistic effect between clove oil and its major compounds and antibiotics against oral bacteria. *Archives of Oral Biology, 56*(9), 907-916.

More, G., Tshikalange, T.E., Lall, N., Botha, F., & Meyer, J.J.M. (2008). Antimicrobial activity of medicinal plants against oral microorganisms. *Journal of Ethnopharmacology, 119*(3), 473-477.

Munuswamy, H., Thirunavukkarasu, T., Rajamani, S., Elumalai, E.K., & Ernest, D. (2013). A review on antimicrobial efficacy of some traditional medicinal plants in Tamilnadu. *Journal of Acute Disease, 2*(2), 99-105.

Nabavi, S.M., Marchese, A., Izadi, M., Curti, V., Daglia, M., & Nabavi, S. F. (2015). Plants belonging to the genus *Thymus* as antibacterial agents: From farm to pharmacy. *Food Chemistry, 173*, 339-347.

Narotzki, B., Reznick, A.Z., Aizenbud, D., & Levy, Y. (2012). Green tea: A promising natural product in oral health. *Archives of Oral Biology, 57*(5), 429-435.

Nordin, M.A.F., Wan Harun, W.H.A., & Abdul Razak, F. (2013). An *in vitro* study on the anti-adherence effect of *Brucea javanica* and *Piper betle* extracts towards oral Candida. *Archives of Oral Biology, 58*(10), 1335-1342.

Ocheng, F., Bwanga, F., Joloba, M., Borg-Karlson, A.K., Gustafsson, A., & Obua, C. (2014). Antibacterial activities of extracts from Ugandan medicinal plants used for oral care. *Journal of Ethnopharmacology, 155*(1), 852-855.

Ochwang'i, D.O., Kimwele, C.N., Oduma, J.A., Gathumbi, P.K., Mbaria, J.M., & Kiama, S.G. (2014). Medicinal plants used in treatment and management of cancer in Kakamega County, Kenya. *Journal of Ethnopharmacology, 151*(3), 1040-1055.

Okumura, K. (2011). Cathelicidins—Therapeutic antimicrobial and anti-tumor host defense peptides for oral diseases. *Japanese Dental Science Review, 47*(1), 67-81.

Oshomoh, E.O., & Idu, M. (2012). Phytochemical screening and antimicrobial activity of ethanol and aqueous extracts of stem of *Glyphaea brevis* (spreng.) monachino on oral microorganisms. *Pharmacognosy Journal, 4*(33), 23-30.

Petti, S., & Scully, C. (2009). Polyphenols, oral health and disease: A review. *Journal of Dentistry, 37*(6), 413-423.

Rasingam, L., Jeeva, S., & Kannan, D. (2012). Dental care of Andaman and Nicobar folks: Medicinal plants use as tooth stick. *Asian Pacific Journal of Tropical Biomedicine, 2*(2), S1013-S1016.

Raut, J.S., & Karuppayil, S.M. (2014). A status review on the medicinal properties of essential oils. *Industrial Crops and Products, 62*, 250-264.

Rivero-Cruz, J.F., Zhu, M., Kinghorn, A.D., & Wu, C.D. (2008). Antimicrobial constituents of Thompson seedless raisins (*Vitis vinifera*) against selected oral pathogens. *Phytochemistry Letters, 1*(3), 151-154.

Rosas-Piñón, Y., Mejía, A., Díaz-Ruiz, G., Aguilar, M.I., Sánchez-Nieto, S., & Rivero-Cruz, J.F. (2012). Ethnobotanical survey and antibacterial activity of plants used in the Altiplane region of Mexico for the treatment of oral cavity infections. *Journal of Ethnopharmacology, 141*(3), 860-865.

Sampaio, F.C., Pereira, M.D.S.V., Dias, C.S., Costa, V.C.O., Conde, N.C., & Buzalaf, M.A. (2009). *In vitro* antimicrobial activity of *Caesalpinia ferrea* Martius fruits against oral pathogens. *Journal of Ethnopharmacology, 124*(2), 289-294.

Sardi, J.C.O., Almeida, A.M.F., & Mendes Giannini, M.J.S. (2011). New antimicrobial therapies used against fungi present in subgingival sites—a brief review. *Archives of Oral Biology, 56*(10), 951-959.

Shi, Q.I.U., Hui, S.U.N., Zhang, A.H., Hong-Ying, X.U., Guang-Li, Y.A.N., Ying, H.A.N., & Xi-Jun, W.A.N.G. (2014). Natural alkaloids: basic aspects, biological roles, and future perspectives. *Chinese Journal of Natural Medicines, 12*(6), 401-406.

Signoretto, C., Canepari, P., Stauder, M., Vezzulli, L., & Pruzzo, C. (2012). Functional foods and strategies contrasting bacterial adhesion. *Current Opinion in Biotechnology, 23*(2), 160-167.

Sousa, R.M.F., de Morais, S.A., Vieira, R.B., Napolitano, D.R., Guzman, V.B., Moraes, T.S., ... & de Oliveira, A. (2015). Chemical composition, cytotoxic, and antibacterial activity of the essential oil from *Eugenia calycina* Cambess. leaves against oral bacteria. *Industrial Crops and Products, 65*, 71-78.

Tong, Z., Ni, L., & Ling, J. (2014). Antibacterial peptide nisin: A potential role in the inhibition of oral pathogenic bacteria. *Peptides, 60*, 32-40.

Vieira, D.R., Amaral, F.M., Maciel, M.C., Nascimento, F.R., Libério, S. A., & Rodrigues, V.P. (2014). Plant species used in dental diseases: Ethnopharmacology aspects and antimicrobial activity evaluation. *Journal of Ethnopharmacology, 155*(3), 1441-1449.

Wade, W. G. (2013). The oral microbiome in health and disease. *Pharmacological Research, 69*(1), 137-143.

Ziech, D., Anestopoulos, I., Hanafi, R., Voulgaridou, G. P., Franco, R., Georgakilas, A. G., ... & Panayiotidis, M. I. (2012). Pleiotrophic effects of natural products in ROS-induced carcinogenesis: The role of plant-derived natural products in oral cancer chemoprevention. *Cancer letters*, *327*(1), 16-25.

Table 5.1: Medicinal plants used for the treatment of dental and oral diseases in Uganda

Plant's scientific name	Plant's local name/ Ugandan tribe	Plant parts and preparation	Oral diseases treated
Bidens pilosa	Enyabarashana/Rukiga	Chew fresh leaves	Toothache
Vernonia amygdalina	Okello-okello/Langi	Stems used to brush teeth; fresh twigs are chewed	Dental caries
Euclea latidens	Amuru-dyek/Langi	Roots used to brush teeth	Dental caries
Hoslundia opposite	Kamunye/Baganda	Chew fresh leaves	Mouth sores
Ocimum gratissimum	Omujaja/Rukiga	Chew fresh leaves	Toothache
Cymbopogon citratus	Kasubi/Baganda	Fresh leaves taken as tea or chewed	Bad breath, toothache
Clematis hirsuta	Adwe/Langi	Fresh leaves are pounded and applied as paste on painful tooth; infusion is drunk	Toothache and sore throat
Tecleanobilis	Nzo/Baganda	Stems used as toothbrush	Dental caries
Zanthoxylum chalybeum	Owucu/Langi Songowowo/ Pokot	Roots used as toothbrush; fresh stem bark is chewed	Dental caries, toothache

Adapted from Ocheng et al. (2014)

6

Natural Products as Anti–Tuberculosis Agents

Introduction

Tuberculosis (TB), a communicable disease, is the leading cause of death in people living with HIV/AIDS. As if that is not enough, the mortality of persons co-infected with TB and HIV has increased due to the emergence of multi-drug resistant tuberculosis (MDR-TB), extensively drug resistant tuberculosis (XDR-TB), and totally drug resistant tuberculosis (TDR-TB). This is because XDR-TB and TDR-TB are often incurable.

Due to the widespread existence of multiple drug resistant strains of *Mycobacterium tuberculosis* and the increase in the prevalence of HIV/AIDS, TB has become one of the deadliest global health emergencies (Holton, Weiss, Tucker, & Wilmanns, 2007). The tubercle bacillus *M. tuberculosis* was discovered by Robert Koch in 1882. By 1998, its genome was completely sequenced, opening the doors to amazing possibilities for target-specific drug development. But post-genomics progress toward novel anti-TB drugs has been slow, mainly hampered by a lack of interest from pharmaceutical and biotechnology companies (Holton et al., 2007).

Corollary to this unfortunate scenario, there is now an urgent need to discover and develop new anti-TB agents (Zumla, Nahid, & Cole, 2013). Writing in the journal *Nature*, Koul, Arnoult, Lounis, Guillemont and Andries (2011) emphasized that the emergence of multi-drug resistant strains of *M. tuberculosis* makes the discovery of new molecular scaffolds a very urgent priority. For this reason, there is now renewed interest in the screening and purification of novel anti-TB agents from natural products (Santhosh & Suriyanarayanan, 2014).

This chapter helps to provide clarity to three fundamental questions:

1. What species of medicinal plants are used as natural remedies for TB?
2. What are the anti-mycobacterial activities of natural products?
3. Which active chemical compounds isolated from natural products confer anti-mycobacterial properties?

To set the stage for a consideration of natural products as anti-TB agents, the first sections of the chapter review the global burden of TB, the growing problem of drug resistant *M. tuberculosis* strains and the twinning of TB to HIV/AIDS.

Global Burden of TB

TB is a contagious (airborne) disease which latently infects over 2 billion people worldwide (Baldwin, Reeves, Powell, Napier, Swimm, & Sun et al., 2015). Mathematical models predict that between the years 2000 and 2020, nearly one billion people would have been newly infected, 200 million would develop TB and 35 million would have died from the disease (WHO, 2000). A major public health problem, TB kills about 2-3 million people in the world every year; over 90% of global TB cases and deaths occur in the developing world (WHO, 2012).

Fyhrquist, Laakso, Garcia Marco, Julkunen-Tiitto and Hiltunen (2014) believe that *M. tuberculosis* is responsible for more human deaths than any other single microbial pathogen. Globally, TB killed more than 1.4 million in 2011 (WHO, 2012). In 2009, an estimated 8.8-9.9 million new TB cases were reported throughout the world. According to WHO estimates, TB is spreading at the rate of one person per second. Mycobacteria have recently increased their virulence and TB is one of the most lethal infections in the world (Askun, Tumen, Satil, & Ates, 2009). Between 1980 and 2005, 90 million cases of TB worldwide were reported to WHO.

In 2005, the global incidence of TB was estimated at 136 cases per 100,000 of the population (Askun et al., 2009). In 2008, WHO estimated that the largest number of new TB cases occurred in South-East Asia, which accounted for 34% of incident cases globally (WHO, 2010a). Around the same time, Africa and the Americas represented a total of 8.8 million new cases of TB and 1.7 million deaths from TB annually (Askun et al., 2009).

Due to the HIV/AIDS epidemic, TB re-emerged as a global emergency, peaking in 2006 to more than 9.9 million cases annually, then falling to an estimated 8.8 million by 2010 (Ralph, Lucas, & Norval, 2013). By 2011, TB was more prevalent in the world than at any other time in human history (Koul et al., 2011). It is estimated that 50% of the population in Sub-Saharan Africa is latently infected with TB (Frothingham, Stout, & Hamilton, 2005).

Approximately half a million people in Africa died of TB in 2004 (Madikizela, Ndhlala, Finnie, & van Staden, 2014a). In 2005, WHO declared TB an emergency in Africa, mainly because the average incidence of TB in African countries more than doubled between 1990 and 2005, largely driven by rising HIV infections (Chaisson & Martinson, 2008). Yet by 2007, Asia had 60% of the global burden of TB (Vermund & Yamamoto, 2007).

For example, in Ethiopia, TB was labelled as one of the major causes of death with 15,700 new cases of infections appearing in 1997 (Cambanis, Yassin, Ramsay, Bertel Squire, Arbide, & Cuevas, 2005). In Tanzania the number of TB cases steadily increased between 1983 and 2000, mainly due to HIV/AIDS (Egwaga, 2003). Thus, among all infectious diseases, TB remains one of the major causes of death (Abuzeid, Kalsum, Koshy, Larsson, Glader, & Andersson et al., 2014).

Pathogenesis of TB

Mycobacterium tuberculosis is an intracellular obligate and aerobic bacillus that multiplies within macrophages. While the bacterium triggers the production of free radicals, it avoids killing by the same radicals (Agarwal, Prasad, & Jain, 2010). During pulmonary inflammation, increased amount of reactive oxygen species and reactive nitrogen intermediates are produced as a consequence of phagocytic respiratory burst, this results in high oxidative stress (Agarwal et al., 2010).

TB commonly infects the lungs and transmits from person to person via droplets from the throat and lungs of people with active disease. Still, the disease may affect different parts of the body. Since it is airborne and because it multiplies in macrophages- stalwart cells of the immune system - TB spreads rapidly in overcrowded settings or in conditions of malnutrition and poverty, where the immune system is already weak (Green, Samie, Obi, Bessong, & Ndip, 2010).

One-third of the world population is latently infected by TB (Xie, Wang, Zeng, Zhou, Duan, & Li et al., 2015). Latent TB infection occurs when pathogenic *M. tuberculosis* bacteria are not active i.e. exist in dormant form and patients do not show any symptoms of the disease (Ganihigama, Sureram, Sangher, Hongmanee, Aree, & Mahidol et al., 2015) Although patients with the dormant form of *M. tuberculosis* cannot transmit the disease, they have a lifelong risk of TB reactivation more especially when co-infected with HIV (Ganihigama et al., 2015).

To gain better insights into the virulence factors of *M. tuberculosis* as well as to unravel the pathogenesis of TB, new tools from systems biology are becoming useful. Chandra, Kumar and Rao (2011) envisage systems biology, which seeks to understand biological systems as a whole, through an integrated approach, is now very helpful in obtaining a global perspective of the TB pathogen and its interactions with the host.

Systems biology has given way to new analyses of the interactome, reactome and pocketome of *M. tuberculosis* (Chandra et al., 2011). The gist of all these global cellular and molecular surveys is to elucidate several factors involved in *M. tuberculosis* pathogenesis and antibiotic resistance. Recently, a publication by Xie et al. (2015) reported that several proteins involved in *M. tuberculosis* virulence, persistence and drug resistance were actually lysine acetylated, what is now known as the acetylome of *M. tuberculosis*.

Suffice to say that considerable insights have already been gleaned from analyzing different aspects of systems biology such as proteins essential for mycobacterial survival, proteins that are highly influential in the network, pathways that are highly connected, host factors responsible for maintaining the TB infection and key factors involved in autophagy and pathogenesis. In addition, systems biology is helping to locate factors that bring about multiple drug resistance.

In many African societies, folks rely on several symptoms to diagnose, correctly or wrongly, individuals with TB. Symptoms of TB are varied but may include coughs lasting more than two months, bloody cough, cough with vomiting, slimy sputum, weight loss, fast or laboured breathing, wheezing, upright body hair, chronic fever, sweating, dehydration, coiled hair, loss of appetite, frequent spitting, malaise, smelly breath, tonsillitis, darkening skin and chest pain (Tabuti, Kukunda, & Waako, 2010).

A common symptom of TB, chest pain, is caused by inflammation of the membranes lining the lungs, leading to the development of lung fibrosis. In the case of pulmonary TB, alveolar macrophages mediate anti-inflammatory responses in the lungs; they do that by producing chemical mediators that lead to granuloma formation (Shinohara, Pantuso, Shinohara, Kogiso, Myrvik, Henriksen, & Shibata, 2009). As a host response to *M. tuberculosis* infection, granuloma formation in addition to inflammatory tissue destruction and repair, represent protective immunity (Shinohara et al., 2009).

Protective immunity against *M. tuberculosis* is based on correct functioning of cell-mediated immunity, especially the secretion of T-helper 1 cytokines by antigen-specific T cells (Sharma, Kalia, Suden, Chauhan, Kumar, & Ram et al., 2014). Cellular immunity plays an important role in protective granuloma formation and stimulation of the antimicrobial activity of infected macrophages. Sharma and co-workers postulate that the main cytokine is interferon-gamma which activates bactericidal effector mechanisms in the macrophage, the mycobacterial host cell.

Modulation of macrophage functions is an important component of the cellular immune response to TB infection. Since many plant products exhibit immuno-modulatory properties, they have the ability to potentiate Th-1 responses involving a variety of T-cell subsets as well as to stimulate the production of cytokines that amplify the immune response against the infectious TB agent. Natural products that cause an uptick of the cellular immune response to TB infection can, therefore, be harnessed as natural medicines for TB.

Drug Resistant TB

Today, one of the most pressing global health challenges involves the growing resistance of *M. tuberculosis* to drugs (Askun et al., 2009). Globally, over 4% of TB patients are infected with *M. tuberculosis* strains that are resistant to first line drugs (Fomogne-Fodjo, Van Vuuren, Ndinteh, Krause, & Olivier, 2014). The increasing rate of MDR-TB, XDR-TB and TDR-TB strains is a major global public health concern because these drug resistant strains have worse disease outcomes. We are not doing nearly enough to take the world away from the precipice of disaster.

MDR-TB refers to strains that resist isoniazid and rifampin, while XDR-TB is resistant to isoniazid, rifampin, fluoroquinolone and the second-line injectable drugs kanamycin, amikacin and capreomycin (Ganihigama et al., 2015). In 2012, estimates suggested 450,000 people developed MDR-TB and 170,000 people died from the same (Ganihigama et al., 2015). South Africa was among the countries with the highest number of MDR-TB and XDR-TB in the world (WHO, 2010b). According to WHO estimates, there were about 500,000 million new cases of MDR-TB in the world in 2011; about 60% of the cases were in the *BRICS* countries- Brazil, Russia, India, China and South Africa.

It was during the 1990s that MDR-TB emerged as a threat to TB control worldwide. A 1997 survey of 35 countries found MDR-TB rates were above 2% in almost a third of the surveyed countries (Pablos-Méndez, Raviglione, Laszlo, Binkin, Rieder, & Bustreo et al., 1998). The highest rates were in Russia and the former Soviet Union, the Baltic States, Argentina, India and China (Toungoussova, Bjune, & Caugant, 2006).

These countries were associated with poorly funded or failing national TB control programmes. Likewise, the appearance of high rates of MDR-TB in New York City in the early 1990s was associated with the dismantling of free public health programmes by the Reagan administration (Barr, Diez-Roux, Knirsch, & Pablos-Méndez, 2001). Neighbourhood poverty was also strongly linked to high incidences of TB in New York City.

Two main factors contribute to drug resistant TB. First, the six months period for TB chemotherapy is too long and leads to poor adherence and non-compliance to treatment by patients. Second, public health institutions and medical staff undertake little or no supervision of patients on TB medication.

Over the long-term, both factors contribute to the increasing rate of MDR-TB, XDR-TB, and TDR-TB (Abuzeid et al., 2014).

Ibekwe, Nvau, Oladosu, Usman, Ibrahim and Boshoff et al. (2014) contend that MDR-TB and XDR-TB, which require therapy for up to two full years with multiple second-line drugs, have confounded TB control programmes due to a high percentage of treatment failure. This is because many of the drugs used in the treatment of MDR-TB and XDR-TB have serious toxic side effects. More often than not, HIV/AIDS patients receiving medication for MDR-TB and XDR-TB do not survive.

The rise in the occurrence of strains of *M. tuberculosis* that are resistant to some or all first and second line antibiotics is so worrisome that new anti-TB drugs are urgently needed. Due to the high incidence of TB cases and the low cure rates of MDR-TB and XDR-TB, the discovery of novel antimycobacterial drugs is essential. The hope is to find drugs that effectively block *M. tuberculosis* virulence factors, drugs that stimulate immunity and an overall anti-TB regimen that is rational and shorter in duration.

HIV/TB Co-epidemics are Difficult to Manage

Nowadays, TB is the most significant AIDS-related opportunistic infection (Frothingham et al., 2005). There is synergy between HIV/AIDS and TB (Raviglione, 2003). The twinning of TB to HIV/AIDS, now referred to as the HIV/TB co-epidemic or dual epidemic, is a serious global health challenge. The AIDS epidemic is expanding and most severe in regions of the world that have the highest rates of latent TB infection (Frothingham et al., 2005).

TB is receiving more attention, particularly in developing countries, because of its direct linkage to HIV/AIDS. It is estimated that one-third of the total number of people living with HIV/AIDS worldwide are co-infected with TB (Amoah, Sandjo, Bazzo, Leite, & Biavatti, 2014). And HIV-positive individuals are up to 50 times more likely to develop TB in a given year than those that are HIV-negative (Amoah et al., 2014).

In Ghana, the influence of HIV on TB is increasing. Whereas 14% of TB cases were attributed to HIV in 1989, almost 59% of TB cases were due to the HIV/AIDS epidemic in 2009 (Amoah et al., 2014). Traditional healers in Uganda also believe TB is a defining symptom and opportunistic infection of HIV/AIDS (Mugisha, Asiimwe, Namutebi, Borg-Karlson, & Kakudidi, 2014). According to Fyhrquist et al. (2014), Sub-Saharan Africa accounts for 80% of all HIV-related TB cases globally (WHO, 2010b).

This is how it works. HIV progressively reduces the effectiveness of the immune system and leaves an individual susceptible to infections such as TB (Asiimwe, Kamatenesi-Mugisha, Namutebi, Borg-Karlsson, & Musiimenta,

2013). Persons with HIV infection, when compared to those without HIV infection, are at increased risk of latent TB infection, progression to active TB disease and suffering from more aggressive forms of TB (Frothingham et al., 2005).

HIV infection also promotes the relapse of TB in previously treated patients (Raviglione, 2003). Persons with HIV infection are also at risk of disseminated infection with *Mycobacterium avium* complex, *Mycobacterium kansasii* and other non-tuberculous mycobacteria. Corollary, HIV infection significantly increases TB-associated mortality.

Similarly, TB hastens immune deterioration in those with HIV infection. It makes HIV-infected persons progress faster to AIDS. Essentially, each disease speeds up the progression of the other and TB considerably cuts the survival of people with HIV/AIDS. This makes TB the leading cause of mortality among people living with HIV (Buwa & Afolayan, 2009). Without proper treatment, approximately 90% of those living with HIV die within months of contracting TB (Frothingham et al., 2005).

TB treatment also complicates HIV treatment. Rifampin, an important drug in TB treatment, reduces the blood levels and bioavailability of many antiretroviral drugs (Frothingham et al., 2005). In addition, immune reconstitution syndrome may occur. The signs and symptoms of immune reconstitution may resemble those of active TB disease, raising the spectre of TB treatment failure.

Adding to the negative impact on the individual patient, HIV/TB co-epidemics are much more difficult to control in the population. TB management strategies that are effective in mostly HIV-negative populations may not always work in populations heavily burdened by HIV infection (Frothingham et al., 2005). However, if started early enough, antiretroviral therapy may reduce the cumulative incidence of TB. Only by starting antiretroviral treatment at a much higher CD4 count and combining it with treatment of latent TB infection, can the TB incidence be reduced by an estimated 70% in HIV-infected populations (Frothingham et al., 2005).

TB Therapy and Management

Before the advent of effective TB chemotherapy, the social stigma of TB was on a par with that of mental disease, as TB was regarded as a disgrace on the entire family (Bryder, 1988). In the 19th century, cod-liver oil was administered in Europe as a preventive measure for childhood TB (Ralph et al., 2013). One or two tablespoons taken 2-4 times daily provided a weight gain benefit to TB patients.

Heliotherapy using filtered sunlight and ultraviolet radiation was the most popular TB treatment method in Europe and the United States of America until the era of antibiotics (Ralph et al., 2013). Vitamin D was also used in the treatment of disseminated TB with a 1948 case report describing success after daily oral administration of cholecalciferol (vitamin D_3). In the second half of the 20th century, vitamin D was replaced by antibiotics.

Since the 1950s, the standard first-line therapy for TB involves a two-month treatment with a combination of rifampicin, isoniazid, ethambutol and pyrazinamide; followed by treatment with a combination of rifampicin and isoniazid for an additional four months (Alvin, Miller, & Neilan, 2014). The patient is considered cured at six months. For latent TB, the standard treatment is 6-9 months of isoniazid alone.

There are also second-line drugs for the treatment of TB: Aminoglycosides, polypeptides, fluoroquinolones, thionamides, cycloserine and p-aminosalicylic acid. A drug is classed as second-line instead of first-line for one of two possible reasons: It may be less effective than the first-line drugs (e.g. p-aminosalicylic acid), or it may have toxic side-effects (e.g. cycloserine).

Unfortunately, stringent supervision to ensure compliance is not always availed to patients receiving TB therapy, particularly in poor and high burden countries in Asia and Africa. In these countries, health infrastructure and staff are too inadequate to meet the humongous demands of TB control. As previously explained, incomplete treatment of the disease causes the development of drug-resistant TB (Alvin et al., 2014).

The push for effective TB treatment reached a head-start in 1993 when WHO declared TB a global emergency. The new declaration was embroidered by the introduction of the Directly Observed Treatment Short-course programmes (DOTS) strategy (De Cock & Chaisson, 1999). Five elements are essential to the success of TB treatment under DOTS: Political commitment, microscopy services, drug supplies, surveillance and monitoring systems, and use of drugs with direct observation of treatment.

However, most TB control programmes fail because one or more of these requirements are missing. In fact, despite successful implementation of most of the elements of this strategy in several African countries and settings, TB case rates continue to escalate where the prevalence of HIV infection is high. Plus, treatment of TB and HIV/AIDS is complicated by adverse drug interactions.

The number of drugs currently in use against *M. tuberculosis* is very limited and most of them were introduced more than 40 years ago. Madikizela et al. (2014a) bemoaned that immunization of neonates with *Bacillus* Calmette Guérin (BCG) mainly protects against TB meningitis and miliary TB. However, the efficacy wanes 10–15 years post-vaccination, thus adults are not protected against pulmonary TB.

Since the release of rifampicin in 1976, only rifabutin and rifapentine have been approved for TB treatment. Unfortunately, these drugs have not yet achieved extended distribution for clinical application (León-Díaz, Meckes-Fischer, Valdovinos-Martínez, Campos, Hernández-Pando, & Jiménez-Arellanes, 2013). In 2012, a new anti-TB drug, TMC207 (or R207910), was approved by the United States of America's Food and Drug Administration (FDA). TMC207 is the first anti-TB drug in four decades with a new mechanism of action, specifically inhibiting ATP synthase (Ganihigama et al., 2015). Since it catalyses the first step in the pathway for the biosynthesis of branched-chain amino acids, acetohydroxyacid synthase is also a potential drug target against *M. tuberculosis* (Wang, Pan, Cao, Lei, Meng, & He et al., 2012).

Ibekwe et al. (2014) concede that though there are many efforts being made to discover new drugs to treat TB, these efforts are not a major focus for many pharmaceutical companies. The reasons for the lack tangible investments by industry are mainly economic, because countries in dire need of new anti-TB drugs are primarily poor, meaning people cannot afford expensive drugs developed by heavily capitalized industries.

To reduce TB cases in developing countries especially in rural communities where healthcare systems are generally weak or inadequate, new models of public-private partnerships have been suggested (Asuquo, Pokam, Adindu, Ibeneme, Ekpereonne, & Obot, 2015). Other reports by Bunalema, Obakiro, Tabuti and Waako (2014) also stress the importance of developing a new battery of drugs to curb resistant TB strains.

An anti-TB drug regime is considered successful if it meets the following requirements: It kills all mycobacteria, prevents patient relapse after cessation of treatment and avoids the development of drug resistant TB (Alvin et al., 2014). As there are naturally occurring drug-resistant mycobacteria at any stage of the infection, it is practically impossible to treat TB with a single drug (Alvin et al., 2014).

The reality on the ground is that majority TB patients only go to hospital after several attempts at self-medication. Inertia to seek hospital-based treatment is exacerbated by the non-specificity of the principal symptoms in addition to the use of traditional medicines (Dodor, 2012). Amoah et al. (2014) found that although a large proportion of people with TB go to the hospitals, many cases are lost due to the inadequacy of diagnostic methods.

In Ghana, for example, the sputum smear microscopy or alcohol-acid resistant bacilli test is the main laboratory method used for the diagnosis of TB but only one laboratory is available per 100,000 people. Elsewhere, to speed up the detection of TB, honeybees and giant African rats have been trained to sense *M. tuberculosis* signature compounds (methyl *p*-anisate and methyl phenylacetate) in sputum (Suckling & Sagar, 2011).

Also, although 1.8% of the new cases of TB and 19% of cases of retreatment are for MDR-TB, there is no second-line treatment as only first-line drugs (rifampicin, isoniazid, pyrazinamide and ethambutol) are available (Amoah et al., 2014). Culture tests and tuberculostatic drugs sensitivity tests are not performed. Therefore, it is difficult to determine if the infectious agent is only *M. tuberculosis* or not (Amoah et al., 2014).

According to Abuzeid et al. (2014), the emergence of multi-drug resistant strains of *M. tuberculosis* underscores the need for continuous development of new and efficient methods to determine the susceptibility of isolates of *M. tuberculosis* in the search for novel antimycobacterial agents. Natural products constitute an important source of new drugs and design and implementation of anti-mycobacterial susceptibility testing methods are necessary to evaluate the different extracts and compounds.

Current challenges surrounding TB treatment regimens, especially growing cases of drug resistance and HIV-TB co-infection, point to the urgent need for novel treatment strategies. Innovative approaches to reduce treatment durations include the development of new anti-mycobacterial agents from natural products, a priority area for any TB research and development initiative (Abuzeid et al., 2014).

In the search for new drugs, the plant kingdom is undoubtedly the most valuable resource to 'pharm' for new anti-TB agents. Pauli, Case, Inui, Wang, Cho, Fischer and Franzblau (2005) submit that the challenge of discovering new anti-TB drugs from natural sources requires an interdisciplinary research enterprise. To operationalize this enterprise, cutting-edge mycobacteriology coupled with innovative tools of natural products chemistry have to be developed and employed in tandem.

Pharmacognosy: The Search for New Anti-TB Drugs

As early as 1985, Norman R. Farnsworth, one of the pioneers of pharmacognosy- the study of traditional medicines, had already stated that 119 compounds extracted from 90 plants were utilized as single entity medicinal agents (Farnsworth, Akerele, Bingel, Soejarto, & Guo, 1985). Above all, 77% of these compounds were obtained through ethnomedicinal knowledge of the plant as used by the traditional knowledge holders. This motif underscores the motivation to analyze traditional medicinal plants for new anti-TB drugs.

The need for new drugs to treat *M. tuberculosis* infection has never been more urgent. The rapid and persistent development of drug-resistant TB has reinvigorated the push for new bioprospecting efforts that may usher in new drugs that can replace the ones to which *M. tuberculosis* has become resistant. Plants hold the promise for the future of TB management.

There are three principle pathways toward the discovery of new pharmacologically significant compounds against TB (Farnsworth et al., 1985): Rational drug design, where the drug is purposefully tailored to fight specific virulence targets in *M. tuberculosis*; combinatorial chemistry, which involves synthesis of a combinatorial library of compounds, which are then tested against the mycobacterial target to determine the most potent compounds; and natural products chemistry whereby bioactive compounds are isolated from biological materials.

The third option is most appealing because nature contains millions of unique and diverse anti-infective chemical agents. Indeed, natural products may pave the way for new anti-TB drug leads, since they provide an unlimited source of chemically diverse compounds (Abuzeid et al., 2014). The record is straight-forward. In the last 20 years, nearly 50% of drugs approved by the FDA in the United States of America have been derivatives of natural products (Uc-Cachón, Borges-Argáez, Said-Fernández, Vargas-Villarreal, González-Salazar, & Méndez-González et al., 2014).

Green, Samie, Obi, Bessong Ndip (2010) assert that chemical compounds isolated from plants play an important role in the discovery of drugs against infectious diseases. Cragg Newman (2013) also suggest that nearly 75% of all the approved anti-infective drugs are derived from medicinal plants. The evidence for anti-infective chemical agents from natural products is unequivocal. Also unequivocal is the successful inhibition of *M. tuberculosis* by extracts from ethnobotanically-selected plants (Boligon, Piana, Kubiça, Mario, Dalmolin, & Bonez et al., 2014).

Natural remedies, especially those derived from ethnomedicinal plants, are still being used worldwide in the management of TB. Data on the efficacy of ethnobotanicals against *M. tuberculosis* are available (Mohamad, Zin, Wahab, Ibrahim, Sulaiman, Zahariluddin, & Noor, 2011). Herbal constituents like iridoids, terpenes, citronellol, nerol and geraniol have shown anti-mycobacterial activities (Kumar, Singh, Sharma, Singh, Dobhal, & Singh, 2013). Suffice to state that experts now support the general motif that selecting plants based on ethnobotanical criteria enhances the probability of finding species with anti-TB activity.

Through the ethnobotanical survey approach, more than 300 novel antitubercular agents were identified and characterized from biological sources between 2003 and 2005 (Copp & Pearce, 2007); another 450 novel compounds were identified from 2006 to 2009 (Salomon & Schmidt, 2012). Ethnobotanical knowledge has led to large-scale bioprospecting programmes and the isolation of novel bioactive compounds. In South Africa, where a large bioprospecting programme is hosted by several research institutions, over 350 plant species used in traditional medicine have been assessed for their anti-TB activities (Eldeen & van Staden, 2007).

According to Alvin et al. (2014), natural products play an essential role in the treatment of TB. The global efforts to decrease the incidence of TB, juxtaposed with the unfortunate development of resistant strains, has increased interest in natural products as sources of novel anti-tubercular compounds, say these authors. Since the year 2000, several new candidate anti-mycobacterial agents including extracts and pure compounds from plants and microorganisms have been added to the anti-TB pharmacopoeia (Newton, Lau, & Wright, 2000).

Plant availability is a limiting factor in the commercial success of some natural products. At times, a large quantity of plant material is required to produce sufficient amounts of the bioactive compounds for clinical use. In other cases, compounds have been isolated from endangered or highly endemic plants. Harvesting of roots and stem bark also threatens the survival of certain plants. These issues bring into the limelight the major conservation concerns surrounding the unsustainable harvesting of medicinal plants. Innovations in plant biotechnology and plant tissue culture offer new hopes of producing anti-TB agents without endangering existing floral diversity, but the cost of such production methods is high, especially in developing countries.

Endophytes: The New Frontier for Non-Cytotoxic Anti-Mycobacterial Agents

There is increasing optimism that novel anti-TB chemical agents could be sourced from endophytes, microorganisms that form a symbiotic relationship with their host plants and function as biological defence agents against foreign phytopathogens (Alvin et al., 2014). Endophytes secrete chemical metabolites to thwart antagonists or lyse pathogen-infected cells. Some of the defensive secondary metabolites secreted by endophytes may have beneficial anti-TB medicinal properties.

The hopes of manufacturing novel anti-TB drugs derived from endophytic secretions are not misplaced because antibiotics and anti-cancer drugs (Taxol from the endophytic fungi *Taxomyces andreanae*) are already being co-produced by endophytes and plants (Strobel, 2003). Undoubtedly, an exciting prospect for mitigating the unstainable and indiscriminate use of plant products as sources of anti-TB agents is the discovery that endophytes could in fact produce bioactive compounds against TB.

From a production standpoint, it is much easier to scale up the fermentation process of endophytic microorganisms, and thus, allowing large-scale production of biologically active compounds to meet large industrial demands for anti-TB drug production. Endophytes, therefore, not only present an exciting opportunity to discover a plethora of anti-mycobacterial compounds but also offer a renewable source of natural products as anti-TB agents.

Vermelhotin, a natural tetramic acid isolated from endophytic fungi, is highly active against clinical strains of MDR-TB, MIC of 1.5-12.5 µg/ml (Ganihigama et al., 2015). In addition, there were 28 novel anti-mycobacterial compounds isolated from endophytic organisms between 2008 and 2012. Of these, 11 were polyketides or polyketide-derived and 10 were small peptides; all of them showed activity against TB.

Nocardithiocin, a peptide produced by the endophyte *Nocardia pseudobrasiliensis* has a MIC value of 0.025 µg/ml against *M. tuberculosis* H37Rv (Mukai, Fukai, Hoshino, Yazawa, Harada, & Mikami, 2009). Extracts of 92 isolates of endophytic fungi inhibited the growth of *M. tuberculosis* H37Ra at MIC values of 0.0625–200 µg/ml (Alvin et al., 2014). The chemical 3-nitropropionic acid is a potent anti-mycobacterial agent isolated from endophytic fungi (Chomcheon, Wiyakrutta, Sriubolmas, Ngamrojanavanich, Isarangkul, & Kittakoop, 2005).

The symbiotic nature of plant-endophyte relationships means that bioactive compounds secreted by endophytes are less likely to be cytotoxic to eukaryotic cells (Alvin et al., 2014). This is significantly important to the pharmaceutical community because drugs developed from such compounds may not adversely affect human cells. The potential of anti-TB drug discovery from endophytes associated with traditional medicinal plants is immense, observed Alvin et al. (2014). Going forwards, if the fight against drug resistant TB is to be won, endophytes should be taken to the battle front.

Common Natural Products

Some common plants contain chemical ingredients which may relieve TB infection. Here, we look at a few common plants whose ingredients have anti-mycobaterial activities: *Hypericum perforatum* (St. John's Wort), green tea, *Curcuma longa*, miswak, champa, marijuana, sweet basil, honey/propolis and *Vernonia* species.

Hyperenone A, present in extracts of the aerial parts of *Hypericum acmosepalum*, a very close relative of *H. perforatum* (St John's Wort), inhibits the growth of *M. tuberculosis* H37Rv and *Mycobacterium bovis* BCG at 75 mg/L and 100 mg/L, respectively (Osman, Evangelopoulos, Basavannacharya, Gupta, McHugh, Bhakta, & Gibbons, 2012). Many *Hypericum* species contain phloroglucinols, anthraquinones, xanthones and filicilic acid derivatives. The last group of compounds has potent antimycobacterial activity (Nogueira, Medeiros, Marcelo-Curto, García-Pérez, Luna-Herrera, & Costa, 2013). Some of these principle chemicals are undergoing clinical trials.

213

Catechins mostly present in green tea may also alleviate TB symptoms. Patients who receive catechins show increased levels of superoxide dismutase (SOD), an enzyme that inhibits the production of hydrogen peroxide through the dismutation reaction. Catechins have strong anti-superoxide formation effect, by scavenging superoxide anion (Agarwal et al., 2010). These findings suggest that crude green tea catechin extracts may play a definite role as adjuvant therapy in pulmonary TB patients.

Curcumin [1,7-bis(4-hydroxy-3-methoxy phenyl)-1,6- heptadiene-3,5-dione] is a phenolic compound. It was originally extracted from the plant *Curcuma longa*, the primary component of the ubiquitous dietary spice turmeric. For centuries, various Asian societies have used curcumin as a traditional medicine to treat numerous disorders. Studies now show that curcumin exhibits anti-mycobacterial activity (Baldwin et al., 2015).

Curcumin has antioxidant, anti-cancer and anti-inflammatory properties but is non-cytotoxic to normal human cells. These properties make curcumin a very attractive chemical ingredient to alleviate TB, though it is relatively unstable and beset by poor bioavailability. The anti-TB action of curcumin is due to its ability to induce the cell death of macrophages (Li, Wang, Huang, Shi, Wan, Wang, & Xi 2014).

Salvadora persica, also known as the miswak plant, is commonly used as a chewing stick for improved oral health. At the School of Traditional Medicine situated at the Shahid Beheshti University of Medical Sciences in Tehran, Iran, scientists have shown that extracts of miswak inhibit the growth of *M. bovis* (Fallah, Fallah, Kamalinejad, Malekan, Akhlaghi, & Esmaeili, 2014). Whether miswak extracts are also effective against *M. tuberculosis* is not exactly clear.

Another excellent anti-mycobacterial agent is plumericin, a phyto-ingredient of *Plumeria bicolor*, commonly known as champa in India (Kumar et al., 2013). Against four MDR strains of *M. tuberculosis*, plumericin performs better than the standard drugs rifampicin and isoniazid; MIC values of 1.3 to 2 μg/ml. *Plumeria bicolor* is also grown in Indonesia, the Philippines and South Africa.

Semenya, Potgieter, Tshisikhawe, Shava, and Maroyi (2012) cite studies where *Cannabis sativa* leaves (marijuana) are used by the Zulu people in South Africa to lighten the burden of TB. Leaves of *C. sativa*, also known as *Mopatse* in the local Pedi language of South Africa, are macerated in warm water overnight and one cup of decoction is taken orally three times a day as a remedy for TB (Semenya et al., 2012). As seen earlier, marijuana has anti-HIV activity, too.

Ocimum basilicum (family Lamiaceae) commonly known as sweet basil and tulsi is a herbaceous, perennial plant native to Asia, Africa and South America but widely cultivated in other parts of the world (Jayaweera, 1981). Siddiqui, Bhatti, Begum and Perwaiz (2012) cite studies where the oil of *O. basilicum* is said to have antibacterial and antifungal properties. Thymol, a well-known anti-septic agent found in mouthwashes, is the main active ingredient of *O. basilicum* (Dikshit & Husain, 1984).

Extracts of *O. basilicum* leaves not only display broncho-dilatory action but also inhibit the proliferation of *Mycobaterium smegmatis* (Boskabady, Kaini, & Haghiri, 2005). Even more, Siddiqui et al. (2012) verified that nine *O. basilicum* compounds inhibit the growth of *M. tuberculosis*. A new compound named Bacilicin inhibits the growth of *M. tuberculosis* H37Rv by at least 49%, MIC 6.25 µg/mL.

In Thailand, honey and propolis, generally used to treat coughs, are natural products that work against drug resistant *Staphylococcus* and *M. tuberculosis* (Chanchao, 2013). Toyang and Verpoorte's (2013) review of the medicinal plants in the genus *Vernonia* shows that traditional healers in India and many African countries harness *Vernonia adoensis* as a natural remedy for TB, cough, gonorrhoea and HIV/AIDS. Many people harvest *Vernonia amygdalina*, *Vernonia cinerea*, *Vernonia kotschyana* and *Vernonia saligna* for use in TB treatment.

African Pharmacopoeia

In Uganda, TB is known by different names in the various languages (Tabuti et al., 2010): *akafuba* (Baganda language), *olukololo* (Basoga language), *ekitundu* (Bafumbira languuage) and *lokudi* (Karimajong language). In general, the disease is locally known as *akakonko*. TB in Uganda is frequently treated using *Albizia coriaria* (Asiimwe et al., 2013) and *V. amygdalina* (Tabuti et al., 2010). Table 6.1 shows plants used in the management of TB in Uganda (Bunalema et al., 2014).

Ugandan traditional healers frequently use the following plants: *Zanthoxylum leprieurii*, *Piptadeniastrum africanum*, *Mangifera indica*, *A. coriaria* and *Rubia cordifolia* (Bunalema et al., 2014; Mugisha et al., 2014). Some of the plants contain active compounds with known anti-TB action. For example, ellagitannin punicalagin isolated from *Combretum molle*, allicin from *Allium sativum* and anthraquinone glycosides (also known as aloin) from *Aloe vera* are active against various strains of *M. tuberculosis*.

Kigelia africana fruit extracts were for the first time shown to have activity against *Mycobacterium aurum* (Fomogne-Fodjo et al., 2014). The fruits of *K. africana* contain several chemical ingredients: iridoids (jiofuran, jioglutide, ajugol and verminoside), phenylpropanoid and phenylethanoid derivatives, a flavonoid glycoside, β-sitosterol and three fatty acids with palmitic acid being the main one. Iridoids, sterols and flavonoids inhibit *M. tuberculosis*.

A couple of studies in South Africa have elucidated the anti-TB activity of local plants: Lall and Meyer (1999); Seidel and Taylor (2004); Mativandlela, Lall and Meyer (2006); Eldeen and van Staden (2007); McGaw, Lall, Meyer and Eloff (2008); and Green, Samie, Obi, Bessong and Ndip (2010).

In KwaZulu-Natal, South Africa, a survey report by York, De Wet and Van Vuuren (2011) revealed the following nine plants were part of the folk remedies for TB: *Acanthospermum glabratum*, *Clematis brachiata*, *Cyperus articulatus*, *Euphorbia tirucalli*, *Helichrysum kraussii*, *Parinari capensis*, *Plectranthus neochilus*, *Senecio deltoideus* and *Terminalia sericea*. The study also showed that other putative anti-TB plants were: *C. molle*, *Ekebergia capensis*, *Lippia javanica*, *Psidium guajava*, *Scadoxis puniceus*, *Senecio serratulloides*, *Syzygium cordatum* and *Tetradenia riparia*.

McGaw et al. (2008) reviewed the potential of South African plants against TB. They stated that about 180 species were employed for alleviating TB and related symptoms. Of those, around 30% had actually been screened for anti-mycobacterial activity. Some of the screened plants are listed in Table 6.2. An ethanol extract of the South African plant *Euclea natalensis* contains a compound called shinanolone, active against *M. tuberculosis* (MIC = 100 µg/ml). Several naphthoquinones and triterpenes isolated from a chloroform extract of *E. natalensis* also showed good anti-mycobacterial activity. The Zulu people in Umtentweni area of KwaZulu-Natal Province use *Boophone disticha* bulb decoctions, endowed with three alkaloids (galanthamine, lycorine, and crinine) to treat TB (Nair & van Staden, 2014).

However, four South African plants have lower MIC values against *M. tuberculosis*: *Berchemia discolor*, 12.5 µg/ml on H37Ra and 10.5 µg/ml on a clinical isolate; *Bridelia micrantha* (25 µg/ml on H37Ra), *Warburgia salutaris* (25 µg/ml on H37Ra) and *T. sericea* (25 µg/ml) on both H37Ra and clinical isolate (Green et al., 2010). Laboratory assays confirmed that acetone extracts of *B. discolor*, *B. micrantha*, *T. sericea* and *W. salutaris* may be important sources of chemical compounds against multidrug-resistant *M. tuberculosis*. York, Van Vuuren and De Wet (2012) observed that *T. sericea* bark had weak activity against *M. smegmatis* (0.67 mg/ml).

Bridelia micrantha contains compounds including friedelin, epi-friedelin and phenolic derivatives such as gallic acid, ellagic acids, anthocyanidin, taraxerol, taraxerone, caffeic acid and flavonoids thought to have anti-TB functions (Green et al., 2010). Compounds isolated from *T. sericea* include termilignan B and arjunic acid. Organic root and bark extracts of *T. sericea* were active against *M. aurum* with MIC ranging from 1.56 to 3.12 mg/ml (Eldeen & van Staden, 2007).

South African plants *Abrus precatorius* subsp. *africanus*, *Ficus sur*, *Pentanisia prunelloides* and *Terminalia phanerophlebia*, with MIC values less than 1.0 mg/ml, have good anti-TB activity (Madikizela, Aderogba, Finnie, & van Staden, 2014b). One compound identified as 1,6-di-O-coumaroyl glucopyranoside, isolated from *T. phanerophlebia* for the first time, inhibited *M. tuberculosis* at a noteworthy MIC value of 63 µg/ml (Madikizela et al., 2014b). The novel compound 1,6-di-O-coumaroyl glucopyranoside can serve as a lead compound for TB drug discovery.

Ntutela, Smith, Matika, Mukinda, Arendse and Allie et al. (2009), working at the Institute of Infectious Disease and Molecular Medicine in Cape Town, South Africa, demonstrated that *Artemisia afra* contains *in vitro* antimycobacterial chemical agents that modulate pulmonary inflammation in early TB infection. An organic fraction of *A. afra* reduces replication of *M. aurum* and *M. tuberculosis* in a dose-dependent manner with IC_{50} values of 1.9 µg/ml and 2.0 µg/ml, respectively; MIC of 10 µg/ml.

There are also exotic plants used as natural medicines for TB by the Bapedi traditional healers of South Africa (Semenya et al., 2012): *Eriobotrya japonica*, has anti-inflammation activity; *Eucalyptus camaldulensis*, anti-proliferative properties; and *Ficus carica* contains phenolic compounds, phytosterols and fatty acids. *Carica papaya* leaves have anti-mycobacterial activity *in vitro*, revealed Green et al. (2010).

TB is managed by using the following natural medicines (Rood, 2013): Infusion of *Pharnaceum lineare*, bark decoction of *Rauvolfia caffra* (quinine tree, kinaboom) and powdered dry leaves of *Asclepias fruticosa* (a poisonous plant commonly called milkweed, melkbos, gansiebos or kapokbossie), used as a snuff for TB treatment. Other anti-TB remedies are *Helichrysum pedunculatum* leaves, brewed like tea and drunk, *Symphytum officinale* (comfrey, rich in vitamin B12 and calcium) extract is drunk, *Nasturtium officinale*, *Acacia nilotica* root extract, *Ceratonia siliqua* (carob) leaf extract is an expectorant or cough remedy, root extract of *Glycyrrhiza glabra* (liquorice root), *Sutherlandia microphylla* (kalkoenbos) leaf powder mixed with syrup is taken to alleviate symptoms and *Perlargonium ramosissimum* weak tincture made from leaf extract is drunk; it has to be weak because strong tincture upsets stomach.

Rood (2013) also noted other natural remedies for TB: Drinking the sap from leaves of *Agave americana* (century plant), root extract of *Bulbine asphodeloides* (copaiva), mixture of honey and olive oil and juice squeezed from *Carpobrotus edulis*, extract of bark and roots of *Ficus sur* (broom cluster-fig), leaf extract from *Nylandtia spinosa* (tortoise berry, formerly *Mundia spinosa*), large doses of root extract of *Thesium hystrix*, and extracts from the leaf tips of *Dodonaea angustifolia* (sand olive).

Tanzanian species of *Terminalia* show antimycobacterial effects when tested on the model organism *M. smegmatis* ATCC 14468 (Fyhrquist et al., 2014). In their study, Fyhrquist and co-workers reported for the first time the antimycobacterial efficacies of root and stem bark extracts of *Terminalia sambesiaca* and *Terminalia kaiserana* as well as the fruit extracts of *Terminalia stenostachya* and leaf extracts of *Terminalia spinosa*.

Terminalia species contain several active chemical compounds including ellagitannins, ellagic acid derivates, gallotannins and condensed tannins that inhibit mycobacteria. But Fyhrquist et al. (2014) sound caution in the use of *Terminalia* as medicinal plants because some condensed tannins from *Terminalia* are very toxic, for example terminalin A, which is present in *Terminalia oblongata*.

Using a luminometry-based method to screen Sudanese plants for antimycobacterial activity, Abuzeid et al. (2014) found that *Khaya senegalensis* (bark and leaves) and *Rosmarinus officinalis* (leaves) were potent at concentrations as low as 6.25 µg/ml. Plants from Central Africa had good antimycobacterial action, MIC values below 130 µg/ml: *Xylopia aethiopica*, *Desmodium velutinum* (stems), *Desmodium salicifolium* (leaves), *Crinum purpurascens*, *Cyathula prostrate* and *Albizia ferruginea* (Fomogne-Fodjo et al., 2014). Again, these species were selected based on the indigenous knowledge by the Bakola pygmies living along the Ngoyang area in Cameroon, who have used these plants for the treatment of respiratory and TB-related symptoms.

Tekwu, Askun, Kuete, Nkengfack, Nyasse, Etoa and Beng (2012), while studying 15 Cameroonian plant extracts with variable activity against *M. tuberculosis* strains, determined that *Echinops giganteus*, whose common name is giant Japanese butterbur, exhibited the most significant antimycobacterial activity with a MIC value of 32 µg/ml and 16 µg/ml against strains H37Ra and H37Rv, respectively. *Echinops giganteus* has known antibacterial activity (Kuete, 2010).

In Nigeria, traditional healers use indigenous ethnomedicinal recipes for the management of TB and related ailments. Ibekwe et al. (2014) studied the antimycobacterial activity of many Nigerian plants. Their results show that *Abrus precatorius*, which contains an isoflavanoid quinone (abruquinone), has a MIC value of 12.5 µg/ml against *M. tuberculosis* strain H37Rv. *Anogeissus leocarpa*, the most commonly used plant among the Nigerian herbalists, contains polyphenols and triterpenoids; it has a MIC value 266 µg/ml against *M. bovis*. Anthraquinone and poly-phenolic flavonoids (1-epicatechol and leucopelargonidol) contribute to the anti-*Mycobaterium* activity of *Cassia siberiana*.

Ibekwe et al. (2014) also found that *C. molle* which contains punicalgin has a MIC value of 600 µg/ml against *M. tuberculosis* strain ATCC 27294 and a drug-resistant clinical isolate. A hydroxycycloartenol glycoside by the name of mollic acid is present in the leaves of *C. molle*. *Erythrina senegalensis* contains isoflavonoids (pasellidin and erythobissin) with MIC values of 8-25 µg/mL against *M. tuberculosis*. *Pterocarpus osun* has glycosides, saponins, steroids and tannins which confer antimycobacterial activity. *Securidaca longepedunculata* methanol and hexane extracts yielded hydroxybenzoic acids and xanthones, with MICs of 312 µg/ml and 1250 µg/ml, respectively, against *M. tuberculosis*.

In Mozambique, *Zanthoxylum capense* (family Rutaceae) is a medicinal plant harvested by the local people to treat TB. Laboratory assays bared promising antimycobacterial potential of *Z. capense* extracts on a range of mycobacterial strains. Luo, Pires, Ainsa, Gracia, Duarte and Mulhovo et al. (2013) have now isolated benzophenanthridine-type alkaloids and neolignans from this plant. Decarine, a benzophenanthridine alkaloid, showed good activity against *M. tuberculosis* H37Rv (MIC of 1.6 µg/ml) and low macrophage cytotoxicity ($IC_{50} >$ 60 µg/ml), indicating considerable selective activity. It goes without saying that the high *in vitro* and *ex vivo* antimycobacterial activity of decarine and the low cytotoxicity towards human macrophages make it a very valuable lead scaffold for the development of new anti-TB drugs.

Still working on Mozambican plants, Luo, Pires, Aínsa, Gracia, Mulhovo and Duarte et al. (2011) discovered that n-hexane extracts of *Maerua edulis* and *S. longepedunculata*, ethyl acetate extract of *Tabernaemontana elegans* and dichloromethane extract of *Z. capense* have considerable activity against *M. bovis* BCG and *M. tuberculosis* H37Ra with MIC values of 15.6–62.5 µg/ml. An ethyl acetate extract of *T. elegans*, though potently cytotoxic, displays strong activity against *M. tuberculosis* H37Rv (MIC 15.6 µg/ml).

In Gabon, where 53% of patients with HIV/AIDS have TB, the scientific (and local) names of plants used to treat TB are (Tchouya, Souza, Tchouankeu, Yala, Boukandou, & Foundikou et al., 2015): *Musanga cecropioides* (*Moghombo*), *Scyphocephalium ochocoa* (*Otsoko*) and *Costus afer* (*Moandu*).

The twinning of HIV/AIDS to TB requires the use of plants that work against dual infection. While studying the secondary data of plants harnessed as anti-HIV/AIDS remedies in Africa, Maroyi (2015) found that several plants with anti-HIV activity also simultaneously alleviate TB symptoms. Notably, anti-HIV plus anti-TB plants were: *Crinum macowani* and *Tulbaghia violacea*, have proven anti-HIV activity and are used to treat TB in South Africa; *Cascabela thevetia* inhibits HIV-1 and treats TB in Uganda; *Warburgia ugandensis*, a known inhibitor of HIV-1 reverse transcriptase and protease, is a natural remedy for TB in Uganda and Tanzania; and *C. papaya* which has proven anti-HIV activity, is a remedy for TB in Tanzania.

Other anti-HIV and anti-TB plants were (Maroyi, 2015): *Maytenus senegalensis* with known anti-HIV action, is also harvested for use in TB treatment in Uganda and Tanzania; *Garcinia buchananii* and *Garcinia livingstonei*, both block HIV-1 protease, are also natural remedies for TB in Namibia and Tanzania (Chinsembu & Hedimbi, 2012); *C. molle*, a known inhibitor of HIV-1 reverse transcriptase, is harnessed as an anti-TB herbal in Uganda; *Euphorbia tirucalli*, has anti-HIV activity, is a natural remedy for TB in Uganda; *Ricinus communis*, a plant with known anti-HIV reverse transcriptase action, is a treatment for TB in South Africa and Tanzania.

219

There are other dual action anti-HIV/TB plants: *Peltophorum africanum*, which inhibits HIV-1 reverse transcriptase is a treatment for TB in South Africa; *Hypoxis hemerocallidea*, blocks HIV-1 reverse transcriptase, is also a remedy for TB in South Africa; *Plectranthus amboinicus*, blocks HIV-1 reverse transcriptase and is a treatment for TB in Uganda; *Morella salicifolia*, blocks HIV-1 transcriptase and protease, also alleviates TB in Tanzania; *P. guajava* has known anti-HIV activity, alleviates TB in Namibia (Chinsembu & Hedimbi, 2010), Uganda and Tanzania; *Flueggea virosa*, a known inhibitor of HIV replication, alleviates TB in Uganda; *S. longipedunculata* inhibits HIV replication, is an anti-TB plant in Ethiopia; and *Zingiber officinale* (ginger), with known anti-HIV activity, is an anti-TB remedy in Uganda (Maroyi, 2015).

Caution should be taken as some of the plants used to treat TB are cytotoxic to human cells. Southern African plants applied as natural remedies for TB yet are known to be toxic include *Asclepias fruticosa*, *Gnidia kraussiana*, *Melianthus comosus* and *T. violacea* (Ndhlala, Ncube, Okem, Mulaudzi, & van Staden, 2013). According to these authors, symptoms of toxicity may include fever, paralysis, respiratory problems, weak heartbeat, irritation of the nose and throat, coughing, sneezing, headache, nausea, salivation, foaming vomit, gastrointestinal disturbance, purging, exhaustion, cardiac arrest and dizziness.

European Pharmacopoeia

In Turkey, Askun et al. (2009) determined that *Thymbra spicata* var. *spicata*, traded under the Turkish name of *Karakekik* (black kekik), exhibits a high level of activity against *M. tuberculosis* (MIC = 196 µg/ml). Carvacrol, rosmarinic acid, hesperidin and naringenin are the major phenolic compounds in *T. spicata* var. *spicata*. Though carvacrol and rosmarinic acid are known to possess antibacterial activity, the latter may be responsible for the anti-mycobacterial efficacy (Askun et al., 2009).

Fifteen *Hypericum* species growing in mainland Portugal, Azores and Madeira were tested for antimycobacterial activity. *Hypericum elodes* and *Hypericum hircinum* subsp. *majus* extracts were the most active against MDR-TB strains with MIC of 25–100 µg/ml (Nogueira et al., 2013). Both *Hypericum* species exhibited significant efficacy against MDR-TB clinical isolates.

Hypericin and pseudo-hypericin (both are anthraquinones) and hyperforin were effective against all the drug-resistant *Mycobacterium* strains and some of the clinical isolates with MIC values of 25-50 µg/ml (Nogueira et al., 2013). However, only hyperforin showed activity against the strain *M. tuberculosis* H37Rv, MIC of 25 µg/ml (Nogueira et al., 2013). Nogueira and co-workers have a patent on *Hypericum* chemical substances useful for the treatment of persistent tuberculosis.

In the United Kingdom, *Arctium lappa* (burdock) is a biennial herbaceous plant traditionally used for its diuretic, carminative, anti-inflammatory, antiseptic and detoxifying properties. *Tussilago farfara* (coughwort) is a perennial herbaceous plant used to treat sore throats and lung ailments such as bronchitis, asthma and chronic cough including TB (Allen & Hatfield, 2004). Zhao, Evangelopoulos, Bhakta, Gray and Seidel (2014) found that the n-hexane extracts of both plants, the ethyl acetate extract of *T. farfara* and the dichloromethane phase derived from the methanol extract of *A. lappa* displayed anti-tubercular activity (MIC 62.5 μg/ml). Best anti-TB actions were exhibited by p-coumaric acid (MIC 31.3 μg/ml) and 4-hydroxybenzoic acid (MIC 62.5 μg/ml) isolated from both plants.

Anti-TB Natural Products in Asia

Indonesia is home to some of the largest tropical rainforests in the world. The country has one of the world's largest floral diversities with 40,000 different plant species- 16,500 of which are endemic and two of the world's 25 biodiversity hotspots found in Sundaland and Wallacea regions. Of these plant species, approximately 10% are believed to possess some medicinal characteristics, thus are utilized as traditional herbal medicine, popularly known as *Jamu* (Schumacher, 1999). Alvin et al. (2014) listed the following Indonesian *Jamu* plants used to treat TB symptoms: *Andrographis paniculata*, *Brucea javanica*, *Caesalpinia sappan*, *Centella asiatica*, *Hibiscus tiliaceus*, *Hibiscus tiliaceus*, *Lantana camara*, *Morinda citrifolia*, *Nasturtium indicum*, *Pluchea indica*, *Rhoeo spathacea*, *R. communis* and *Vitex trifolia*.

In Taiwan, work by Chen, Huang, Sun, Chiang, Chiang, Tsai and Weng (2011) revealed that cinnamic acid, a natural occurring phenolic plant compound, decreased the viability of MDR-TB bacilli in a dose-dependent way. Their results showed the anti-tuberculosis activity of cis-cinnamic acid was approximately 120-fold that of trans-cinnamic acid. Against TB, cis-cinnamic acid exhibited higher synergistic effect with isoniazid and rifampicin than trans-cinnamic acid.

The plants *Albizia lebbeck*, *Artemisia absinthium*, *Ephedra gerardiana*, *Ephedra intermedia*, *Fragaria indica*, *Inula obtusifolia* and *Punica granatum* are employed in the treatment of TB in the communities of Gallies Abbottabad, northern Pakistan (Kayani, Ahmad, Zafar, Sultana, Khan, & Ashraf et al., 2014).

Ayurveda, the ancient practice of medicine developed in India, considers TB as the king of diseases (Raja-yakshma in Sanskrit). In other parts of the world, malaria is the king of diseases. Whatever is the case, many Indian plants are used to manage TB. Ethyl p-methoxycinnamate isolated from the essential oil of *Kaempferia galanga* rhizomes is an anti-TB compound (Lakshmanan,

Werngren, Jose, Suja, Nair, & Varma et al., 2011). Ethyl p-methoxycinnamate inhibits both drug susceptible and MDR clinical isolates of *M. tuberculosis* (MIC 0.242–0.485 mM).

The roots of *Vetiveria zizanioides* (family Poaceae), popularly known as *Khas Khas*, *Khas* or *Khus* grass in India; inhibit *M. tuberculosis* H37Rv and H37Ra strains. Ethanolic extract of roots produce potent anti-*M. tuberculosis* activity, MIC = 500 μg/ml (Saikia, Parveen, Gupta, & Luqman, 2012). The hexane fraction also shows antimycobacterial action by producing a continuous decline in the growth index of *M. tuberculosis* at 50 μg/ml.

Sharma et al. (2014) in their report indicate that plants such as *Viscum album* (European mistletoe), *Tinospora cordifolia* (*Guduchi* and *Giloy*) and *Withania somnifera* (*Ashwagandha* or Indian ginseng) potentiate immune functions during TB infection. The authors say piperine, a trans-trans isomer of 1-piperoyl-piperidine isolated from black pepper (*Piper longum*), is an inhibitor of human p-glycoprotein and CYP3A4.

That is not all. Piperine also enhances bioavailability and has potential immuno-modulatory activity. Plus, there are indications piperine shuts down microbial virulence proteins. Sharma et al. (2014) cite studies where piperine inhibits the NorA efflux pump of *Staphylococcus aureus*. One study showed that murine splenocytes exposed to piperine exhibited proliferation of T- and B-lymphocytes, increased Th-1 cytokines and enhanced macrophage activation. All these properties of piperine are helpful in diminishing TB infection.

In their study, Sharma et al. (2014) found that piperine (1 mg/kg) in mice infected with *M. tuberculosis* activates the differentiation of T cells into a Th-1 sub-population which increases the secretion of Th-1 cytokines interferon-gamma and interleukin-2. Their results also show that piperine is synergistic to the action of antibiotics. Compared to rifampicin alone, a combination of piperine and rifampicin (1 mg/kg) exhibits better efficacy of and leads to further reductions of mycobacteria in the lungs. The results of Sharma and colleagues point to one thing: Up-regulation of Th-1 immunity by piperine may be synergistically combined with rifampicin to potentiate its therapeutic efficacy in immunocompromised TB patients.

The Lamiaceous plant, *Premna odorata*, also known as *Alagaw* in Filipino, is a small tree abundant in low-altitude thickets and secondary forests in Albay Province, the Philippines (Lirio, Macabeo, Paragas, Knorn, Kohls, & Franzblau et al., 2014). A water decoction of the leaves is used to treat patients with TB. The results of Lirio et al. (2014) demonstrated that the ethnomedicinal plant *P. odorata* possesses antimycobacterial compounds thus supporting the traditional use of this plant in the treatment of TB. Purification of a dichloromethane fraction active against *M. tuberculosis* H37Rv strain led to the isolation of 1-heneicosyl formate, whose MIC value against H37Rv was 8 μg/ml.

Macabeo, Vidar, Chen, Decker, Heilmann and Wan et al. (2011) while studying the plant *Voacanga globose* in the Phillipines discovered the presence of globospiramine, a new spirobisindole alkaloid with potent activity against *M. tuberculosis* H37Rv in microplate Alamar blue assay (MIC = 4 µg/ml) and low-oxygen recovery assay (MIC = 5.2 µg/ml).

In India, *Citrullus colocynthis* (family Cucurbitaceae) is a folk herbal remedy for TB. Fractions of *C. colocynthis* inhibited 16 clinical isolates of *M. tuberculosis* including 7 drug-susceptible strains, 8 MDRs and one XDR (Mehta, Srivastva, Kachhwaha, Sharma, & Kothari, 2013). Mehta and co-workers elucidated that ursolic acid and cucurbitacin E2-0-β-D-glucopyranoside were the main active biomarkers against *M. tuberculosis* H37Rv with MIC values of 50 and 25 µg/ml, respectively. Tawde, Gacche and Pund (2012) established that Indian plants like *Acacia catechu*, *Ailanthus excels*, *Andrographis paniculata*, *Aegle marmelos* and *Datura metel* had *in vitro* anti-mycobacterial efficacy.

Using a colorimetric microplate-based assay, 36 Malaysian plant species exhibited anti-TB activity with MIC values ranging from 1600–400 µg/ml (Mohamad et al., 2011). Notable activity was recorded for the leaf extract of *Angiopteris evecta* which exhibited the highest activity, MIC of 400 µg/ml. Five other extracts, namely, *Costus speciosus* (stem and flower), *Piper sarmentosum* (whole plant), *Pluchea indica* (leaf), *Pluchea indica* (flower) and *Tabernaemontana coronaria* (leaf) produced anti-mycobacterial activity, each with MIC of 800 µg/ml.

In Thailand, a study by Sureram, Senadeera, Hongmanee, Mahidol, Ruchi-rawat and Kittakoop (2012) showed that *Tiliacora triandra*, an appetizing plant added as an ingredient in local Thai cuisines, contains three bisbenzylisoquino-line alkaloids: Tiliacorinine, 2'-nortiliacorinine and tiliacorine. When the three natural compounds were tested against 59 clinical isolates of *M. tuberculosis*, they were all active, MIC values ranging from 0.7 to 6.2 µg/ml. The three bisbenzyl-isoquinoline alkaloids exhibit a MIC value of 3.1 µg/ml against most MDR-TB isolates. Since tiliacorinine, 2'-nortiliacorinine and tiliacorine have better inhibi-tory profiles against MDR-TB than some of the current first-line drugs, these plant chemical compounds have the potential to become natural scaffolds for novel anti-MDR-TB drugs. The use of the Thai spice plant *T. triandra* in the fight against TB looks promising.

Anti-TB Plants in South America

Brazil, with 82,755 TB cases in 2012, is a leading South American hub for anti-TB natural products. The plants *Struthanthus concinnus* and *Struthanthus mar-ginatus* are sold in open-air markets and used to manage TB infections in Brazil, which records about 72,000 new TB cases and 4,700 TB-related deaths every year (Leitão, Leitão, de Almeida, Cantos, Coelho, & da Silva, 2013). Bioassay-guided fractionation of hexane extracts from both species has led to the isolation and identification of steroids and terpenoids. In anti-tubercular assays, the MIC of the extracts and isolated compounds ranged from 25 to 200 µg/ml. Fractions and sub-fractions of *Tabernaemontana catharinensis*, a Brazilian plant with high levels of steroids, alkaloids and phenolic compounds were effective against *M. smegmatis* (MIC = 19.53–156.25 µg/ml).

Moreira, Martins, Pietro, Sato, Pavan and Leite et al. (2013) observed that Brazil is also home to plants called the 'everlasting flowers' (also known as 'sempre-vivas' in Portuguese, since they maintain their appearance and colour after drying). Many of these plants are exported to Europe, Japan and North America as ornamental flowers, giving the people of Minas Gerais State in Brazil a source of income. Moreira et al. (2013) studied the anti-mycobacterial activity of two of the 'sempre-vivas' plants, namely *Paepalanthus latipes* and *Paepalanthus bromelioides*.

The scientists found that two methoxylated flavonoids (flavonoid 7-methylquercetagetin and 7-methylquercetagetin-4'-O-β-D-glucopyranoside) isolated from *P. latipes* and naphthopyranone fractions from *P. bromelioides* had no noteworthy anti-mycobacterial activity, MIC value of 500-2000 µg/ml for all compounds tested against H37Rv and *M. avium* ATCC 15769. However, the compounds induced innate immunity through the production of high levels of hydrogen peroxide which aids in macrophage killing of mycobacteria (Moreira et al., 2013). It was concluded that despite poor activity *in vitro*, the compounds are quite potent *in vivo* (inside the macrophage).

Brazil is home to five genera and approximately 500 species of Piperaceae whose benzoic acid derivatives frequently exhibit antimicrobial, molluscicidal, antifungal and leishmanicidal activities (Regiane, Espelho, Pires, Garcia, Cardozo-Filho, & Cortez et al., 2015). A new benzoic acid derivative called 4-methoxy-3-[(E)-3-methyl- 1,3-butadien-1-yl]-5-(3-methyl-2-buten-1-yl)-benzoic acid was isolated from *Piper diospyrifolium*. This new compound has moderate activity against *M. tuberculosis* H37Rv, MIC value of 125 mg/ml.

Piper regnellii var. *pallescens*, popularly known as *Caapeba* or *Pariparoba* in Brazil, contains the anti-mycobacterial compound neolignans eupomatenoid-5, MIC 1.9 µg/ml on H37Rv and a good selectivity index of 20.0 (Scodro, Pires, Carrara, Lemos, Cardozo-Filho, & Souza et al., 2013). Therefore, neolignans eupomatenoid-5 is a good candidate for the future development of anti-TB drugs.

Celastrus vulcanicola (plant family Celastraceae) is a subtropical woody vine distributed in the Caribbean and South American countries of Peru and El Salvador. One of its chemical constituents is a dihydro-β-agarofuran sesquiterpene called 1α-Acetoxy-6β,9β-dibenzoyloxy-dihydro-β-agarofuran which has activity against H37Rv and MDR strains, MIC value of 6.2 µg/ml (Torres-Romero, Jiménez, Rojas, Gilman, López, & Bazzocchi, 2011). The antimycobacterial ability of this sesquiterpene is similar to or even better than isoniazid or rifampin, two of the best first-line drugs commonly used in the treatment of TB (Torres-Romero et al., 2011).

In vitro assays demonstrated that (-)-licarin A isolated from the Mexican plant *Aristolochia taliscana* had antimycobacterial activity against mono- and MDR *M. tuberculosis* (León-Díaz et al., 2013). The plant genus *Diospyros* is one of the most important sources of 1,4 naphthoquinones which confer potent anti-TB activity (Uc-Cachón et al., 2014). Isolated from *Diospyros anisandra* growing in Mexico, the three naphthoquinones plumbagin, maritinone and 3,3'-biplumbagin are some of the most active against *M. tuberculosis* (Uc-Cachón et al., 2014).

In fact, against the pan-resistant *M. tuberculosis* strain, the bioactivity of maritinone and 3,3'-biplumbagin was 32-times more potent than the TB drug rifampicin. Both compounds were non-toxic to PBMC and Vero cells. These findings, according to the Mexican scientists, make maritinone and 3,3'-biplumbagin uniquely suitable for the development of a new type of anti-TB drug which can overcome resistance to first- and second-line anti-TB medications.

Canadian First Nations' Anti-TB Plants

Juniperus communis, or the common juniper, is the eighth most extensively used medicinal plant by the indigenous peoples of North America. Carpenter, O'Neill, Picot, Johnson, Robichaud, Webster and Gray (2012) explain that the First Nations of the Canadian Maritimes use infusions of juniper primarily as a tonic and for the treatment of TB. Research at the University of New Brunswick, Saint John, New Brunswick, Canada, has shown that isocupressic acid, communic acid and deoxypodophyllotoxin isolated from aerial parts of juniper were active against *M. tuberculosis*.

In another study, Gordien, Gray, Franzblau and Seidel (2009) attribute the antimycobacterial activity of *J. communis* to a sesquiterpene (longifolene) and two diterpenes (totarol and trans-communic acid). Totarol showed the best activity against *M. tuberculosis*. Totarol was also most active against the isoniazid-, streptomycin- and moxifloxacin-resistant variants of TB. Longifolene and totarol were most active against the rifampicin-resistant strains of TB. Gordien and co-workers conclude that the presence of anti-mycobacterial terpenoids in the *J. communis* plant justifies the ethnomedicinal use of this species as a traditional remedy for TB.

Li, O'Neill, Webster, Johnson and Gray (2012), writing on ethnomedicinal knowledge of the people of the Canadian First Nations, aver that extracts from *Aralia nudicaulis* rhizomes taken as tea significantly inhibit mycobacterial activity. They identified two C17 polyacetylenes, falcarinol and panaxydol as the most important ingredients responsible for the antimycobacterial activity of *A. nudicaulis* rhizomes thus corroborating the ethnopharmacological applications of this plant by the indigenous people of Canada. Despite having low solubilities, falcarinol and panaxydol showed MIC values of 25.6 μM and 36.0 μM and IC$_{50}$ values of 15.3 μM and 23.5 μM against *M. tuberculosis* H37Ra, respectively.

The First Nations of Canada and Native American communities also use infusions of *Heracleum maximum* (or cow parsnip) roots for the treatment of TB (O'Neill, Johnson, Webster, & Gray, 2013). O'Neill and colleagues found that a polyacetylene called (3R,8S)-falcarindiol and a furanocoumarin named 6-isopentenyloxyisobergapten exhibited MIC values of 24 μM and 167 μM and IC$_{50}$ values of 6 μM and 27 μM against H37Ra, respectively. Their experiments lend much credence to the ethnopharmacological application of *H. maximum*, often prepared as a tea after soaking the roots in hot water, in the treatment of TB.

A Closer Look at Natural Products as Anti-TB Agents

In recent decades, TB has re-emerged as a major disease of global importance mainly due to HIV/AIDS. TB and HIV are co-evolving together in what is being dubbed the HIV/TB co-epidemic or the dual epidemic. But it is the increasing caseloads of drug resistant TB that brings into sharp focus the urgent need for novel and new anti-TB drugs to counter the growing plague.

Disappointingly, research and development of new anti-TB drugs has not kept pace with the growing global prevalence of TB. There have been no new anti-TB drugs over the past 50 years. The last time a drug was specifically researched and developed for the treatment of TB was in the late 1960s. That drug was rifampicin.

This being the case, the global community should take a wider view and urgent approach toward new treatments for TB. Such a strategy should include a return to Mother Nature and a call to action the use of anti-TB natural products. Therefore, with respect to TB, the study of medicinal plants is aimed at ushering in a new generation of innovative anti-TB drugs. This is important for several reasons.

Globally, TB cases and mortality are increasing. TB pathogenesis has become complicated because the disease is twinned to HIV infection. There are also challenges surrounding the current DOTS therapy because the duration of treatment is long. And, all too often, some drugs are becoming ineffective partly because of the proliferation of drug resistant strains of *M. tuberculosis*.

Since TB became a global emergency in 1993, the current treatment strategy based on DOTS, though helpful in securing treatment for many patients, is still fraught with problems such as poor administration, lack of laboratory facilities for diagnosis, lack of surveillance and monitoring systems and inadequate drug supplies. There is more bad news as drug resistant mycobacteria produce severe disease outcomes, TB/HIV dual epidemics are stubborn to DOTS treatment and the probability of mortality for HIV/TB co-infected persons is high.

TB cure rates ebb in settings characterized by poverty, deplorable living conditions, inadequate nutrition, lack of funding for TB prevention programmes and poor organization of public treatment programmes. Adherence to treatment is also hampered by the lack of strict supervision by health staff, shortages of drugs, drug toxicity and side effects and strong beliefs in the use of traditional medicines or self-medication through natural products.

Advances in post-genomics and systems biology have not yet yielded the new and innovative treatments against TB. Capitalist greed, not the lack of breakthrough scientific ideas, is in reality the far more fundamental obstacle to the development of new and novel drugs against TB. Research and development of innovative and more efficacious medicines is not a priority - at least for now - for pharmaceutical industries that consider TB a disease of the poor.

In 2003, the estimated average cost of bringing a new drug to the market was US$ 802 million (DiMasi, Hansen, & Grabowski, 2003). But big pharmaceutical companies fear to invest millions of dollars in the development of new anti-TB drugs because TB is mostly a disease for poor countries. TB drugs, like those for malaria, are classified as 'less profitable drugs'. So, pharmaceutical companies are wary that they may not reap enough profits to account for their huge investments.

In the wake of all these shortcomings, natural products especially medicinal plants still present a unique ray of hope to rejig the situation, especially to lower the cost of research and development. For example, pharmacognosy and ethnobotanical studies may unravel plant leads from which novel anti-TB chemical ingredients may be isolated. Novel drugs for TB may also be developed from secondary chemical secretions of endophytic fungi that live symbiotically with plants.

The advantage is that many secondary metabolites of endophytes which may have anti-mycobacterial activity may also be non-cytotoxic to eukaryotes including human cells. Besides providing drug leads, natural products that inhibit the growth of mycobacteria may help the human body to stonewall TB infection and reactivation. Interestingly, common plants like green tea and spices like turmeric contain anti-TB chemical agents. But it is still not clear whether marijuana, a known anti-HIV plant, has bioactivity against mycobacteria.

In all the African countries mentioned in this chapter (Cameroon, Central African Republic, Gabon, Ethiopia, Mozambique, Namibia, Nigeria, Uganda, South Africa and Tanzania), at least 60 listed plant species are known to display anti-TB activity. In South Africa, where more rigorous bioprospecting and antimicrobial studies have been done, at least 20 plants have been shown to inhibit *M. tuberculosis* (see Table 6.2). Some of the African plant species that putatively lessen TB symptoms include *A. precatorius*, *A. afra*, *C. molle*, *F. sur*, *K. africana*, *P. africanum*, *S. longipedunculata* and *T. sericea*.

Several African plants also block HIV replication, hence may be important in maintaining the lid on the dual epidemics of HIV and TB. Some of these dual anti-HIV/TB functional plants are *C. macowani*, *T. violacea*, *Cascabela thevetia*, *W. ugandensisis*, *M. senegalensis*, *G. buchananii*, *G. livingstonei*, *C. molle*, *R. communis*, *P. africanum*, *H. hemerocallidea*, *P. amboinicus*, *F. virosa*, *S. longipedunculata* and *Z. officinalis*. Further studies are required to isolate and characterise the main anti-mycobacterial active compounds from African plants. Unfortunately, many scientists in Africa lack cutting-edge equipment in their laboratories. As a result, plant materials from Africa are shipped to developed countries where anti-mycobacterial testing and isolation of active compounds is done and patented.

From selected African plants, the following antimycobacterial chemical compounds have been isolated: ellagitannin punicalagin, allicin, anthraquinone glycosides, iridoids, phenylpropanoids, beta-sitosterol, galanthimine, lycorine, crinine, friedelin, epi-friedelin, gallic acid, ellagic acids, anthocyanidin, taraxerol, taraxerone, caffeic acid, termilignan B, arjunic acid, glucopyranosides, terminalin A, 1-epicatechol, leucopelargonidol, hydroxybenzoic acids, xanthones, benzophenanthridine alkaloids, neolignans and decarine.

Characterization of active compounds from almost half of the plants that are used to manage TB in African countries has not yet been done. More resources and research efforts should be directed not only at bioprospecting but also at antimycobacterial testing and characterization of active chemical compounds. Given the high burden of TB in African countries, governments and private initiatives should invest more in the search and development of new anti-TB drugs, especially those that are effective against resistant strains.

The main African hope for the development of a new anti-TB drug may lie in South Africa, the only African country with a coordinated research effort in bioprospecting, antimicrobial testing and isolation of active chemical ingredients through various state-of-the-art techniques like high-performance liquid chromatography, thin-layer chromatography and mass spectroscopy.

European plants from three countries (Turkey, Portugal and United Kingdom) have been evaluated for anti-mycobacteria action. *Thymbra spicata*, *Hyperricum* species, *A. lappa* and *T. farfara* inhibit mycobacteria *in vitro*. Several active ingredients: Carvacrol, rosmarinic acid, hesperidin, naringenin, hypericin, hyperforin, p-coumaric acid and 4-hydroxybenzoic acid are potent against mycobacteria.

In Asia, some of the countries that have conducted research on natural products for TB include Indonesia, Taiwan, India, Pakistan, the Philippines, Malaysia and Thailand. At least 30 plant species are used to manage TB in these seven countries. Anti-TB active compounds include cinnamic acid, ethyl p-methoxycinnamate, piperine, 1-heneicosyl formate, globospiramine, ursolic acid, cucurbitacin, and bisbenzylisoquinoline alkaloids. Although TB is very widespread in Asia, research on anti-TB natural products has not matched the high prevalence levels of the disease. Lamentably, very few active chemical compounds have been characterized, not least from the huge reserves of putative medicinal plants that lie in the forests of Indonesia.

About 13 plants in the South and North American countries of Brazil, Peru, El Salvador, Mexico and Canada are applied as remedies for TB. Some of the active chemical compounds from these plants include benzoic acid derivatives, neolignans eupomatenoid-5, sesquiterpenes, licarin A and naphthoquinones. Anti-TB plants used by the indigenous people of Canada have yielded interesting antimycobacterial chemical agents, namely, isocupressic acid, communic acid, deoxypodophyllotoxin, longifolene, totarol, falcarinol, panaxydol and furanocoumarin.

Conclusion and Way Ahead

This chapter has provided an incisive indication of plant species and other natural products that contain chemical substances that stymie TB. Antimycobacterial activities of putative anti-TB plants and other natural products used in different parts of the world, and some of the active chemical ingredients of these natural products have been presented. The chapter has affirmatively answered the question of whether natural products inhibit mycobacterial infections. In fact, research shows that some chemical ingredients of plants are even more effective than standard anti-TB drugs.

To reiterate, many natural products may be anti-TB in nature, very anti-TB; but their extracts and active compounds should be evaluated for human cytotoxicity. So, this chapter provides the clearest look yet at the antimicrobial powers of natural products against TB. Plants and other natural products may contain the secret chemical ingredients that could *ceteris paribus* turn the page to a new and happier frontier of anti-TB drugs. This way, the global TB tragedy may go the way of smallpox, the only infectious human disease ever to be erad-icated, in 1980.

Hopefully, the next decade will see unprecedented progress in the re-search and development of new anti-TB drugs. By converting natural products into new and more potent drugs for TB, and getting these novel drugs to the patients at the right time, it may be possible to wipe TB off the face of the earth by 2050. Therefore, this chapter represents what is best about plants and other natural products: The power to heal the world from TB. Indeed, the hope is that natural products may become part of the strategy for 'The Stop TB Partnership' whose pushy target is to eliminate TB to less than one case per 1 million by the year 2050.

If the world's scientific and business communities put more attention and resources - tantamount to the huge investments feeding into the current hun-ger for smart phones - humanity could make a giant leap in the development of new anti-TB drugs. For now, the enthusiasm in the global scientific efforts to harness the power of natural products and turn them into novel anti-TB drugs, including the wealth of potent anti-mycobacterial plant extracts, points to one trend: The global ambition to eliminate TB by the year 2050 is an achievable goal.

References

Abuzeid, N., Kalsum, S., Koshy, R.J., Larsson, M., Glader, M., Andersson, H., ... & Lerm, M. (2014). Antimycobacterial activity of selected medicinal plants traditionally used in Sudan to treat infectious diseases. *Journal of Ethnopharmacology, 157*, 134-139.

Agarwal, A., Prasad, R., & Jain, A. (2010). Effect of green tea extract (catechins) in reducing oxidative stress seen in patients of pulmonary tuberculosis on DOTS Cat I regimen. *Phytomedicine, 17*(1), 23-27.

Allen, D.E., & Hatfield, G. (2004). *Medicinal Plants in Folk Tradition: An Ethnobotany of Britain and Ireland.* Timber Press, Portland.

Alvin, A., Miller, K.I., & Neilan, B.A. (2014). Exploring the potential of endophytes from medicinal plants as sources of antimycobacterial compounds. *Microbiological Research, 169*(7), 483-495.

Amoah, S.K., Sandjo, L.P., Bazzo, M.L., Leite, S.N., & Biavatti, M.W. (2014). Herbalists, traditional healers and pharmacists: a view of the tuberculosis in Ghana. *Revista Brasileira de Farmacognosia, 24*(1), 89-95.

Asiimwe, S., Kamatenesi-Mugisha, M., Namutebi, A., Borg-Karlsson, A. K., & Musiimenta, P. (2013). Ethnobotanical study of nutri-medicinal plants used for the management of HIV/AIDS opportunistic ailments among the local communities of western Uganda. *Journal of Ethnopharmacology, 150*(2), 639-648.

Askun, T., Tumen, G., Satil, F., & Ates, M. (2009). *In vitro* activity of methanol extracts of plants used as spices against Mycobacterium tuberculosis and other bacteria. *Food Chemistry, 116*(1), 289-294.

Asuquo, A.E., Pokam, B.T., Adindu, A., Ibeneme, E.O., Ekpereonne, E., & Obot, V. (2015). A public–private partnership model to reduce tuberculosis burden in Akwa Ibom State–Nigeria. *International Journal of Mycobacteriology, 4*(1), 20-21.

Baldwin, P.R., Reeves, A.Z., Powell, K.R., Napier, R.J., Swimm, A.I., Sun, A., ... & Kalman, D. (2015). Monocarbonyl analogs of curcumin inhibit growth of antibiotic sensitive and resistant strains of *Mycobacterium tuberculosis. European Journal of Medicinal Chemistry, 92*, 693-699.

Barr, R.G., Diez-Roux, A.V., Knirsch, C.A., & Pablos-Méndez, A. (2001). Neighborhood poverty and the resurgence of tuberculosis in New York City, 1984-1992. *American Journal of Public Health, 91*(9), 1487-1493.

Boligon, A.A., Piana, M., Kubiça, T.F., Mario, D.N., Dalmolin, T.V., Bonez, P.C., ... & Athayde, M.L. (2014). HPLC analysis and antimicrobial, antimycobacterial and antiviral activities of *Tabernaemontana catharinensis* A. DC. *Journal of Applied Biomedicine, 13*(1), 7-18.

Boskabady, M.H., Kaini, S., Haghiri, B. (2005). Relaxant effects of *Ocimum basilicum* on guinea pig tracheal chains and its possible mechanism. *DARU Journal of Pharmaceutical Sciences*, *13*, 28–33.

Bryder, L. (1988). *Below the magic mountain: A social history of tuberculosis in twentieth-century Britain.* Oxford University Press.

Bunalema, L., Obakiro, S., Tabuti, J.R., & Waako, P. (2014). Knowledge on plants used traditionally in the treatment of tuberculosis in Uganda. *Journal of Ethnopharmacology*, *151*(2), 999-1004.

Buwa, L.V., & Afolayan, A.J. (2009). Antimicrobial activity of some medicinal plants used for the treatment of tuberculosis in the Eastern Cape Province, South Africa. *African Journal of Biotechnology*, *8*, 6683–6687.

Cambanis, A., Yassin, M.A., Ramsay, A., Bertel Squire, S., Arbide, I., & Cuevas, L.E. (2005). Rural poverty and delayed presentation to tuberculosis services in Ethiopia. *Tropical Medicine and International Health*, *10*(4), 330-335.

Carpenter, C.D., O'Neill, T., Picot, N., Johnson, J.A., Robichaud, G.A., Webster, D., & Gray, C.A. (2012). Anti-mycobacterial natural products from the Canadian medicinal plant *Juniperus communis*. *Journal of Ethnopharmacology*, *143*(2), 695-700.

Chaisson, R.E., & Martinson, N.A. (2008). Tuberculosis in Africa—combating an HIV-driven crisis. *New England Journal of Medicine*, *358*(11), 1089-1092.

Chanchao, C. (2013). Bioactivity of honey and propolis of *Tetragonula laeviceps* in Thailand. In *Pot-Honey* (pp. 495-505). Springer New York.

Chandra, N., Kumar, D., & Rao, K. (2011). Systems biology of tuberculosis. *Tuberculosis*, *91*(5), 487-496.

Chen, Y.L., Huang, S.T., Sun, F.M., Chiang, Y.L., Chiang, C.J., Tsai, C. M., & Weng, C.J. (2011). Transformation of cinnamic acid from *trans-* to *cis-* form raises a notable bactericidal and synergistic activity against multiple-drug resistant *Mycobacterium tuberculosis*. *European Journal of Pharmaceutical Sciences*, *43*(3), 188-194.

Chinsembu, K.C. & Hedimbi, M. (2010). An ethnobotanical survey of plants used to manage HIV/AIDS opportunistic infections in Katima Mulilo, Caprivi region, Namibia. *Journal of Ethnobiology and Ethnomedicine*, 6:25.

Chinsembu, K.C., & Hedimbi, M. (2012). Ethnomedicinal study of plants used to manage HIV/AIDS-related disease conditions in the Ohangwena region, Namibia. *International Journal of Medicinal Plant Research*, *1(1)*, 4-11.

Chomcheon, P., Wiyakrutta, S., Sriubolmas, N., Ngamrojanavanich, N., Isarangkul, D., Kittakoop, P. (2005). 3-Nitropropionic acid (3-NPA), a potent antimycobacterial agent from endophytic fungi: is 3-NPA in some plants produced by endophytes? *J. Nat. Prod.*, *68*, 1103-1105.

Copp, B.R., & Pearce, A.N. (2007). Natural product growth inhibitors of Mycobacterium tuberculosis. *Natural Product Reports, 24*(2), 278-297.

Cragg, G.M., & Newman, D.J. (2013). Natural products: a continuing source of novel drug leads. *Biochimica et Biophysica Acta, 1830*, 3670–3695.

De Cock, K.M., & Chaisson, R.E. (1999). Will DOTS do it? A reappraisal of tuberculosis control in countries with high rates of HIV infection [Counterpoint]. *The International Journal of Tuberculosis and Lung Disease, 3*(6), 457-465.

Dikshit, A., Husain, A., (1984). Antifungal activities of some essential oils against animal pathogens. *Fitoterapia*, 55, 171–176.

DiMasi, J.A., Hansen, R.W., & Grabowski, H.G. (2003). The price of innovation: new estimates of drug development costs. *Journal of Health Economics, 22*(2), 151-185.

Dodor, E.A., 2012. The feelings and experiences of patients with tuberculosis in the Sekondi-Takoradi metropolitan district: implications for TB control efforts. *Ghana Med. J., 46*, 211-218.

Egwaga, S.M. (2003). The impact of HIV on transmission of tuberculosis in Tanzania. *Tuberculosis, 83*(1), 66-67.

Eldeen, I.M.S., & van Staden, J. (2007). Antimycobacterial activity of some trees used in South African traditional medicine. *South African Journal of Botany, 73*(2), 248-251.

Fallah, M., Fallah, F., Kamalinejad, M., Malekan, M. A., Akhlaghi, Z., & Esmaeili, M. (2014). The Antimicrobial Effect of Aquatic Extract of Salvadora Persica on *Mycobacterium Bovis in vitro*. *International Journal of Mycobacteriology, 4*(1), 167-168.

Farnsworth, N.R., Akerele, O., Bingel, A.S., Soejarto, D.D., & Guo, Z. (1985). Medicinal plants in therapy. *Bulletin of the World Health Organization, 63*, 965–81.

Fomogne-Fodjo, M.C.Y., Van Vuuren, S., Ndinteh, D. T., Krause, R. W. M., & Olivier, D.K. (2014). Antibacterial activities of plants from Central Africa used traditionally by the Bakola pygmies for treating respiratory and tuberculosis-related symptoms. *Journal of Ethnopharmacology, 155*(1), 123-131.

Frothingham, R., Stout, J.E., & Hamilton, C.D. (2005). Current issues in global tuberculosis control. *International Journal of Infectious Diseases, 9*(6), 297-311.

Fyhrquist, P., Laakso, I., Garcia Marco, S., Julkunen-Tiitto, R., & Hiltunen, R. (2014). Antimycobacterial activity of ellagitannin and ellagic acid derivate rich crude extracts and fractions of five selected species of *Terminalia* used for treatment of infectious diseases in African traditional medicine. *South African Journal of Botany, 90*, 1-16.

Ganihigama, D.U., Sureram, S., Sangher, S., Hongmanee, P., Aree, T., Mahidol, C., ... & Kittakoop, P. (2015). Antimycobacterial activity of natural products and synthetic agents: Pyrrolodiquinolines and vermelhotin as anti-tubercular leads against clinical multidrug resistant isolates of *Mycobacterium tuberculosis*. *European Journal of Medicinal Chemistry*, *89*, 1-12.

Gordien, A.Y., Gray, A.I., Franzblau, S.G., & Seidel, V. (2009). Antimycobacterial terpenoids from *Juniperus communis* L. (Cuppressaceae). *Journal of Ethnopharmacology*, *126*(3), 500-505.

Green, E., Samie, A., Obi, C.L., Bessong, P.O., & Ndip, R.N. (2010). Inhibitory properties of selected South African medicinal plants against Mycobacterium tuberculosis. *Journal of Ethnopharmacology*, *130*(1), 151-157.

Holton, S.J., Weiss, M.S., Tucker, P.A., & Wilmanns, M. (2007). Structure-based approaches to drug discovery against tuberculosis. *Current Protein and Peptide Science*, *8*(4), 365-375.

Ibekwe, N.N., Nvau, J.B., Oladosu, P.O., Usman, A.M., Ibrahim, K., Boshoff, H.I., ... & Okogun, J.I. (2014). Some Nigerian anti-tuberculosis ethnomedicines: A preliminary efficacy assessment. *Journal of Ethnopharmacology*, *155*(1), 524-532.

Jayaweera, D.M.A. (1981). *Medicinal Plants, Part 3*. National Science Council of Sri Lanka Publication, Colombo, pp. 101.

Kayani, S., Ahmad, M., Zafar, M., Sultana, S., Khan, M.P.Z., Ashraf, M. A., ... & Yaseen, G. (2014). Ethnobotanical uses of medicinal plants for respiratory disorders among the inhabitants of Gallies–Abbottabad, Northern Pakistan. *Journal of Ethnopharmacology*, *156*, 47-60.

Koul, A., Arnoult, E., Lounis, N., Guillemont, J., & Andries, K. (2011). The challenge of new drug discovery for tuberculosis. *Nature*, *469*(7331), 483-490.

Kuete, V. (2010). Potential of Cameroonian plants and derived products against microbial infections: a review. *Planta Medica*, 76, 1479–1491.

Kumar, P., Singh, A., Sharma, U., Singh, D., Dobhal, M. P., & Singh, S. (2013). Anti-mycobacterial activity of plumericin and isoplumericin against MDR *Mycobacterium tuberculosis*. *Pulmonary Pharmacology and Therapeutics*, *26*(3), 332-335.

Lall, N., & Meyer, J.J.M. (1999). *In vitro* inhibition of drug-resistant and drug-sensitive strains of *Mycobacterium tuberculosis* by ethnobotanically selected South African plants. *Journal of Ethnopharmacology*, 66, 347–354.

Lakshmanan, D., Werngren, J., Jose, L., Suja, K.P., Nair, M.S., Varma, R. L., ... & Kumar, R.A. (2011). Ethyl p-methoxycinnamate isolated from a traditional anti-tuberculosis medicinal herb inhibits drug resistant strains of *Mycobacterium tuberculosis in vitro*. *Fitoterapia*, *82*(5), 757-761.

Leitão, F., Leitão, S.G., de Almeida, M.Z., Cantos, J., Coelho, T., & da Silva, P. E. A. (2013). Medicinal plants from open-air markets in the State of Rio de Janeiro, Brazil as a potential source of new antimycobacterial agents. *Journal of Ethnopharmacology*, *149*(2), 513-521.

León-Díaz, R., Meckes-Fischer, M., Valdovinos-Martínez, L., Campos, M. G., Hernández-Pando, R., & Jiménez-Arellanes, M.A. (2013). Antitubercular Activity and the Subacute Toxicity of (−)-Licarin A in BALB/c Mice: A Neolignan Isolated from *Aristolochia taliscana*. *Archives of Medical Research*, *44*(2), 99-104.

Li, H., O'Neill, T., Webster, D., Johnson, J.A., & Gray, C.A. (2012). Antimycobacterial diynes from the Canadian medicinal plant Aralia nudicaulis. *Journal of Ethnopharmacology*, *140*(1), 141-144.

Li, M.Y., Wang, H.L., Huang, J., Shi, G.C., Wan, Y.G., Wang, J.X., & Xi, X.E. (2014). Curcumin inhibits 19-kDa lipoprotein of *Mycobacterium tuberculosis* induced macrophage apoptosis via regulation of the JNK pathway. *Biochemical and Biophysical Research Communications*, *446*(2), 626-632.

Lirio, S.B., Macabeo, A.P.G., Paragas, E.M., Knorn, M., Kohls, P., Franzblau, S.G., ... & Aguinaldo, M.A.M. (2014). Antitubercular constituents from Premna odorata Blanco. *Journal of Ethnopharmacology*, *154*(2), 471-474.

Luo, X., Pires, D., Ainsa, J.A., Gracia, B., Duarte, N., Mulhovo, S., ... & Ferreira, M.J.U. (2013). *Zanthoxylum capense* constituents with antimycobacterial activity against Mycobacterium tuberculosis in vitro and ex vivo within human macrophages. *Journal of Ethnopharmacology*, *146*(1), 417-422.

Luo, X., Pires, D., Aínsa, J.A., Gracia, B., Mulhovo, S., Duarte, A., ... & Ferreira, M.J.U. (2011). Antimycobacterial evaluation and preliminary phytochemical investigation of selected medicinal plants traditionally used in Mozambique. *Journal of Ethnopharmacology*, *137*(1), 114-120.

Macabeo, A.P.G., Vidar, W.S., Chen, X., Decker, M., Heilmann, J., Wan, B., ... & Cordell, G.A. (2011). Mycobacterium tuberculosis and cholinesterase inhibitors from Voacanga globosa. *European Journal of Medicinal Chemistry*, *46*(7), 3118-3123.

Madikizela, B., Aderogba, M.A., Finnie, J.F., & van Staden, J. (2014b). Isolation and characterization of antimicrobial compounds from Terminalia phanerophlebia Engl. & Diels leaf extracts. *Journal of Ethnopharmacology*, *156*, 228-234.

Madikizela, B., Ndhlala, A.R., Finnie, J.F., & van Staden, J. (2014a). Antimycobacterial, anti-inflammatory and genotoxicity evaluation of plants used for the treatment of tuberculosis and related symptoms in South Africa. *Journal of Ethnopharmacology*, *153*(2), 386-391.

Maroyi, A. (2015). Alternative medicines for HIV/AIDS in resource-poor settings: Insights from use of traditional medicines in Sub-Saharan Africa. Available on: http://scholar.google.com/scholar?hl=en&q=Maroyi%2C+ (downloaded on 8 February, 2015).

Mativandlela, S.P.N., Lall, N., & Meyer, J.J.M. (2006). Antibacterial, antifungal and antitubercular activity of (the roots of) Pelargonium reniforme (CURT) and Pelargonium sidoides (DC) (Geraniaceae) root extracts. *South African Journal of Botany, 72,* 232–237.

McGaw, L.J., Lall, N., Meyer, J.J.M., & Eloff, J. N. (2008). The potential of South African plants against Mycobacterium infections. *Journal of Ethnopharmacology, 119*(3), 482-500.

Mehta, A., Srivastva, G., Kachhwaha, S., Sharma, M., & Kothari, S.L. (2013). Antimycobacterial activity of Citrullus colocynthis (L.) Schrad. against drug sensitive and drug resistant Mycobacterium tuberculosis and MOTT clinical isolates. *Journal of Ethnopharmacology, 149*(1), 195-200.

Mohamad, S., Zin, N.M., Wahab, H.A., Ibrahim, P., Sulaiman, S.F., Zahariluddin, A.S.M., & Noor, S.S.M. (2011). Antituberculosis potential of some ethnobotanically selected Malaysian plants. *Journal of ethnopharmacology, 133*(3), 1021-1026.

Moreira, R.R., Martins, G.Z., Pietro, R.C., Sato, D.N., Pavan, F.R., Leite, S.R., ... & Leite, C.Q. (2013). *Paepalanthus* spp: Antimycobacterial activity of extracts, methoxylated flavonoids and naphthopyranone fractions. *Revista Brasileira de Farmacognosia, 23*(2), 268-272.

Mugisha, M.K., Asiimwe, S., Namutebi, A., Borg-Karlson, A.K., & Kakudidi, E.K. (2014). Ethnobotanical study of indigenous knowledge on medicinal and nutritious plants used to manage opportunistic infections associated with HIV/AIDS in western Uganda. *Journal of Ethnopharmacology, 155*(1), 194-202.

Mukai, A., Fukai, T., Hoshino, Y., Yazawa, K., Harada, K., Mikami, Y., et al. (2009). Nocardithiocin, anovel thiopeptide antibiotic, produced by pathogenic *Nocardia pseudobrasiliensis* IFM 0757. *Journal of Antibiotics, 62,* 613–9.

Nair, J. J., & van Staden, J. (2014). Traditional usage, phytochemistry and pharmacology of the South African medicinal plant *Boophone disticha* (Lf) Herb. (Amaryllidaceae). *Journal of Ethnopharmacology, 151*(1), 12-26.

Ndhlala, A.R., Ncube, B., Okem, A., Mulaudzi, R.B., & van Staden, J. (2013). Toxicology of some important medicinal plants in southern Africa. *Food and Chemical Toxicology, 62,* 609-621.

Newton, S.M., Lau, C., & Wright, C.W. (2000). A review of antimycobacterial natural products. *Phytotherapy Research, 14*(5), 303-322.

Nogueira, T., Medeiros, M.A., Marcelo-Curto, M.J., García-Pérez, B.E., Luna-Herrera, J., & Costa, M.C. (2013). Profile of antimicrobial potential of fifteen Hypericum species from Portugal. *Industrial Crops and Products, 47,* 126-131.

Ntutela, S., Smith, P., Matika, L., Mukinda, J., Arendse, H., Allie, N., ... & Jacobs, M. (2009). Efficacy of *Artemisia afra* phytotherapy in experimental tuberculosis. *Tuberculosis, 89*, S33-S40.

O'Neill, T., Johnson, J.A., Webster, D., & Gray, C.A. (2013). The Canadian medicinal plant Heracleum maximum contains antimycobacterial diynes and furanocoumarins. *Journal of Ethnopharmacology, 147*(1), 232-237.

Osman, K., Evangelopoulos, D., Basavannacharya, C., Gupta, A., McHugh, T.D., Bhakta, S., & Gibbons, S. (2012). An antibacterial from *Hypericum acmosepalum* inhibits ATP-dependent MurE ligase from Mycobacterium tuberculosis. *International Journal of Antimicrobial Agents, 39*(2), 124-129.

Pablos-Méndez, A., Raviglione, M.C., Laszlo, A., Binkin, N., Rieder, H. L., Bustreo, F., ... & Nunn, P. (1998). Global surveillance for antituberculosis-drug resistance, 1994–1997. *New England Journal of Medicine, 338*(23), 1641-1649.

Pauli, G.F., Case, R.J., Inui, T., Wang, Y., Cho, S., Fischer, N.H., & Franzblau, S. G. (2005). New perspectives on natural products in TB drug research. *Life Sciences, 78*(5), 485-494.

Ralph, A.P., Lucas, R.M., & Norval, M. (2013). Vitamin D and solar ultraviolet radiation in the risk and treatment of tuberculosis. *The Lancet Infectious Diseases, 13*(1), 77-88.

Raviglione, M.C. (2003). The TB epidemic from 1992 to 2002. *Tuberculosis, 83*(1), 4-14.

Regiane, B.D.L., Espelho, S.C., Pires, C.T.A., Garcia, V.A.D.S., Cardozo-Filho, L., Cortez, L.E., ... & Cortez, D.A. (2015). A new benzoic acid derivative from Piper diospyrifolium and its anti-*Mycobacterium tuberculosis* activity. *Phytochemistry Letters, 11*, 18-23.

Rood, B. (2013). *Nature's own pharmacy*. Pretoria, South Africa: Protea Book House.

Saikia, D., Parveen, S., Gupta, V.K., & Luqman, S. (2012). Antituberculosis activity of Indian grass Khus (*Vetiveria zizanioides* L. Nash). *Complementary Therapies in Medicine, 20*(6), 434-436.

Salomon, C., & Schmidt, L. (2012). Natural products as leads for tuberculosis drug development. *Current Topics in Medicinal Chemistry, 12*(7), 735-765.

Santhosh, R.S., & Suriyanarayanan, B. (2014). Plants: a source for new antimycobacterial drugs. *Planta Medica*, 80, 9–21.

Schumacher, T. (1999). *Plants used in medicine*. In: Whitten T, Whitten J, editors. Indonesian heritage: plants. Singapore: Archipelago Press; p. 68–9.

Scodro, R.B.L., Pires, C.T.A., Carrara, V.S., Lemos, C.O.T., Cardozo-Filho, L., Souza, V.A., ... & Cortez, D.A.G. (2013). Anti-tuberculosis neolignans from *Piper regnellii*. *Phytomedicine, 20*(7), 600-604.

Seidel, V., Taylor, P.W., 2004. In vitro activity of extracts and constituents of *Pelargonium* against rapidly growing mycobacteria. *International Journal of Antimicrobial Agents, 23,* 613–619.

Semenya, S., Potgieter, M., Tshisikhawe, M., Shava, S., & Maroyi, A. (2012). Medicinal utilization of exotic plants by Bapedi traditional healers to treat human ailments in Limpopo province, South Africa. *Journal of Ethnopharmacology, 144*(3), 646-655.

Sharma, S., Kalia, N.P., Suden, P., Chauhan, P.S., Kumar, M., Ram, A.B., ... & Khan, I.A. (2014). Protective efficacy of piperine against *Mycobacterium tuberculosis. Tuberculosis, 94*(4), 389-396.

Shinohara, T., Pantuso, T., Shinohara, S., Kogiso, M., Myrvik, Q.N., Henriksen, R.A., & Shibata, Y. (2009). Persistent inactivation of macrophage cyclooxygenase-2 in mycobacterial pulmonary inflammation. *American Journal of Respiratory Cell and Molecular Biology, 41*(2), 146-154.

Siddiqui, B.S., Bhatti, H.A., Begum, S., & Perwaiz, S. (2012). Evaluation of the antimycobacterium activity of the constituents from *Ocimum basilicum* against Mycobacterium tuberculosis. *Journal of Ethnopharmacology, 144*(1), 220-222.

Strobel, G.A. (2003). Endophytes as sources of bioactive products. *Microbes and Infection, 5*(6), 535-544.

Suckling, D.M., & Sagar, R.L. (2011). Honeybees *Apis mellifera* can detect the scent of Mycobacterium tuberculosis. *Tuberculosis, 91*(4), 327-328.

Sureram, S., Senadeera, S. P., Hongmanee, P., Mahidol, C., Ruchirawat, S., & Kittakoop, P. (2012). Antimycobacterial activity of bisbenzylisoquinoline alkaloids from *Tiliacora triandra* against multidrug-resistant isolates of *Mycobacterium tuberculosis. Bioorganic and Medicinal Chemistry Letters, 22*(8), 2902-2905.

Tabuti, J.R., Kukunda, C.B., & Waako, P.J. (2010). Medicinal plants used by traditional medicine practitioners in the treatment of tuberculosis and related ailments in Uganda. *Journal of Ethnopharmacology, 127*(1), 130-136.

Tawde, K.V., Gacche, R.N., & Pund, M.M. (2012). Evaluation of selected Indian traditional folk medicinal plants against *Mycobacterium tuberculosis* with antioxidant and cytotoxicity study. *Asian Pacific Journal of Tropical Disease, 2,* S685-S691.

Tchouya, G.R.F., Souza, A., Tchouankeu, J.C., Yala, J.F., Boukandou, M., Foundikou, H., ... & Lebibi, J. (2015). Ethnopharmacological surveys and pharmacological studies of plants used in traditional medicine in the treatment of HIV/AIDS opportunistic diseases in Gabon. *Journal of Ethnopharmacology, 162*(1), 306-316.

Tekwu, E.M., Askun, T., Kuete, V., Nkengfack, A.E., Nyasse, B., Etoa, F. X., & Beng, V.P. (2012). Antibacterial activity of selected Cameroonian dietary spices ethno-medically used against strains of *Mycobacterium tuberculosis*. *Journal of Ethnopharmacology*, *142*(2), 374-382.

Torres-Romero, D., Jiménez, I.A., Rojas, R., Gilman, R.H., López, M., & Bazzocchi, I.L. (2011). Dihydro-β-agarofuran sesquiterpenes isolated from *Celastrus vulcanicola* as potential anti-*Mycobacterium tuberculosis* multidrug-resistant agents. *Bioorganic and Medicinal Chemistry*, *19*(7), 2182-2189.

Toungoussova, O.S., Bjune, G., & Caugant, D.A. (2006). Epidemic of tuberculosis in the former Soviet Union: Social and biological reasons. *Tuberculosis*, *86*(1), 1-10.

Toyang, N.J., & Verpoorte, R. (2013). A review of the medicinal potentials of plants of the genus *Vernonia* (Asteraceae). *Journal of Ethnopharmacology*, *146*(3), 681-723.

Uc-Cachón, A.H., Borges-Argáez, R., Said-Fernández, S., Vargas-Villarreal, J., González-Salazar, F., Méndez-González, M., ... & Molina-Salinas, G. M. (2014). Naphthoquinones isolated from *Diospyros anisandra* exhibit potent activity against pan-resistant first-line drugs *Mycobacterium tuberculosis* strains. *Pulmonary Pharmacology and Therapeutics*, *27*(1), 114-120.

Vermund, S.H., & Yamamoto, N. (2007). Co-infection with human immunodeficiency virus and tuberculosis in Asia. *Tuberculosis*, *87*, S18-S25.

Wang, D., Pan, L., Cao, G., Lei, H., Meng, X., He, J., ... & Liu, Z. (2012). Evaluation of the *in vitro* and intracellular efficacy of new monosubstituted sulfonylureas against extensively drug-resistant tuberculosis. *International Journal of Antimicrobial Agents*, *40*(5), 463-466.

WHO (2010b). Multidrug and extensively drug-resistant TB (M/XDR-TB) (Global Report on Surveillance and Response. WHO/HTM/TB/2010.3). World Health Organization, Geneva.

WHO (2010a). WHO Tuberculosis Fact sheet No. 104, Available at: http://www.who.int/ mediacentre/factsheets/fs104/en/ (accessed 01.05.10).

WHO (2012). Global Tuberculosis Report 2012. Retrieved from http://www.who.int/tb/publications/global_report/en/index.

WHO (2000). Global tuberculosis control. WHO report 2000, Geneva, http://www.who.int/gtb/publications/globrep00/index.html)(accessed 4 February 2010).

Xie, L., Wang, X., Zeng, J., Zhou, M., Duan, X., Li, Q., ... & Xie, J. (2015). Proteome-wide lysine acetylation profiling of the human pathogen Mycobacterium tuberculosis. *The International Journal of Biochemistry and Cell Biology*, *59*, 193-202.

York, T., De Wet, H., & Van Vuuren, S. F. (2011). Plants used for treating respiratory infections in rural Maputaland, KwaZulu-Natal, South Africa. *Journal of Ethnopharmacology*, *135*(3), 696-710.

York, T., Van Vuuren, S.F., & De Wet, H. (2012). An antimicrobial evaluation of plants used for the treatment of respiratory infections in rural Maputaland, KwaZulu-Natal, South Africa. *Journal of Ethnopharmacology*, *144*(1), 118-127.

Zhao, J., Evangelopoulos, D., Bhakta, S., Gray, A. I., & Seidel, V. (2014). Antitubercular activity of Arctium lappa and Tussilago farfara extracts and constituents. *Journal of Ethnopharmacology*, *155*(1), 796-800.

Zumla, A., Nahid, P., Cole, S.T., 2013. Advances in the development of new tuberculosis drugs and treatment regimens. *Nature Review Drug Discovery*, *12*(5), 388–404.

Table 6.1: Plants for managing tuberculosis in Uganda

Scientific name of plant	Plant family	Local name of plant	Plant parts used
Combretum molle	Combretaceae	*Ndagi*	Stem bark
Phaseolus vulgaris	Fabaceae	*Bijanjaro*	Husks
Mangifera indica†	Anacardiaceae	*Muyembe*	Stem bark
Rubia cordifolia	Rubiaceae	*Kasalabakesi*	Leaves, whole plant
Dracaena steudneri	Asparagaceae	*Kajjolyenjovu*	Stem bark
Canarium schweinfurthii	Burseraceae	*Muwafu*	Stem bark, seeds
Callistemon citrinus	Myrtaceae	*Mwambala butonya*	Stem bark, leaves
Erythrina abyssinica	Fabaceae	*Eggirikiti*	Stem bark
Hibiscus fuscus	Malvaceae	*Lusaala*	Leaves
Garcinia buchananii	Clusiaceae	*Musaali*	Stem bark
Blighia unijugata	Sapindaceae	*Enkuza nyana*	Stem bark
Vernonia amygdalina	Asteraceae	*Mululuza*	Leaves
Moringa oleifera†	Moraceae	*Moringa*	Fruits, seeds
Maytenus senegalensis†	Celastraceae	*Naligwalimu, Muwaiswa*	Leaves, fruits
Aloe vera	Xanthorrhoeaceae	*Kigaji*	Leaves
Allium sativum	Amaryllidaceae	*Katungulu chumu*	Fruits
Eucalyptus sp. †	Myrtaceae	*Kalitunsi, Ekalitus*	Stem bark
Warburgia salutaris	Canellaceae	*Mwiha, Abaki*	Stem bark
Ocimum suave	Lamiaceae	*Muhumuzanganda*	Leaves
Zanthoxylum chalybeum†	Rutaceae	*Ntale ya dungu, Eusugu*	Roots
Momordica foetida	Cucurbitaceae	*Luiwula/Mwishwa*	Leaves
Persea americana	Lauraceae	*Ovacado*	Leaves
Azadirachta indica†	Meliaceae	*Neem*	Seeds
Allium sativum†	Alliaceae	*Garlic*	Leaves
Bidens pilosa†	Asteraceae	*Nyabarashana*	Flowers
Acacia hockii	Mimosaceae	*Kashiono*	Stem bark

Carica papaya†	Caricaceae	Leaves
	Amapapali	
Helichrysum odoratissimum†	Asteraceae	leaves
	Lweza	
Achyranthes aspera†	Amaranthaceae	Flowers
	Muhurura	

Adapted from Bunalema et al.. (2014) and Tabuti et al. (2010); †denotes plants that have proven activity against Mycobacteria tuberculosis and other Mycobacteria species

Table 6.2: Anti-mycobacterial activity of selected South African plants

Scientific name of plant	Bioactive compounds	Anti-mycobacterial activity
Arctotis auriculata	Tannins, flavonoids, alkaloids, and cyanogenic glucosides	Petroleum ether leaf extract, MIC of 8.5 mg/ml against *M. smegmatis*
Artemisia afra	Volatile oil, terpenoids, coumarins and acetylenes	Ethanol leaf extract, MIC = 1.56 mg/ml against *M. smegmatis*
Helichrysum spp.	Flavonoids, sesquiterpenoids, acylated phloroglucinols, tannins, saponins, cyanogenic glucosides, caespitate from *Helichrysum caespititium*	*Helichrysum melanacme* acetone extract, MIC = 0.1 mg/ml and water extract, MIC = 1 mg/ml against *M. tuberculosis*; *Helichrysum odoratissimum* acetone extract, MIC = 0.5 mg/ml; *Helichrysum caespitatum* acetone extract, MIC = 0.1 mg/ml; caespitate, MIC = 0.1 mg/ml against *M. tuberculosis*
Warburgia salutaris	Drimane sesquiterpenoids including warburganal and polygodial	Dichloromethane bark extract, sesquiterpene mixture and 11α-hydroxycinnamosmolide were active against *M. tuberculosis* and *M. bovis* BCG
Combretum imberbe	Pentacyclic triterpenes, triterpene acids and related glycosides	Pentacyclic triterpenes, MIC = 1.56–25 μg/ml against *Mycobacterium fortuitum*
Terminalia sericea	Roots contain termilignan B and arjunic acid	Bark and root ethanol, ethyl acetate and dichloromethane extracts active, MIC = 1.56–3.12 mg/ml against *M. aurum*; Termilignan B and arjunic acid not active against *M. aurum*
Acacia nilotica	Hydroxyproline, serine, dimethyltriptamine, β-amyrin, and betulin	Leaf, bark and root ethanol and ethyl acetate extracts active, MIC = 0.195–1.56 mg/ml against *M. aurum*
Acacia sieberiana	Hydroxyproline, serine, dimethyltriptamine, β-amyrin, and betulin	Leaf, bark and root ethanol, ethyl acetate and dichloromethane extracts active, MIC = 0.78–6.25 mg/ml against *M. aurum*
Faidherbia albida	Tannins	Leaf and bark ethanol and ethyl acetate extracts active, MIC = 3.12–12.5 mg/ml against *M. aurum*
Pelargonium reniforme *Pelargonium sidoides*	Tannins, phenolic compounds, umckalin and related coumarins in *P. reniforme* tubers; essential oils, flavonoids and phytosterols, fatty acids	Unsaturated fatty acids active against *Mycobacterium aurum, M. smegmatis, Mycobacterium fortuitum, Mycobacterium abscessus,* and *Mycobacterium phlei*
Orthosiphon labiatus	Labdane diterpenoids	Labdane diterpenoid, MIC = 157 μM against

		M. tuberculosis
Salvia radula *Salvia verbenaca* *Salvia dolomitica*	Carnosol, rosmadial, carnosic acid, 7-O-methylepirosmanol, oleanolic acid and ursolic acid	Extracts of *Salvia radula*, *Salvia verbenaca* and *Salvia dolomitica*, MIC = 0.1 mg/ml against *M. tuberculosis*
Syzygium gerrardii	Tannins	Ethanol extract of leaves, MIC = 6.25 mg/ml against *M. smegmatis*; not active against *M. tuberculosis*
Polysiphonia virgata	Fatty acids	Fatty acid mixture active against *M. smegmatis* and *M. tuberculosis*
Prunus africana	β-sitosterol and terpenoids	Leaf and bark ethyl acetate and dichloromethane extracts active, MIC = 0.78–6.25 mg/ml against *M. aurum*; ethanol extract of leaves not active against *M. smegmatis* and *M. tuberculosis*
Coleonema album	Phenolic acids, flavonoids, coumarins, prenylated coumarins and terpenoids	Acetone and ethanol leaf extracts active, MIC = 3.1 mg/ml on *M. aurum*
Salix mucronata	-	Leaf, bark and root ethanol, ethyl acetate and dichloromethane extracts active, MIC = 1.56–.25 mg/ml on *M. aurum*
Dodonaea angustifolia	Dodonic acid, hautriwaic acid and structurally similar diterpenoids, β-sitosterol and stigmasterol, and several flavonoids including santin	Ethanol extract of leaves, MIC = 3.13 mg/ml against *M. smegmatis*, MIC = 5 mg/ml against *M. tuberculosis*; aqueous decoctions and infusions of leaves and stems and ethyl acetate extract, MIC = 5 mg/ml on *M. smegmatis*; ethanol and methanol extracts, MIC = 1.25 mg/ml against *M. smegmatis*

Adapted from McGaw, Lall, Meyer, and Eloff (2008)

7 The World of Malaria: Antimalarial Medicines from Mother Nature

Introduction

Malaria is an old disease whose treatment can benefit from new scientific interventions. Today, the burden of malaria remains worrisome mainly because of the emergence of parasite resistance to available antimalarial drugs. In the face of mounting drug resistance, scientists have ramped up bioprospecting efforts in the hope of discovering new antimalarial medicines from Mother Nature.

Because two antimalarial drugs- quinine and artemisinin, were discovered through improved understanding of indigenous knowledge of plants in Peru and China, respectively, there is a nostalgic sense of desire that, today, pharmacognosy and ethnopharmacology can help unravel new and better drugs to treat malaria.

In this chapter, we turn the spotlight onto some of the medicinal plants and natural chemical agents that may provide leads or better still be converted into more efficacious drugs for the treatment of malaria. And, as we shall soon discover, we do not need to look very far away for antimalarial plants. Common food plants like avocado, cocoa, guava, ginger, mango, sorghum, pumpkins, pawpaw, pineapple and tea are considered effective natural remedies for malaria. Nature's pharmacy is never too far away. Interestingly, because some of the antimalarial plants are edible, their ingestion as food makes them good prophylactic agents for malaria. Food is the best medicine.

By way of preamble, the initial sections of the chapter delve into malaria aetiology and symptoms, global burden and control of malaria, association of malaria and HIV/AIDS, and synthetic drugs for the treatment of malaria. Later, the chapter describes pharmacopoeias of plants used in the treatment of malaria in Africa, Asia, Amazonia and Old Europe. For the first time in recent years, this monograph is unique because it comprehensively details antimalarial therapies in various parts of the world. It also describes antimalarial plants used as single and combined treatment regimens. In certain cases, active ingredients against *Plasmodium* are highlighted.

The hope is that after detailed *in vitro* and *in vivo* antiplasmodial, toxicological and dosage evaluations, some of these natural products may be harnessed for use as antimalarial therapies especially in rural populations where synthetic drugs are high-priced and unavailable, and where public health facilities are faraway.

Malaria Aetiology and Symptoms

Malaria is also known as the king of diseases (Alemu, Shiferaw, Addis, Mathewos, & Birhan, 2013). It is caused by unicellular protozoan parasites belonging to the genus *Plasmodium*. Malaria is one of the leading causes of morbidity and mortality in the world. For a long time, four *Plasmodium* species were known to cause malaria in humans: *Plasmodium falciparum*, *Plasmodium vivax*, *Plasmodium malariae* and *Plasmodium ovale*. But there is now a fifth human malaria parasite, the hitherto monkey malaria parasite *Plasmodium knowlesi* (White, 2008).

The most lethal form of malaria is caused by the parasite *P. falciparum*, transmitted to humans by the female *Anopheles* mosquito, during a blood meal (Diou, Gauthier, Tardif, Fromentin, Lodge, Sullivan, & Tremblay, 2009). *P. falciparum* is the most deadly human malaria parasite, responsible for about 90% of all malaria deaths. Extant strains evolved from a single host transfer event, most likely from gorillas (Liu, Li, Learn, Rudicell, Robertson, & Keele et al., 2010). It goes without saying that there are potential *Plasmodium* reservoirs in apes.

Textbook symptoms of malaria have changed over time, much like the malaria parasite itself. Stangeland, Alele, Katuura and Lye (2011) itemized, in decreasing order of magnitude, the symptoms of malaria as recounted by local people at risk of the disease. The symptoms include: high body temperature, shivering, chills, headache, vomiting, pale eyes, loss of appetite, weakness, not being active, abdominal pain, diarrhoea, jaundice/yellow skin and yellow eyes. Patients usually distinguish a unique fever associated with malaria.

Other clinical indications of malaria are: Goose pimples, fast heart rate, blisters on mouth, thirst, fluctuating temperature, anaemic, pale skin/hands, mental confusion/hallucinations, backache/stiff neck, dry lips, yellow placenta, red eyes, constipation, change in colour/physical appearance, urinating yellow urine, cold feet, dizziness, weakness but no fever, nausea, vomiting yellow stuff, bitter taste in the mouth, sweating and convulsions. Mischaracterization of malaria is common.

Abbah, Amos, Chindo, Ngazal, Vongtau and Adzu et al. (2010) also stated malaria commonly presents as fever, headache, generalized body pains, shivering, arthralgia, vomiting, anorexia and anaemia. Malnutrition and a deficiency in iron, vitamin A and zinc are linked to increased malaria incidence, mortality, still births and underweight babies. Gestational malaria is responsible for low birth weight and maternal anaemia in endemic areas.

Childs, Abuelezam, Dye, Gupta, Murray, Williams and Buckee (2015) believe most infected individuals in endemic regions harbour multiple *Plasmodium* clones resulting from a complex history of exposure. They postulated that repeated and simultaneous infections with different antigenically diverse parasites may lead to a semi-immune status. In older children and adults living in endemic regions, this semi-immunity may be protective against severe disease.

Cabrera, Neculai and Kain (2014) submit that erythrocyte disorders such as the sickle cell haemoglobin variant and glucose 6-phosphate dehydrogenase (G6PD) deficiency are prominent in malaria endemic regions and correlate with resistance to severe disease. White, Pukrittayakamee, Hien, Faiz, Mokuolu and Dondorp (2014) agreed that because the geographic distributions of sickle cell anaemia, haemoglobins C and E, ovalocytosis, thalassaemias and G6PD deficiency are almost similar to that of malaria before the introduction of control measures, these disorders confer survival advantage to people in malaria endemic areas. However, the role of CD36 (cluster of differentiation 36) in malaria pathobiology is controversial. Some studies implicate CD36 as a central receptor that mediates severe disease. Other studies say CD36 functions as a key element in innate defense (Cabrera et al., 2014).

Global Burden and Control of Malaria

Over 40% of the world's population lives in malaria-endemic areas covering 104 countries of the world. Overall, mathematical models suggest 3.4 billion people are at risk of malaria infection in 97-109 countries and territories (Diarra, van't Klooster, Togola, Diallo, Willcox, & de Jong, 2015). Malaria is the world's most prevalent vector-borne disease, with mosquitoes killing one person every 30 seconds in Africa (Fowler, 2006). In 2012, over 627,000 people died from malaria. The Democratic Republic of Congo (DRC), in particular, encumbers one of the highest burdens of malaria in Sub-Saharan Africa. Over a third of adults in the DRC have malaria parasites in their blood (Hay, Okiro, Gething, Patil, Tatem, Guerra, & Snow, 2010). DRC accounts for up to 15% of the global malaria deaths.

By 2009, malaria inflicted about 300–500 million people worldwide, killing about 1 million people annually (Hay et al., 2010). More human death and disease are caused by *Plasmodium* than by all other eukaryotic pathogens combined (Conway, 2015). In 2010, about 216 million malaria attacks occurred worldwide and the number of malaria-related deaths was estimated at 600,000 (Danno, Rerolle, de Sigalony, Colas, Terzan, & Bordet, 2014). In 2012, there were an estimated 207 million cases of malaria; out of about 3.4 billion people at risk of the disease (World Health Organization, 2014).

It seems malaria control efforts are bearing fruit; thus the declining global prevalence of malaria cases during the years leading up to 2012. For example, a few African countries like Eritrea, Rwanda and Zambia have reduced malaria deaths by 50% mostly due to adequate coverage of key interventions such as insecticide treated bed nets, indoor residual spraying with DDT and intensified treatment of cases (Stangeland et al., 2011).

However, rollback malaria control efforts are being hampered by the movement of people across the landscape; this helps malaria parasites to skip over long and extended geographic spaces and exchange genetic material with parasites located at great distances (Carrel, Patel, Taylor, Janko, Mwandagalir-wa, & Tshefu et al., 2014). Medical geographers and spatial epidemiologists could contribute valuable knowledge to the control of malaria.

A categorization of countries as malaria free, eliminating malaria, or con-trolling malaria was provided by Cotter, Sturrock, Hsiang, Liu, Phillips and Hwang et al. (2013) and the WHO (2008a; 2008b). Despite improvements in malaria control, almost 81% of malaria attacks still occur in Africa, where chil-dren and pregnant women are at increased risk of the disease. Daily, malaria kills 1,200 children in Sub-Saharan Africa and more than 200 children in Ugan-da. Shortages of coartem (artemether–lumefantrine) at Macha Hospital in southern Zambia are always accompanied by increases in paediatric hospitaliza-tions for malaria (Mharakurwa, Thuma, Norris, Mulenga, Chalwe, & Chipeta et al., 2012).

Malaria is a major obstacle to social-economic progress in Sub-Saharan Africa, accounting for 40% of public health subventions. The disease causes premature deaths, can leave patients with permanent neurological damage, slashes productivity and increases school absenteeism. In endemic countries, about 25-40% of out-patients turn up with malaria. Affected families some-times spend up to 25% of their income on malaria treatment and prevention, a massive cost for poor households.

Malaria is usually associated with poverty and stagnant water. In Thailand, malaria is linked to rubber plantations (Bhumiratana, Sorosjinda-Nunthawarasilp, Kaewwaen, Maneekan, & Pimnon, 2013). The heavy toll ex-acted by malaria is not only compounded by the growing problem of parasite resistance to synthetic drugs. It is also fuelled by increasing insecticide re-sistance of mosquito vectors. These challenges continue to invite the search for new antimalarial drugs from plants, especially because there is no evidence of resistance to whole-plant extracts.

In addition, despite increased donor funds for research and control pro-grammes to roll back malaria, the disease remains a major public health challenge, especially in tropical and subtropical regions of Africa and Asia. In many African countries, donor funds are often misused by government and malaria control project officials. Despite donor-funded interventions in Luapula Province of Zambia, malaria increased from 32.9 to 50.5% between 2006 and 2010, respectively (Mharakurwa et al., 2012).

Artemisinin-based combination therapy and widespread use of impregnated bed nets have reduced the morbidity and mortality due to malaria. But parasite resistance to the current arsenal of drugs, combined with the fact that the cost of the current antimalarial drugs is prohibitive in poor settings, justify the pressing need to characterise new antimalarial agents that are cheaper and more effective. It is also important to discover new drugs with less toxicity and side-effects. Effective and cheaper treatment of malaria will contribute to the attainment of Millennium Development Goal number 6, *viz.*, combating malaria and HIV/AIDS.

Association of Malaria and HIV/AIDS

Malaria and HIV are among the two most important public health problems facing developing countries today. In 2010, Sub-Saharan Africa is said to have experienced 1.8 million and 1.2 million deaths attributable to HIV/AIDS and malaria, respectively (Vamvaka, Twyman, Christou, & Capell, 2014). Nine out of ten malaria deaths occur in Africa and the rest occur in Asia and Latin America (Alemu et al., 2013).

By the year 2009, both malaria and HIV/AIDS caused more than 4 million deaths a year (Diou et al., 2009). This mortality situation has now changed partly due to substantial scaling up of prevention and treatment strategies more especially antiretroviral therapy for HIV/AIDS. Thus, in the years leading up to 2015, the three diseases of malaria, HIV, and tuberculosis, while infecting more than a third of the global population, were responsible for nearly three million deaths each year (Childs et al., 2015).

However, in terms of biogeography, there is a superimposition between *P. falciparum* and HIV-1 infections. This spatial overlap produces a much higher concentration in the burden of both diseases within the same territories. Malaria made up about 14% of opportunistic infections prevalent in persons with HIV/AIDS in Gabon. In recent years, mortality due to malaria has risen due to HIV/AIDS.

Malaria and HIV co-infection is a major public health problem in tropical and sub-tropical regions of the world. Their geographical overlap translates into significant co-morbidity and higher mortality particularly in malaria endemic areas of Southern Africa, the epicentre of HIV/AIDS.

Few experiments contest the role of malaria as a risk factor in HIV infection (Cuadros, Branscum, & Crowley, 2011a; Cuadros, Branscum, & Garcia-

Ramos, 2011b). However, a growing corpus of experimental results shows malaria parasites increase susceptibility to HIV infection and escalate progression to AIDS. In endemic areas, frequent and severe episodes of malaria are generally held as a nadir of immune suppression.

In agreement with Borkow and Bentwich (2004), chronic protozoal infections increase the risk of HIV infection through a process of chronic immune activation. Chronic malaria infection may result in increased HIV plasma viral load. Vamvaka et al. (2014) stated that acute malaria induces a temporary increase in the HIV viral load.

Dual infection with malaria and HIV fuels the spread of both diseases in Sub-Saharan Africa (Abu-Raddad, Patnaik, & Kublin, 2006). Following Alemu et al. (2013), malaria and HIV/AIDS increase the severity of each other's symptoms and do worsen complications to both clinical diagnosis and treatment.

De Ridder, Kooy and Verpoorte (2008) asserted that if HIV progresses and immunosuppression worsens, the manifestations of malaria also worsen. The symptoms, severity and consequences of malaria in HIV patients are worse than in patients who only have malaria. Due to diminished immunity, the malaria treatment failure rates are also higher. Patients with complicated *P. falciparum* malaria are also profoundly immunosuppressed and susceptible to opportunistic infections (Traoré, Baldé, Camara, Baldé, Diané, & Diallo et al., 2015).

Vamvaka et al. (2014) opine that the immunosuppressive effects of HIV escalate the risk of malaria infection in individuals living in malaria endemic areas. HIV/AIDS infected persons show severe malaria symptoms and longer or frequent durations of malaria bouts. HIV also tends to promote opportunistic feverish conditions, which makes it difficult to arrive at an accurate clinical malarial diagnosis.

In Zambia, HIV infection increases malaria-related mortality in children (Chintu, Luo, Bhat, DuPont, Mwansa-Salamu, Kabika, & Zumla, 1995). In Uganda, HIV increases the risk of placental malaria as new-borns of HIV-positive women show higher rates of parasitaemia (Brahmbhatt, Kigozi, Wabwire-Mangen, Serwadda, Sewankambo, & Lutalo et al., 2003). HIV also increased the risk of malaria in Kenyan women (Van Eijk, Ayisi, Ter Kuile, Misore, Otieno, & Rosen et al., 2003).

Without laboratory diagnosis, opportunistic conditions during HIV infection are usually misdiagnosed as malaria (Vamvaka et al., 2009). This leads to wastage and misuse of antimalarial drugs and a failure to correctly treat either HIV or malaria infections. Brentlinger, Behrens and Micek (2006) argued that co-morbidity nullifies the effectiveness of both antimalarial and antiretroviral drugs.

On the other hand, co-administration of drugs may increase the risk of drug-related toxicity (Brentlinger et al., 2006). HIV patients easily develop adverse effects to antimalarial drugs. The risk of cytotoxicity when antiretroviral and antimalarial drugs are taken by the same patient at the same time is high. For this reason, recognition of the linkages between malaria and HIV infection is important and synergistic approaches involving the control of malaria as a strategy to combat HIV/AIDS and vice versa are needed in co-endemic areas.

Preparations from *Artemisia annua* (a known antimalarial plant) and *Moringa oleifera* may be combined and used to treat HIV-positive patients that have contracted malaria because extracts from both plants have been shown to inhibit HIV (Hirt, Lindsey, & Balagizi, 2008).

Pharmaceuticals for the Treatment of Malaria

Antimalarial drugs stem from seven drug classes: 4-aminoquinolines (chloroquine, amodiaquine and piperaquine), 8-aminoquinolines (primaquine and tafenoquine), arylaminoalcohols (quinine, mefloqine and lumefantrine), antifolates, artemisinin derivatives, respiratory chain inhibitors and antibiotics.

In many malaria endemic countries of Africa and Asia, chloroquine and sulfadoxine–pyrimethamine (Fansidar®) are no longer efficacious because the parasites have developed resistance. These two drugs are oftentimes substituted by artemisinin-based combination therapy, believed to produce better outcomes. Artemisinin-based combination therapy is the first line of treatment for uncomplicated malaria.

However, chloroquine is still effective against *Plasmodium vivax*. In addition, it is still used, though not officially recommended, in some rural areas in developing countries. Fansidar® is still used singly in preventive intermittent treatment of pregnant women in Africa and in combination with artemisinin derivatives in several parts of the world. Yes, there is increasing resistance, but chloroquine and Fansidar® are still used.

In 1971, Chinese scientists isolated artemisinin, a sesquiterpene lactone, which was highly unusual because it contained an endoperoxide moiety in contrast to known antimalarial drugs (Wright, 2005). Many African countries have embraced the use of artemisinin-combined therapy as first-line treatment for uncomplicated malaria. Southern Africa implemented a shift in drug policy in 2003, from chloroquine (to which *P. falciparum* was resistant) to artemether–lumefantrine as the first line treatment (Mharakurwa et al., 2012). Widespread adoption of artemisinin-combined therapy is challenged by several problems including toxicity, high costs and production of artemisinin derivatives to match standards of good manufacturing practice.

Failure of artemisinin-based combination therapy has been reported in Cambodia and Thailand (Alker, Lim, Sem, Shah, Yi, & Bouth et al., 2007), East

Africa (Holmgren, Hamrin, Svärd, Mårtensson, Gil, & Björkman, 2007) and Mali (Djimdé, Fofana, Sagara, Sidibe, Toure, & Dembele, 2008). Indeed, artemisinin-resistant malaria parasites were detected at the Thailand-Cambodia border (Maude, Socheat, Nguon, Saroth, Dara, & Li et al., 2012; Maude, Pontavornpinyo, Saralamba, Aguas, Yeung, & Dondorp et al., 2009). Artemisinin resistance has also been documented in the Greater Mekong sub-region consisting of Burma, Laos, Vietnam and the Yunnan Province of China (Dondorp, Yeung, White, Nguon, Day, Socheat, & von Seidlein, 2010; Dondorp, Nosten, Yi, Das, Phyo, & Tarning et al., 2009).

Despite the cost and adverse effects, a standard treatment for severe malaria in Africa is the intravenous administration of quinine. Resistance against quinine in Africa has not been reported. Quinine is the only medicine authorized for the treatment of acute malaria in pregnant women irrespective of term (Danno et al., 2014). Available under the trade name Quinimax®, quinine is administered orally or by injection.

The usual dose of quinine used in medical centres and recommended by WHO is 24 mg/kg per day in three doses for 7 days (Danno et al., 2014). The dosage for pregnant women is the same for adults. However, quinine is associated with various side-effects: hypoglycaemia, cardiotoxicity, allergic reactions, anaemia and signs of cinchonism characterized by tinnitus, dizziness, headaches, visual problems, decline in hearing acuity, nausea and diarrhoea.

To circumvent the dangers of malaria in gravid women, WHO recommends three main control measures: the use of mosquito bed nets impregnated with insecticides, good management of cases of malaria, and intermittent preventative treatment which consists of administering a curative dose of an antimalarial drug twice during pregnancy.

Drugs for malaria prevention need to be active against liver stages of the parasites. Prevention of malaria is done by monthly doses of amodiaquine–sulfadoxine–pyrimethamine during the rainy season in children aged between 3 months and 5 years across the sub-Sahel region (White et al., 2014). Primaquine, the only drug licenced for malaria prophylaxis, is considered to be toxic. Although it is the only drug specifically developed to inhibit liver infection, primaquine has been curtailed by the associated toxicity, poor compliance and increased risk of haemolysis when administered to persons with G6PD, a common phenotype in Africa (Carraz, Jossang, Franetich, Siau, Ciceron, & Hannoun et al., 2006). It causes haemolytic anaemia in people with G6PD.

Singh, Kaushik, Mohanakrishnan, Tiwari and Sahal (2015) claim that chemotherapeutic attempts to eliminate malaria have failed largely due to the emergence of drug resistant forms of *Plasmodium* that have rendered quinolones like chloroquine, quinine, primaquine and mefloquine ineffective in the vast majority of malaria-endemic areas.

Molecular and Nanotechnolgical Tools against Malaria

Sequencing of the entire *Plasmodium* genome through the Malaria Genome Project may open new vistas to identify *Plasmodium* specific targets for drug discovery. The WHO Initiative for Vaccine Research (IVR) and Malaria Vaccine Advisory Committee (MALVAC) provide guidance to WHO member countries on priorities in malaria vaccine research and development. Sadly, the use of vaccines to prevent malaria is immunologically hampered by the parasite's constant changes of the variable surface glycoproteins. Parasites escape the host immune system, making the development of a reliable vaccine a very big challenge (Stanisic, Barry, & Good, 2013).

Ahead of World Malaria Day on 25 April 2015, The RTS,S Clinical Trials Partnership reported that a vaccine candidate (RTS,S/AS01), developed over 30 years by GloxoSmithKline, prevented a substantial number of cases of clinical malaria over a 3–4 year period in young infants and children when administered with or without a booster dose (RTS,S Clinical Trials Partnership, 2015). According to their results, efficacy was enhanced by the administration of a booster dose. They envisage the vaccine has the potential to make a substantial contribution to malaria control when used in combination with other effective control measures, especially in areas of high transmission.

Recent developments in parasite genomics and increasingly large amounts of data from population studies are helping to identify antigens that are promising lead targets for candidate vaccines. Advances in systems immunology could accelerate efforts to unravel the mechanisms of acquired immunity to malaria (Tran, Samal, Kirkness, & Crompton, 2012). Metabolomics may also add a unique dimension in our endeavours to better understand malaria parasite biology in the hope of discovering novel therapeutic and vaccine targets (Lakshmanan, Rhee, & Daily, 2011).

Moreover, transgenic fungi can express antiplasmodial effector molecules that can target the parasite inside its vector (Abdul-Ghani, Al-Mekhlafi, & Al-absi, 2012). Encouraging as these research efforts may be, turning their results into real-life therapeutics is a still a herculean task. Plus, discovery and characterization of effective vaccines need to be coupled with more innovation and funding to translate findings into newly designed vaccine products for clinical trials (Conway, 2015).

Santos-Magalhães and Mosqueira (2010) lamented that despite the fact that we live in an era of advanced technology, infectious diseases like malaria continue to elude our imagination; they are not yet unamenable to innovative public health treatment and control strategies. According to these authors, the main drawbacks of conventional malaria chemotherapy are the development of multiple drug resistance and the non-specific targeting to intracellular parasites, resulting in high dose requirements and subsequent intolerable toxicity.

Santos-Magalhães and Mosqueira (2010) submitted that nanosized carriers were receiving special attention with the aim of minimizing the side effects of drug therapy, such as poor bioavailability and the selectivity of drugs. Several nanosized delivery systems have already proved their effectiveness in animal models for the treatment and prophylaxis of malaria. Writing on advances in nanotechnology and nanomedicines for malaria treatment, Aditya, Vathsala, Vieira, Murthy and Souto (2013) also mentioned research focussing on the development of new biocompatible systems capable of incorporating drugs, de-escalating resistance and contributing to new methods of diagnosis, control and treatment of malaria by target delivery. But these efforts are still at basic research level and exactly when these nanomedicines and nano-drug carriers will reach the bedsides of malaria patients in developing countries with limited resources and infrastructure is still a pipedream.

Antiplasmodial Activity Assay

The *in vitro* antimalarial activity of extracts against the 3D7 strain of *P. falciparum* is measured by parasite survival using the parasite lactate dehydrogenase (pLDH) assay (Makler, Ries, Williams, Bancroft, Piper, Gibbins, & Hinrichs, 1993). The measurement of pLDH has a correlation with parasitemia and may offer a method that can be developed into a simple test for the detection of parasitemia. The assay is based on the observation that the lactate dehydrogenase (LDH) enzyme of *P. falciparum* has the ability to rapidly use 3-acetyl pyridine NAD (APAD) as a coenzyme in the reaction leading to the formation of pyruvate from lactate (Makler & Hinrichs, 1993). The test uses the parasite's lactate dehydrogenase which is different from the host lactate dehydrogenase.

Lactate dehydrogenase is an enzyme found in all the cells and speeds up the formation of pyruvate from lactate reducing a co-enzyme NAD (nicotinamide adenine dinucleotide) to NADH. In parasites, the NAD analogue APAD (3-acetylpyridine adenine nucleotide) is reduced to APADH and upon this reduction the yellow NBT/PES (nitro blue tetrazolium + phenazine ethosulphate) is converted to purple formazan crystals. The absorbance is then read at 620 nm using a multiwell spectrophotometer (Infinite F500). The formation of these crystals indicates the pLDH activity and therefore the survival of parasites.

The percentage survival of parasites is a measure of the plant extracts' inhibitory activity against *P. falciparum*. This inhibitory activity is determined by the IC_{50} value, measured by making 10 three-fold serial dilutions of the test samples in duplicates in a transparent 96-well flat bottom plate. The plate is put in an airtight box, gassed and incubated for 48 hours followed by developing with NBT/PES reagent. The IC_{50} is expressed as the % parasite survival relative to the control, calculated from fitted sigmoidal dose-response curves.

Dose-response curves are obtained by plotting percentage parasite survival against the logarithm of the concentration using the GraphPad Prism software package (GraphPad software, Inc, California, USA). IC_{50} values are calculated graphically by interpolation from these curves. The criteria for a dose response curve are that there should be at least two points at the lower and upper level of the curve. The percentage survival for the lower level should be between 0 and 20% while that for the upper level should be above 80%.

IC_{50} is defined as the extract concentration that causes 50% inhibition of the malaria parasites. Lower IC_{50} values depict relatively more potent extracts. At the Council for Scientific and Industrial Research (CSIR) in Pretoria, South Africa, crude extracts or test compounds that show IC_{50} of ≤ 10 µg/ml are considered active. Therefore, test compounds with $IC_{50} > 10$ µg/ml are considered inactive, those with 7 µg/ml $\leq IC_{50} \leq 10$ µg/ml show marginal activity and those with 4 ug/ml $\leq IC_{50} \leq 6$ µg/ml show moderate activity. Test compounds with $IC_{50} \leq 3$ µg/ml are considered highly active. Previously, some publications classified antiplasmodial activity in the following categories: high ($IC_{50} < 5$ µg/ml), promising ($5 < IC_{50} < 15$ µg/ml), moderate ($15 < IC_{50} < 50$ µg/ml), and inactive ($IC_{50} > 50$ µg/ml). Note that what is 'active' in one lab may be deemed 'inactive' in another lab and the context should be taken into consideration.

The ratio of cytotoxicity to biological activity is defined as selectivity index and is generally considered that biological efficacy is not due to the *in vitro* cytotoxicity when selectivity index is equal to or greater than 10. For example, methanolic extracts of antimalarial preparations of *Dorstenia klaineana* used in Kenya have poor selectivity indexes of 0.87 to 0.95.

That being said, it is important to prompt that lack of antimalarial activity of plant extracts *in vitro* is not synonymous to lack of activity *in vivo*, for several reasons. Some biological and phytochemical tests are limited in terms of distribution and availability of active ingredients taking part in the reactions. Besides, efficacy may be altered because of differences in the extraction procedures and reconstitution of the herbal remedies via methods different from those by the local people.

Ethnobotany

Ethnobotany is the study of how indigenous people utilize plants for nutrition, healing diseases, shelter, clothing and other uses. A vast majority of prescription drugs used in the world today contain compounds that are directly or indirectly, via semi-synthesis, derived from plants (Oksman-Caldentey & Inze´, 2004). Even the synthetic drugs and compounds used in modern medicine owe their active chemical compounds to bioactive compounds in plants. The structures of active chemical compounds in plants are often identified and copied.

Be that as it may, natural products and particularly microorganisms and medicinal plants remain important sources of new drugs. Over the past 60 years, natural products have provided a direct source of therapeutic agents and a basis for drug development. This is despite the many improvements in rational drug design and synthetic chemistry methods by big pharmaceutical companies.

Given that there are many opportunities in the discovery of new molecules from natural origin, a simple, robust and cost-effective colorimetric assay based on the inhibition of beta-hematin has been adapted to routinely screen plant extracts with the ultimate goal of identifying novel antimalarial ingredients (Vargas, Ioset, Hay, Ioset, Wittlin, & Hostettmann, 2011). This test gives good correlations and positive antiplasmodial values comparable to *Plasmodium* growth inhibition assays.

Indigenous knowledge, coupled with a history of safe use and ethnopharmacological efficacy, present a faster approach to discover new antimalarial agents. This new approach, now called reverse pharmacology (Chinsembu, 2009), promises to shorten the classical drug discovery process from say 20 to 5 years. Ethnobotany, pharmacognosy and ethnopharmacology can quicken the drug discovery process.

Simoes-Pires, Hostettmann, Haouala, Cuendet, Falquet, Graz and Christen (2014) reckon that reverse pharmacology, termed bedside-to-bench, is a research approach based on indigenous knowledge and relates to reversing the classical laboratory to clinic pathway to a clinic to laboratory practice. They opine that reverse pharmacology is a trans-disciplinary approach focused on indigenous knowledge, experimental observations and clinical experiences.

Tapping into the rich vein of ethnobotanical knowledge can unveil traditional medicines that could provide crucial leads to the development of new drugs against malaria. Plants continue to be a very important resource for new medicines and beneficial compounds. However, given rampant drug shortages in poor countries, even qualified western-trained medical doctors sometimes prescribe herbal remedies.

The remarkable antimalarial properties of Peruvian bark (*Cinchona calisaya* and *Cinchona succirubra*), known for more than 383 years, resulted in the discovery of quinine. Infusions of the *Cinchona* plant bark have been used to treat human malaria from as early as 1632. The development of artemisinin derivatives from the traditionally used Chinese plant *qing hao* (*Artemisia annua*), also reaffirms the potential of ethnobotanicals to provide effective drugs for the treatment of malaria.

Natural products have made and continue to make an immense contribution to malaria chemotherapy, either directly as antimalarial agents, or as important lead compounds for the discovery of more potent antimalarials (Kumar, Mahajan, & Chibale, 2009). Natural agents have provided templates for the development of structurally simpler analogues that serve as effective antimalarials. Still, while most people living in malaria endemic areas use traditional medicine, no new antimalarial drugs have recently emerged from ethnopharmacology-oriented research.

Plants as Self-reliant Antimalarial Remedies

According to De Ridder et al. (2008), the first description of the Chinese herb *Artemisia annua* dates back to the year 168 B.C. *Ging hao* means green herb, used as a medicinal tea infusion to treat intermittent fevers. There is still slight confusion regarding the Chinese nomenclature of *Artemisia*. Two species, *A. annua* (*qing hao*) and *Artemisia apiacea* (*huang hua hao*), were distinguishable by 1518. But, according to the history of *qing hao* in the Chinese *materia medica*, *A. annua* is *huang hua hao* and not, as is commonly assumed, *qing hao* (Hsu, 2006). In the history of *qing hao*, *A. annua* and *A. apiacea* (contains small amounts of artemisinin), were not recognized as different species.

The use of *A. annua* as a self-reliant treatment for malaria in developing countries was reviewed by De Ridder et al. (2008). Self-reliant treatment involves the local production practices of *A. annua* including the use of traditionally-prepared teas as an effective treatment for malaria. Alas, self-sufficiency is negatively affected because *A. annua* is not native to Africa. Also, artemisinin is not soluble in water (Jansen, 2006), so its administration as a tea is not effective to cure malaria. The concentration of artemisinin in *A. annua* tea is far too low to cure malaria and opens the floodgates for parasites to develop resistance to artemisinin.

Common dietary constituents and encapsulation affect the bioavailability and therapeutic efficacy of oral consumption of the dried leaf herbal medicine (Weathers, Jordan, Lasin, & Towler, 2014). When dried leaves were encapsulated into either hydroxymethyl-cellulose or gelatin capsules, there was >50% decrease in released artemisinin but no change in released flavonoids (Weathers et al., 2014).

In the presence of millet or corn meal, the amount of released artemisinin declined, but there was no change in released flavonoids (Weathers et al., 2014). By 2013, Van Der Kooy and Sullivan (2013) wrote that very little scientific work had been conducted on the *A. annua* formulation. They also argued that available literature contained many discrepancies being selectively championed by scientists on either side of an often polarized and heated debate. Recrudescence and cure rate are topical issues in this controversy.

One side of the debate underlines the possible role of synergism and prodrugs. On the other side of the argument, there are claims the effectiveness of the flavonoid-rich *A. annua* formulation is misleading given the low content of artemisinin in *A. annua*, the low bioavailability of artemisinin when the traditional formulation is administered and the high levels of recrudescence in patients using the infusion (Jansen, 2006). It is feared that high rates of recrudescence of *P. falciparum* may lead to the development of artemisinin resistant strains.

Other Plant Remedies against Malaria

Many plant remedies are used to treat malaria in Africa, Asia and the Americas. Previous studies have shown that more than 1200 medicinal plants from 160 families are used worldwide to treat malaria (Willcox & Bodeker, 2004). But it is the African countries which have had a lion's share of antimalarial herbs. In Cotonou, Benin, the homeopathic medicine *China rubra 7CH* supplied by Boiron Laboratories (China Group) reduced side-effects associated with quinine treatment of malaria in pregnant women (Danno et al., 2014). Whether *China rubra 7CH* inhibits *Plasmodium* is not clear.

Tea (*Camellia sinensis*) leaves contain gallocatechins, flavonoid compounds that inhibit *P. falciparum* more potently than the antimalarial drug mefloquine (Tegar & Purnomo, 2013). Gallocatechins inhibit the parasite's lactate dehydrogenase enzyme. The inhibitory action of gallocatechins on lactate dehydrogenase was illustrated through molecular docking experiments.

African pumpkin (*Momordica balsamina*), is an extensively cultivated vegetable consumed in many tropical and subtropical regions of the world. This species has also been widely used in traditional medicine, especially in Africa, to treat diabetes and malaria. Ramalhete, da Cruz, Mulhovo, Sousa, Fernandes, Prudêncio and Ferreira (2014) found that 16 triterpenoids isolated from *M. balsamina* exhibited *in vitro* antimalarial activity against blood and liver stages of chloroquine-resistant strains of *P. falciparum*.

Azadirachta indica (neem tree) is used to manage malaria symptoms in Kenya, Ivory Coast, Ghana, Madagascar and Sudan (Muthaura, Keriko, Derese, Yenesew, & Rukunga, 2011). *Strychnopsis thouarsii* and *Ampelozyziphus amazonicus* have been used for malaria prophylaxis in Madagascar and countries in the Amazon, respectively (Carraz et al., 2006; Andrade-Neto, Brandão, Nogueira, Rosário, & Krettli, 2008). *Vernonia amygdalina* holds the most promise for development into a nutraceutical against diabetes and malaria (Toyang & Verpoorte, 2013).

Mongalo, McGaw, Finnie and van Staden (2015) found that *Securidaca longepedunculata* is an antimalarial plant in many countries. In their review, they quote studies where the dichloromethane extract of the leaves showed antiplasmodial activity, IC_{50} = 6.9 µg/ml, against *P. falciparum*. The methanol extract of the roots also suppressed *Plasmodium berghei* by 82% at a dose of 0.56 mg/kg. Against a chloroquine-resistant *P. falciparum* strain, methanol and chloroform extracts of the roots exhibited an IC_{50} of 250 µg/ml.

In Burkina Faso, Kenya and Tanzania, the plant *Cassia singueana* is used as a traditional treatment for malaria, sometimes working as an adjuvant (Hiben, Sibhat, Fanta, Gebrezgi, & Tesema, 2015). Leaf sap and a hot decoction of powdered leaves are taken orally to treat malaria. The methanolic extracts of the root bark, known to contain lupeol, has significant activity against *P. berghei* and chloroquine-resistant *P. falciparum*.

Jain, Sood and Gowthamarajan (2013) report that curcumin had moderate antimalarial activity, IC_{50} of 5–18 µM and was effective in treating cerebral malaria. Curcumin is small molecular weight polyphenolic compound isolated from the rhizomes of turmeric (*Curcuma longa*), a plant traditionally used as a spice. In addition to its direct killing effect of *Plasmodium*, curcumin is also able to prime the immune system. Curcumin-artemisinin combination therapy for malaria was reported (Nandakumar, Nagaraj, Vathsala, Rangarajan, & Padmanaban, 2006).

Curcumin inhibits chloroquine-resistant *P. falciparum* growth in culture in a dose dependent manner with an IC_{50} of 5 µM. Oral administration of curcumin to mice infected with *P. berghei* reduces blood parasitemia by 80–90% and enhances host survival significantly. However, since most experiments are done in mice, the results are not necessarily applicable to humans. Further, the *in vivo* antimalarial efficacy of curcumin is reduced because 90% of curcumin is metabolized within 30 minutes. Due to its poor absorption, rapid metabolism and excretion, it is also unlikely that substantial concentrations of curcumin are pharmacologically active in the body after ingestion.

Species in the plant family Acanthaceae, for example, *Andrographis paniculata*, *Hypoestes rosea* and *Clinacanthus siamensis*, contain terpenes and xanthones with antiplasmodial activities (Lekana-Douki, Bongui, Liabagui, Edou, Zatra, & Bisvigou et al., 2011). *Artocarpus rigidus* and *Ficus fistulosa* exhibit antiplasmodial activities attributable to three flavonoids: Artonin F, 7-demethylartonol E and a cycloartobiloxanthone (Verrucarin L acetate). Likewise, lignans of *Pycnanthus angolensis* have strong antiplasmodial activity. The bark and roots of *Nauclea latifolia* (Rubiaceae), also known as African peach or fig, are a common remedy for malaria in Savannah Africa. The plant is imbued with monoterpenes, triterpenes, indole alkaloids, saponins and traces of inorganic compounds in the roots (Abbah et al., 2010).

Leaf poultices of *Acalypha fruticosa* in Yemen, *Acalypha torta* in Nigeria and *Acalypha wilkesiana* in many countries are used to treat malaria. These multi-use medicinal plants are known to contain several active ingredients including 2-acetylfuran, myo-inositol, daucosterol, emodin, β-sitosterol, ursolic acid, rutin, quercetin 7-rutinoside, n-hexadecanoic acid and 1,2-benzenedicarboxylic acid (Seebaluck, Gurib-Fakim, & Mahomoodally, 2015).

Sebastiania chamaelea and *Chrozophora senegalensis* are used by traditional healers to treat malaria in Nigeria and Senegal (Garcia-Alvarez, Moussa, Soh, Nongonierma, Abdoulaye, & Nicolau-Travers et al., 2013). The aqueous crude extract of *C. senegalensis* leaves showed the most significant antiplasmodial activity *in vitro* (IC_{50} < 2 μg/ml). *In vitro* potentiation assays revealed strong synergistic activity of *S. chamaelea* extract with chloroquine against chloroquine-resistant *P. falciparum* strain W2-Indochina. Ellagic acid was the main antiplasmodial principle in both plants.

Interestingly, 93% of nature-derived antimalarials referenced by the WHO and 62% of antimalarial natural species in a MEDLINE search had anticancer activity (Duffy, Wade, & Chang, 2012). It is plausible to speculate that antimalarial natural products may possess anticancer properties or at least offer leads to scientists working in the field of anticancer drug discovery.

Kaur, Jain, Kaur and Jain (2009) provide a detailed 1998-2008 review of the chemical structures of antimalarials from plant and marine organisms. The antimalarial compounds include alkaloids (naphthylisoquinoline, bisbenzylisoquinoline, protoberberine and aporphine, indole, and manzamine), terpenes (sesquiterpenes, triterpenes and diterpenes), quassinoids, flavonoids, limonoids, chalcones, peptides, xanthones, quinones and coumarins. Their review also illustrated miscellaneous natural antimalarial molecules such as sarachine, plakortones, aigialomycin D, dehydrodiconiferyl dibenzoate, justicidin B, ellagic acid, uveosides, syncarpamide, pentothenic acid, lupeol, pycnidione, allicin, curcumin, (+)-catechin 3-gallate, mucochloric acid, endothall, anisomycin and cerulenin.

McCracken, Kaiser, Boshoff, Boyd and Copp (2012) also state that 4-methoxy-6-styryl-2H-pyran-2-ones are antiplasmodial polyketides derived from fungi and rudimentary angiosperms. Dihydrostyryl- and styryl-pyrones, isolated from a number of sources, including the flowering plants *Alpinia speciosa* and *Polygala sabulosa*, exhibit activity towards infectious diseases such malaria; 6-styryl-pyran-2-ones exhibited moderate activity towards *P. falciparum* with IC_{50} values varying between 1.3 and 17 μM.

Fungi as Antimalarial Agents

Natural antimalarials are not only restricted to plants. Scientists in Australia found the fungus *Ramaria subaurantiaca* produces potent antiplasmodial chemical compounds including spermatinamine (IC_{50} = 0.23 µM) and the polyamine alkaloid, pistillarin (IC_{50} = 1.9 µM, selectivity index >53) (Choomuenwai, Schwartz, Beattie, Andrews, Khokhar, & Davis, 2013). Spermatinamine, originally isolated from the sponge *Pseudoceratina* sp., is highly toxic to human cells (selectivity index = 9).

Cortinarius species produced the chemical compound (1*S*,3*S*)-austrocortirubin which displayed promising antiplasmodial activity. This compound was identified as a natural product scaffold that could be used in the generation of an antimalarial tetrahydroanthraquinone (Choomuenwai, Andrews, & Davis, 2012).

The fumagillin family of natural products, including its new synthetic analog fumarranol, potently inhibit the growth of both chloroquine-sensitive and drug-resistant *P. falciparum* strains *in vitro* and *in vivo* (Chen, Xie, Bhat, Kumar, Shapiro, & Liu, 2009). Fumagillin is a complex biomolecule used as an antimicrobial agent, even to control the microsporidian *Nosema apis* disease in honey bees. It was first isolated in 1949 from *Aspergillus fumigatus*, one of the most ubiquitous airborne saprophytic fungi.

Marine Microbial Metabolites as AntiPlasmodial Agents

Maskey, Helmke, Kayser, Fiebig, Maier, Busche and Laatsch (2004) worked on trioxacarcins, complex antibiotics produced by marine Streptomyces derived from the Gulf of Mexico. All trioxacarcins exhibited high antibacterial and some of them showed higher anti-tumour and anti-malaria activities. Manivasagan, Kang, Sivakumar, Li-Chan, Oh and Kim (2014) write that some trioxacarcins from marine actinobacteria have extremely high antiplasmodial activity, comparable to the activity of artemisinin.

Studies have identified the 3,6-dialkyl-4-hydroxy-pyran-2-one marine microbial metabolites pseudopyronines A and B to be modest growth inhibitors of *P. falciparum* (McCracken et al., 2012). In 2009, symplostatin 4 (Sym4) was isolated from two marine cyanobacterial species *Symploca* and *Schizothrix* (Stolze, Deu, Kaschani, Li, Florea, & Richau et al., 2012). Experiments revealed that Sym4 was a potent nanomolar growth inhibitor of *P. falciparum* strains 3D7 and W2 (IC_{50} = 36–100 nM). New evidence suggests Sym4 is an inhibitor of the food vacuole falcipains in *P. falciparum*.

Pharmacopoeias of Antimalarial Plants

Many different plant species have been used to treat malaria in various parts of the world. Here, we look at some of the antimalarial plants in the following countries and regions: Benin, Burkina Faso, Cameroon, Ethiopia, Gabon, Ghana, Guinea, Kenya, Mali, Namibia, Nigeria, Uganda, Senegal, South Africa, Rwanda, Zambia, Zimbabwe, India, Malaysia, Amazon region and Renaissance Europe. Memvanga, Tona, Mesia, Lusakibanza and Cimanga (2015) also reviewed antimalarial activity of medicinal plants from the Democratic Republic of Congo.

In his extensive study published in the esteemed journal *Acta Tropica*, Chinsembu (2015) details plants used as antimalarial agents in Sub-Saharan Africa.

Benin

Malaria presents in about 40% of all patients seeking treatment at health centres in Benin (Danno et al., 2014). Yetein, Houessou, Lougbégnon, Teka and Tente (2013) documented a total of 82 plant species used as antimalarials in the plateau of Allada situated in the south of Benin, West Africa. Plants are used to heal 70% of malaria cases in Benin. *Dichapetalum madagascariense, Acanthospermum hispidum, Sarcocephalus latifolius, Dialium guineense, Carica papaya* or pawpaw and *Citrus limon* or lemon were frequently used for malaria treatment.

Other plant species used to alleviate malaria symptoms were: *Adansonia digitata, Cleome gynandra, Chamaecrista rotundifolia, Hibiscus surratensis, Lantana camara* (has lantanine, a quinine-like alkaloid), *M. oleifera, Khaya senegalensis, Kigelia africana, Cassia occidentalis, Uvaria chamae, Vernonia amygdalina, Xylopia aethiopica* and *Zingiber officinale* (ginger). Yetein et al. (2013) cited studies conducted elsewhere which showed that *D. madagascariense, C. limon, U. chamae, S. latifolius, C. rotundifolia, A. hispidum, C. papaya, D. guineense* and *C. occidentalis* have varying levels of antiplasmodial activity.

Bero, Ganfon, Jonville, Frédérich, Gbaguidi, DeMol, Moudachirou and Quetin-Leclercq (2009) evaluated twelve plant extracts on antiplasmodial activity using the measurement of the plasmodial lactate dehydrogenase activity on chloroquine-sensitive (3D7) and resistant (W2) strains of *P. falciparum* in Benin. Their results revealed that all the plant extracts had low cytotoxicity.

Inhibition of *P. falciparum* was observed with the dichloromethane extracts of *A. hispidum* (IC_{50} =7.5 µg/ml on 3D7 and 4.8 µg/ml on W2), *Keetia leucantha* leaves and twigs (IC_{50} = 13.8 µg/ml and 11.3 µg/ml on 3D7 and IC_{50} = 26.5 µg/ml and 15.8 µg/ml on W2, respectively), *Carpolobia lutea*, (IC_{50} = 19.4 µg/ml on 3D7 and 8.1 µg/ml on W2) and *Strychnos spinosa* leaves (IC_{50} = 15.6 µg/ml on 3D7 and 8.9 µg/ml on W2).

Burkina Faso

Ilboudo, Basilico, Parapini, Corbett, D'Alessandro and Dell'Agli et al. (2013) observed that extracts of the leaves and twigs of the shrub *Canthium henriquesianum* are a frequent treatment for malaria in Burkina Faso. Known as *Laagui Fofana* in the local language, *C. henriquesianum* plant parts are used to make a tepid decoction. The preparation is applied singly or in combination with other plant extracts to alleviate malaria.

A common remedy for malaria is a decoction of *Gardenia sokotensis*, whose organic fraction has an *in vivo* activity of ED_{50} of 116 mg/kg against *P. berghei*, and *Vernonia colorata*, whose twigs also have good antiplasmodial action (IC_{50} = 14.1 µg/ml for a 1:1 dichlormethane/methanol extract). *Vernonia colorata* is also found in Zimbabwe. Roots of *Canthium multiflorum* contain a derivative of ursenoic acid, 19-hydroxy-3-oxo- ursa-1,12-dien-20,28-oic acid, with low antiplasmodial activity (IC_{50} = 26 µg/ml).

Water preparations of *G. sokotensis* and *V. colorata* had no antiplasmodial activity. And sadly, decoctions of these plants were toxic to normal human fibroblasts *in vitro*. These results call into doubt the efficacy of some plants used as traditional medicines; this justifies the need to conduct scientific validation.

In another study, good antimalarial activities were displayed by extracts of *Dicoma tomentosa*, *Psorospermum senegalense* leaves and *G. sokotensis* leaves (Jansen, Angenot, Tits, Nicolas, De Mol, Nikiéma, & Frédérich, 2010). Preparations of these three plants had IC_{50} values of 7.0-14.0 µg/ml. Moderate antiplasmodial actions, IC_{50} values ranging from 15-50 µg/ml, were found for *Boswellia dalzielii* leaves, *Waltheria indica* roots, *Bergia suffruticosa* whole plant, *Vitellaria paradoxa* bark and *Jatropha gossypiifolia* leaves.

Jatrophone, a product of *Jatropha isabelli*, exerts significant activity against *P. falciparum* strains 3D7 and K1 (Hadi, Hotard, Ling, Salinas, Palacios, Connelly, & Rivas, 2013). Jatrophone belongs to a large family of terpenes that were isolated from *Jatropha* diterpenes. It has a broad range of biological activities including anti-tumour, cytotoxic, anti-inflammatory, molluscidal, and fungicidal properties.

Cameroon

Resistance to antimalarial drugs is a leading cause of morbidity and mortality in Cameroon, a West African country that lies closer to the equatorial rainy forests. In their search for more effective and new treatments, Titanji, Zofou and Ngemenya (2008) revealed that researchers in Cameroon had by

June 2007 identified nearly 217 different plant species used by traditional healers as antimalarial remedies. Table 7.1 presents some antimalarial plants used in Cameroon. Almost a hundred phytochemicals had been isolated from 26 species some of which were good potential leads for the development of new antimalarial drugs.

Crude extracts and essential oils prepared from 54 other species showed a wide range of activity on *Plasmodium* species. These developments show that a lot of research is being done on antimalarial plants. *Khaya ivorensis* and *Alstonia boonei* are used for malaria treatment in central Cameroon. Antiplasmodial activity in BALB/c mice was observed when aqueous extracts from the stem bark of the two plants were prepared and tested separately and in combination against *P. berghei* (Tepongning, Lucantoni, Nasuti, Dori, Yerbanga, & Lupidi et al., 2011).

Several studies have revealed that *Khaya grandifoliola* and *K. ivorensis* contain active antiplasmodial constituents called limonoids. Some of the limonoids are proceranolide, mexicanolide, khivorin, angolensate, gedunin, khayanolide, khayalactone and swietenine. Gedunin was the most active showing IC_{50} values of 0.02–1.25 µg/ml on various strains of *P. falciparum* strains.

Parasite growth in mice treated with *K. ivorensis* extracts at daily dosages of 400 mg/kg was inhibited by 35%. Administration of *A. boonei* at 400 mg/kg to mice reduced parasitemia by 21%. Assays for liver and kidney enzymes demonstrated that the *K. ivorensis* and *A. boonei* plant extracts were mildly toxic after 14 days, though this was reversible.

Boyom, Kemgne, Tepongning, Ngouana, Mbacham and Tsamo et al. (2009) found that extracts of plants in the family Annonaceae, namely, *Uvariopsis congolana* (stems), *U. congolana* (leaf), *Polyalthia oliveri* (stem bark) and *Enantia chlorantha* (stem bark and stems) displayed high activity of less than 5 µg/ml against *P. falciparum* W2 strain which is resistant to chloroquine and other antimalarials.

In previous experiments, *E. chlorantha* water and ethanol extracts, in addition to purified alkaloids from the stem bark, had remarkable antiplasmodial activities *in vitro* and *in vivo* (Agbaje & Onabanjo, 1994; Vennerstrom & Klayman, 1988). *Enantia polycarpa* from Côte d'Ivoire also showed good potency *in vitro* against the K1 strain of *P. falciparum* (Atindehou, Schmid, Brun, Koné, & Traore, 2004). *Cymbopogon giganteus* is also active against chloroquine-resistant *Plasmodium* (Kimbi & Fagbenro-Beyioku, 1996).

Acetogenins (a fatty acid-derived class of secondary metabolites), the principle active chemical ingredients of *Uvariopsis congensis*, may also be present in the chemo-taxonomically similar species *U. congolana*- a plant often eaten by sick wild chimpanzees and known to have antibacterial, antimalarial and antileishmanial properties (Boyom et al., 2009). Plants in the Moraceae family, that is, *Artocarpus communis* stem bark and leaf and *Dorstenia convewa* twigs showed high potency against W2 *in vitro,* IC_{50} < 5 µg/ml. *A. communis* and *D. convewa* contain prenyl flavonoids and geranyl flavonoids, the latter group of compounds are cytotoxic to cancer cells. A related species to *A. communis* is *Artocarpus integer* which contains prenylated stilbene, IC_{50} = 1.7 µg/ml against *P. falciparum.*

Croton zambesicus is imbued with diterpenes having considerable activity against *P. berghei* in mice. In another study, 21 species in the family Annonaceae were used in the treatment of malaria in four areas of Cameroon (Tsabang, Fokou, Tchokouaha, Noguem, Bakarnga-Via, Nguepi, & Nkongmeneck, 2012). *Annickia chlorantha*, sold in many markets, was the main plant species utilized for malaria treatment. Boniface, Verma, Shukla, Cheema, Srivastava and Khan et al. (2015) reported that *Conyza sumatrensis* leaves are formulated into an antimalarial remedy in Cameroon. The soft aerial part of the plant is taken as a decoction alongside *Rauvolfia vomitoria* stem bark, lime fruit, *C. papaya* mature leaves and *Cymbopogom citratus* leaves.

Together with the leaves of *Commelina benghalensis,* stem bark extracts of *Steganotaenia araliacea* - also used to induce labour in Zambia, were found to have antiplasmodial properties in Cameroon.

Ethiopia

Mesfin, Giday, Animut and Teklehaymanot (2012) documented medicinal plants that are traditionally used for the treatment of malaria in Shinile District, eastern Ethiopia. *Aloe* sp., *A. indica* and *Tamarindus indica* were the most commonly used plants for malarial treatment. In mice, ethanol and water leaf extracts of *Aloe* caused 73.94% and 58.10% parasitaemia suppression, respectively, at a dose of 650 mg/kg. Ethanol extract of *A. indica* leaves produced 54.79% parasitaemia suppression at the dose of 650 mg/kg but its water extract gave a lower parasite suppression (21.47%) at a similar dose. Water extract of the fruits of *T. indica*, believed to contain tannins, saponins, sesquiterpenes, alkaloids and phlobatannins, showed the highest parasitaemia suppression (81.09%) at the dose of 650 mg/kg. Leaves of *Salvadora persica* are powdered, boiled and drunk after adding sugar. Dried roots of *Withania somnifera* are crushed, boiled and drunk after adding goat/camel milk. *Acokanthra schimperi* leaves are pounded, mixed in water, sieved through thin cloth and filtrate is drunk.

According to the Ethiopian scientists, an infusion of the fruit/pulp of *T. indica* is kept overnight and drunk after taking goat soup. Fresh leaves of *Aloe* are squeezed and diluted with water and drunk. Syrup prepared from dried *Aloe* leaves and that of *Asparagus africanus* plus *Cassia italica* is also drunk. In the case of *A. indica*, fresh apical leaves and buds are pounded, mixed with water (soaked) and the filtrate is drunk. Lemon and salt (sometimes sugar) are added. Pounded leaves of *Maerua oblongifolia* (sometimes mixed with *W. somnifera* leaves) are boiled with goat milk and drunk. Unlike water extracts, limonoids and alcoholic extracts of the leaves and seeds of *A. indica* were effective against *P. falciparum in vivo.*

Mekonnen (2015) described the use of *Croton macrostachyus* root and fruit extracts for the treatment of malaria. Both extracts significantly inhibited parasitemia and increased survival time in infected mice. The plant has promising activity against *P. berghei* in a dose-dependent manner and this supports the folkloric use of the plant for treating malaria.

Gabon

People in Haut-Ogooué Province, south-eastern Gabon, use several plants to treat malaria. Here, findings of Lekana-Douki et al. (2011) are described. Gabonese patients harvest the stems and leaves of *Adhatoda latibracteata*, boil them and drink the solution to alleviate malaria. A dichloromethane extract of alkaloid-rich *A. latibracteata*, weakly cytotoxic to human cells, had very high antimalarial activities, with IC_{50} values of 0.7 and 1.6 µg/ml on *Plasmodium* strains FCB and W2, respectively.

The leaves of *Aframomum giganteum* are boiled and the decoction is orally taken to treat headache and fever. Known for their deworming and purgative powers, extracts of *A. giganteum* are also applied to easy toothache. A dichloromethane extract of *A. giganteum* showed promising antiplasmodial activities (IC_{50} = 8 and 13.5 µg/ml on strains FCB and W2, respectively). Terpenes, flavonoids, diaryl heptanoids and sesquiterpenes give *A. giganteum* and related species strong antiplasmodial efficacy.

A nicely fragrant plant applied as a cosmetic, *Culcasia lancifolia* has moderate antimalarial activity, most likely due to sesquiterpenes. It is a known analgesic and anti-inflammatory remedy. *Dorstenia klaineana* has moderate antiplasmodial activity (IC_{50} around 17 µg/ml) but strong cytotoxicity (0.43 µg/ml), with a selectivity index of 0.03.

On the authority of Lekana-Douki et al. (2011), *Leonotis africana* infusions and baths are a common treatment for malaria, diarrhoea, and postcircumcision healing. The plant has moderate antiplasmodial activities (IC_{50} =27.1 and 15.2 µg/ml on strains FCB and W2, respectively), and weak cytotoxicity (LD_{50} = 439.1 µg/ml; selectivity indexes = 16.20 to 28.89). Flavonoids and terpenes are candidate compounds from this species.

The same authors go on to say an infusion of *Monodora myristica*, sometimes in combination with *N. latifolia*, kills worms and heals headaches and constipation. A methanolic extract of *M. myristica* had high antimalarial activity

(IC$_{50}$ = 5.5 and 6.1 µg/ml on strains FCB and W2, respectively) and weak cyto-toxicity (LD$_{50}$ = 95.7 µg/ml), producing good selectivity indexes of 17.40 and 15.69). Antiplasmodial efficacy may be due to the terpenes and alkaloids found in this species and its close relatives.

To manage malaria, patients in Libreville sip infusions of *Staudtia gabonensis*, often mixed with *E. chlorantha* or *Combretodendron africanum*. A red-sap plant whose leaf decoction heals eye pain, gonorrhoea and rheumatism, a methanolic extract of *S. gabonensis* has high antimalarial value (IC$_{50}$ of 0.8 µg/ml on strains FCB and W2) and great selectivity indexes (58.25 for both strains).

Lekana-Douki et al. (2011) found that whereas dichloromethane extracts of *N. latifolia* showed promising antimalarial activities (IC$_{50}$ = 6.6 and 8.0 µg/ml on strains FCB and W2, respectively), the methanolic extracts displayed moderate antiplasmodial actions (IC$_{50}$ = 17.1 and 18.4 µg/ml on strains FCB and W2, respectively). But both organic extracts of *N. latifolia* were indiscriminate for host and parasite cells, with selectivity indexes for both around 3. In their studies of plants used in the treatment of HIV/AIDS opportunistic diseases in Gabon, Tchouya, Souza, Tchouankeu, Yala, Boukandou and Foundikou et al. (2015), citing other studies, documented the use of *Sarcocephalus latifolius* as an antimalarial plant.

Ghana

In Dangme West District, several plants were used to treat malaria. The four most frequently cited species of plants were *A. indica, Cassia siamea, Citrus aurantifolia* and *N. latifolia* (Asase, Akwetey, & Achel, 2010). Other frequently cited antimalarial plants were *A. hispidus, V. amygdalina, C. papaya, K. senegalensis, M. oleifera* and *Theobroma cacao* (cocoa). The following plants were documented for the first time: *Bambusa vulgaris, Deinbollia pinnata, Elaeis guineensis* and *Solanum torvum*. Many plants used in Ghana have known antiplasmodial efficacies, namely: *A. hispidus, A. indica, Lippia multiflora, Mangifera indica, Morinda lucida, N. latifolia, Securinega virosa, Cassia alata, C. occidentalis, C. siamea* and *V. amygdalina*.

Asase, Hesse and Simmonds (2012) also found 33 plant species were utilized for malaria treatment in southern Ghana. The most frequently cited plants were: *Anopyxis klaineana, Annona muricata, A. boonei, Cocos nucifera, Citrus sinensis* and *C. aurantifolia*. A combined formulation consisting of *Jatropha curcas, Gossypium hirsutum, Physalis angulata* and *Delonix regia* was also used for the treatment of malaria. An antimalarial phyto-remedy called *phyto-laria*, based on *Cryptolepis sanguinolenta*, has been developed and is widely used in Ghana (Bourdy, Willcox, Ginsburg, Rasoanaivo, Graz & Deharo, 2008). Regrettably, arsenic contamination, beyond the WHO permissible level of 1.0 parts per million, was a major pollutant in ready-to-use antimalarial water preparations of *C. sanguinolenta, V. amygdalina, Momordica charantia, N. latifolia, Alstonia boonei, A.*

indica, *Monodora myristica* and *Xylopia aethiopica* (Affum, Shiloh, & Adomako, 2013). To avoid harming the health of patients, it is important to monitor herbal products for toxic metal pollution.

Guinea

An ethnobotanical survey on medicinal plants used by Guinean traditional healers in the treatment of malaria was reported by Traore, Baldé, Diallo, Baldé, Diané and Camara et al. (2013). With 53% prevalence in rural areas, malaria represents the first cause of hospital admissions in Guinea. In 2013, the average cost of one dosage of artemisinin-combined therapy ranged from €5 to €8.5. For the local people, this was quite expensive, compelling affected populations to use herbal medicines to manage malaria. Some of the plant species, plant parts and antiplasmodial activities are listed in Table 7.2.

Traore et al. (2013) cited empirical reports of antiplasmodial active ingredients, namely: ellagic acid from *Alchornea cordifolia* which exhibited an IC_{50} value of 0.11 µg/ml on *P. falciparum* strain FcM29, fagaronine from *Fagara zanthoxyloides* had an IC_{50} value of 0.018 µg/ml on *P. falciparum* strain NF54, vismione H from *Vismia guineensis* displayed an IC_{50} of 0.088 µg/ml on strain NF54 and an alkaloid strictosamide from *Nauclea* species. Clinical trials involving *Cochlospermum planchonii* and *Nauclea pobeguinii* showed that these species were promising candidates for the development of drugs against uncomplicated malaria.

Kenya

Gathirwa, Rukunga, Njagi, Omar, Mwitari and Guantai et al. (2008) and Gathirwa, Rukunga, Njagi, Omar, Guantai, Muthaura and Mwitari (2007) analyzed the antimalarial efficacy of plants used in the Meru community. Their results showed that a methanolic extract of *Turraea robusta* was the most active against *P. falciparum* D6 strain. Aqueous extracts of *Lannea schweinfurthii* had the highest anti-plamodial activity followed by *T. robusta* and *Sclerocarya birrea* (marula). In mice, *L. schweinfurthii* extracts had the highest antimalarial activity, followed by *T. robusta* and *S. birrea,* with the methanol extracts being more active than aqueous ones.

Five different plant extract combinations consisting of *Boscia salicifolia* and *S. birrea*; *Rhus natalensis* and *T. robusta*; *R. natalensis* and *B. salicifolia*; *T. robusta* and *S. birrea*; and *L. schweinfurthii* and *B. salicifolia* suppressed >90% of the parasites in mice. The use of plant combinations in traditional medicine is clinically important because it reduces the emergency of drug resistant parasite strains.

Rukunga, Gathirwa, Omar, Muregi, Muthaura and Kirira et al. (2009) found that extracts of the following plants were active against *P. falciparum* ENT30, a resistant strain: *Zanthoxylum chalybeum*, IC_{50} = 2.32; *Cyperus articulatus*, IC_{50} = 8.59 µg/ml; and *Cissampelos pareira*, IC_{50} = 7.705 µg/ml. Scientists at the Kenya Medical Research Institute also studied medicinal plants from Maasai communities (Kigondu, Rukunga, Gathirwa, Irungu, Mwikwabe, & Amalemba et al., 2011). Their results revealed that leaves and roots of *Fuerstia africanaa* had high antiplasmodial activities against the chloroquine-sensitive antiplasmodial strain D6, IC_{50} = 1.5 and 4.6 µg/ml, respectively, with a selectivity index of 44 against Vero cells.

Another plant, *Manilkara discolor*, exhibited promising antiplasmodial action, 26.6 µg/ml. Ethyl acetate extracts of the roots of *Pentas lanceolata* (known to contain asperuloside, an iridoid monoterpene and a series of iridoid glucosides) and the leaves of *Sericocomopsis hildebrandtii* showed moderate activities against *Plasmodium* strains, IC_{50} values of 14.3 and 16.51 µg/ml, respectively (Kigondu et al., 2011). It was recommended that *F. africana* could be studied further with the hope of developing its active chemical determinants into new antimalarial drugs.

Nguta and Mbaria (2013) screened crude plant extracts which displayed low chemo-suppression of parasitaemia as follows: *A. indica*, 3.1%; *Dichrostachys cinerea*, 6.3%; *T. indica*, 25.1%; *Acacia seyal*, 7.8%; and *Grewia trichocarpa*, 35.8%. With an LC_{50} of 285.8 µg/ml, *A. indica* root bark extract was moderately cytotoxic while *T. indica* stem bark and *G. trichocarpa* root extracts, with LC_{50} values of 516.4 and 545.8 µg/ml, respectively, were weakly toxic. However, *A. seyal* and *D. cinerea* root extracts were non-toxic, LC_{50} = 5915.6 µg/ml and 8298.5 µg/ml, respectively. Lower LC_{50} values denote more cytotoxicity than higher values. Disparities in the presence and concentrations of bioactive and cytotoxic chemical ingredients are mostly due to the genetic makeup of the plant, within species variation, age of the plant, season, locality, extraction method and length of storage time of the plant material.

Musila, Dossaji, Nguta, Lukhoba and Munyao (2013) found aqueous extract of the stem bark of *A. digitata* exhibited high chemosuppression of parasitaemia, about 60% in *P. berghei* infected mice. Aqueous extracts *Canthium glaucum* showed 32% chemosuppression of parasitaemia. Organic extracts of *Launaea cornuta* (rich in sesquiterpene lactones) and *Zanthoxylum chalybeum*, though active against *Plasmodium*, were toxic in brine shrimp assays.

Luo and Kuria ethnic groups use several plants to treat malaria. Selected plant extracts were screened against two *P. falciparum* strains, chloroquine sensitive D6 and chloroquine resistant W2 (Owuor, Ochanda, Kokwaro, Cheruiyot, Yeda, Okudo, & Akala, 2012). Promising antiplasmodial results were observed with extracts of *Tylosema fassoglensis*, *Ageratum conyzoides* and *Ocimum kilimandscharicum*.

Analysis of medicinal plants traditionally used for the treatment of malaria in Kenya was reviewed by Muthaura et al. (2011). The plants *Boscia angustifolia, Cyperus articulatus, Gutenbergia cordifolia, Schkuhria pinnata, Ludwigia erecta, Fagaropsis angolensis, Sericocomopsis hildebrandtii* and *Zanthoxylum usambarense* were some of the plants applied as antimalarial remedies. *C. articulatus* is used to treat cerebral malaria in Guinea and ordinary malaria in Nigeria (Akendengue, 1992). Other antimalarial plants used in Kenya are shown in Tables 7.3 and 7.4.

There are several antiplasmodial active compounds from plants: An alkaloid, nitidine, was extracted from *Toddalia asiatica*; coumarins such as 2'epicycloisobrachycoumarinone epoxide and cycloisobrachycoumarinone epoxide were isolated from *Vernonia brachycalyx*; flavonoids such as acacetin, genkwanin and 7-methoxyacacetin were identified from *Artemisia afra*. Flavonoids from *A. afra* have moderate *in vitro* antiplasmodial activities (IC_{50} = 4.3–12.6 μg/ ml). Chemical constituents in *A. annua*, terpenoids and flavonoids, produce a potent synergistic effect against *Plasmodium* parasites. Several studies show the total antiplasmodial activity of *A. annua* is also a result of several polymethoxyflavones such as casticin, artemetin, chrysosplenetin, chrysosplenol-D and circilineol (Muthaura et al., 2011). Other antiplasmodial agents were flavonones like 5-deoxyabyssinin II, abyssinin III, abyssinone IV and V and sigmoidin A from *Erythrina abyssinica*; terpenoids such as diterpene ajugarin-1 and tritepene ergosterol-5,8-endoperoxide from *Ajuga remota* and triterpenoid limonoid-deacetoxy-7-oxogedunin from *Ekebergia capensis*.

Cocquyt, Cos, Herdewijn, Maes, Van den Steen and Laekeman (2011) discovered that *A. remota*, prescribed for malaria by 66% of Kenyan herbalists, contains ergosterol-5,8-endoperoxide, ajugarin-I, 8-O-acetylharpagide and several phytoecdysteroids. Their assays confirm some of these constituents display a concentration-dependent inhibition of chloroquine-sensitive and chloroquine-resistant *P. falciparum* and *Mycobacterium tuberculosis*. The Belgian authors, who provided detailed illustrations of biological models of action on *Plasmodium*, hypothesized that *A. remota* has direct antiplasmodial and immune-stimulatory or adjuvant properties.

Two sesquiterpenes, mustakone and corymbolone, were isolated from *Cyperus articulatus*. According to Muthaura et al. (2011), antiplasmodial spermine alkaloids like budmunchiamine K1, 5-Normethylbudmunchiamine K3, 6-Hydroxybudmunchiamine K2, 6-Hydroxy-5-normethylbudmunchiamine K4, and 9-Normethylbudmunchiamine K5 were all characterized from *Albizia gummifera*. These results show that some Kenyan plants contain chemical ingredients that may be further developed into novel antimalarial drugs.

Mali

In Mali, malaria is still the leading cause of medical consultation, accounting for about 37.4% of consultations. Diarra et al. (2015) identified 97 plants used to treat malaria. *Trichilia emetica, Mitragyna inermis, Sarcocephalus latifolius, Cassia sieberiana, Cochlospermum tinctorium, Anogeissus leiocarpa, Guiera senegalensis* and *Entada africana* were quoted as the most used in the treatment of malaria. *Trichilia emetica*, IC_{50} = 12 μg/ml against *P. falciparum*, contains kurubasch aldehyde with antiplasmodial activity of 76 μM. A decoction of *Argemone mexicana* had clinical antimalarial efficacy comparable to artesunate–amodiaquine (Simoes-Pires et al., 2014). Three alkaloids selective for *P. falciparum* were isolated from *A. mexicana*: allocryptopine, protopine and berberine. The plant originated from the USA-Mexico border, then spread to tropical and sub-tropical regions including Mali. It has a long history in folk medicine, used to heal cancers, warts, skin diseases, inflammation, rheumatism, jaundice, leprosy, microbial infections and malaria.

Namibia

Plants used to treat malaria in Namibia are listed in Table 7.5. Some of these plants were reported by Chinsembu and Hedimbi (2012); Chinsembu, Hedimbi, and Mukaru (2011); and Chinsembu and Hedimbi (2010). Chinsembu, as principal researcher and his doctoral student, Nailoke Pauline Kadhila-Muandingi, are screening indigenous Namibian mushrooms for antimalarial activities, an effort funded by Namibia's National Commission on Research, Science and Technology.

Nigeria

Adebayo and Krettli (2011) reviewed antimalarial plants found and used in Nigeria. Nigerian antimalarial phyto-therapies and their biological activities are listed in Table 7.6. Decoctions, teas and steamy baths of *Alstonia boonei*, a tall tree of 33 metres, are administered as antimalarial cures. Antimalarial pills have been made from the stem bark extracts of this plant. *Tithonia diversifolia* aqueous and alcohol leaf extracts are 50 and 74% effective against *Plasmodium*, respectively. However, the aqueous extracts have high toxicity in mice.

Dike, Obembe and Adebiyi (2012)'s ethnobotanical survey revealed 22 species were used as antimalarials. Some of these include: *Anacardium occidentale, Allamanda cathartica, Alstonia congensis, Bixa orellana, Dacryodes edulis, Canna indica, Dioscorea dumetorum, Mallotus oppositifolius, Persea americana, Ficus exasperata* (fig tree) and *Ludwigia peruviana*. Others were *Axonopus compressus, C. citratus* and *N. latifolia*.

In Ogbomoso, south-west Nigeria, 40 plant species belonging to 32 different families are administered as antimalarial remedies (Olorunnisola, Adetutu, Balogun, & Afolayan, 2013). Notable among these are fruits of onion (*Allium cepa*), unripe fruits of pineapple (*Ananas comosus*), stem barks and leaves of cashew trees (*A. occidentale*), leaves of pawpaw (*C. papaya*), and leaves or stem barks of guava trees (*Psidium guajava*). Other antimalarials were leaves of cotton plants (*Gossypium barbadense*), rhizomes of ginger (*Z. officinale*), fruits of kolanut (*Garcinia kola*), leaves of pigeon pea (*Cajanus cajan*), leaves of avocado (*Persea americana*) and grains of sorghum (*Sorghum bicolor*).

Harungana madagascariensis extracts are remedies for tuberculosis, diarrhoea, dysentery, syphilis, gonorrhea, parasitic skin diseases and wounds. Its active phytochemicals include anthraquinone, anthranoids, courmarins and triterpenoids. Stem barks of *H.* madagascariensis have activity against *Plasmodium, in vivo* and *in vitro* (Iwalewa, Omisore, Adewunmi, Gbolade, Ademowo, & Nneji et al., 2008).

Olorunnisola et al. (2013) mention several antimalarial recipes and dosages. Four yellow *C. papaya* leaves and 30 leaves of *V. amygdalina* are soaked in a bottle of water. To clear malaria, a glassful is taken orally thrice daily for 20 days. Leaves of *V. amygdalina*, bark and leaves of *A. indica* (neem tree) and the bark of *M. indica* are boiled in water for 40 minutes. A full cup is taken orally thrice daily until malaria symptoms vanish. The bark of *E. chlorantha*, leaves of *M. lucida, Picralima nitida*, leaves of *Physalis angulate* and *Piper guineense* are boiled in water for an hour. One glass cup is taken orally twice daily after meals. Patients also bath in plant extracts.

The rhizomes of *C. longa* and leaves of and *H. madagascariensis, R. vomitoria, M. indica, P. guajava* and the bark of *E. chlorantha* are boiled with aqueous extract from fermented maize starch. A cup of the concoction is taken orally thrice daily. The concoction is also used for bathing and steam inhalation. Care should be taken as this natural remedy has side-effects like vomiting and cardiac problems.

Among traditional healers in Lagos State, Ishola, Oreagba, Adeneye, Adirije, Oshikoya and Ogunleye (2014) found 41 plant species belonging to 27 families were employed as antimalarial herbal recipes. *Enantia chlorantha, C. papaya, A. indica, C. citratus, M. lucida, M. indica,* and *A. boonei* were the most frequently used plants, with at least 20% frequency. Traditional healers have devised multiple plant combinations to manage malaria. Two plant recipes include: *A. boonei, Capsicum frutescens; E. chlorantha, C. citratus; C. papaya, P. guajava; A. indica, A. boonei;* and *V. amygdalina* plus *Citrus aurantium*. Three plant mixtures were: *Gossypium barbadense, Ocimum gratissimum, C. aurantium; C. papaya, Citrus paradisi, A. comosus;* and *C. citratus, Curcuma longa* and *C. aurantifolia.* Four plant combinations were: *C. papaya, C. citratus, A. comosus, A. indica; Citrus aurantifolia,*

A. indica, M. indica, M. lucida; Cajanus cajana, A. indica, A. boonei, R. vomitoria; and *Gossypium barbadense, C. longa, C. citratus* and *A. boonei.*

There were also five plant mixtures made up of: *O. gratissimum, A. occidentale, Lecaniodiscus cupanioides, C. longa* and *C. aurantifolia.* Six plant antimalarial concoctions were made from *M. lucida, N. latifolia, C. citratus, M. oleifera, G. kola* and *P. guajava.* Leaves of *M. lucida* (half of the whole blend) are mixed with the leaves of *N. latifollia, C. citratus, C. papaya* and *M. oleifera,* then added to leaves and bark of mango, in equal quantities. A cup of the six-plant brew is taken twice a day. Vomiting and allergic reactions may occur. A nine plant mixture was the highest concoction applied against malaria, consisting of *E. chlorantha, N. latifolia, C. citratus, C. longa, C. paradisi, C. papaya, C. aurantifolia, A. boonei* and *A. comosus.*

It may seem weird to administer a medicinal potion of nine plants. But inventive as many Nigerian traditional doctors are, and given the allegations of fake antimalarial drugs in the country, the multiple plant combinations have been carefully selected to circumvent the increasing problem of *Plasmodium* resistance encountered when a single plant remedy is used. Plant combinations and methods of preparation may also reduce toxicity *in vivo.* Multiple medicinal plant preparations, unlike single ones, may be more efficacious due to the synergistic effects produced by diverse compounds, in addition to encumbering the development of resistant strains of the parasite.

Uganda

Stangeland, Alele, Katuura and Lye (2011) studied plants used to manage malaria in in Nyakayojo Sub-County in south-western Uganda. Their study identified 48 plants used to treat malaria. A literature cross-check showed that more than two-thirds of the plant species in western Uganda had known antimalarial functions and nearly half had documented antiplasmodial activity. The most commonly used species were *V. amygdalina, Vernonia adoensis,* the indigenous *Aloe* species, *Justicia betonica* and *T. diversifolia. Vernonia amygdalina,* the mainstay of malaria treatment, is a known antiplasmodial remedy which contains steroid glucosides, coumarins and sesquiterpene lactones.

However, in Mbarara District, Kamatenesi-Mugisha and Oryem-Origa (2007) found that *V. amygdalina* is traditionally applied to induce labour, which may indicate that the plant has abortifacient effects, and therefore unsafe for malaria treatment in pregnant women. It is therefore urgent to test antimalarial plants used by pregnant women for their effects on the smooth muscles to discern plants that are harmless. *V. amygdalina* has high antiplasmodial activity but exhibits strong cytotoxicity towards cell lines. Like that of *Vernonia adoensis,* the antiplasmodial activity of *V. amygdalina* is credited to the presence of glaucolides, glycocides, and polysaccharides.

Several African *Aloe* species have antiplasmodial action, too. This is mostly due to the presence of anthrone C-glucoside homonataloin, polysaccharides, mannans, anthraquinones, lectins, proteins ((Van Zyl & Viljoen, 2002). Aerial parts of *Justicia betonica* have antiplasmodial efficacy and justetonin, a quinoline alkaloid glycoside, is believed to be the main antiplasmodial agent (Bbosa, Kyegombe, Lubega, Musisi, Ogwal-Okeng, & Odyek, 2013). Another Ugandan plant, *T. diversifolia*, has firm antiplasmodial action ascribed to two main active compounds: tagitinin C and sesquiterpene lactones.

In Budiope County, the most frequent antimalarial plants *V. amygdalina*, *Momordica foetida*, *Zanthoxylum chalybeum*, *Lantana camara* and *M. indica* (Tabuti, 2008). Other plants were *Chenopodium ambrosioides*, *Chenopodium opulifolium*, *A. indica*, *M. oleifera*, *Leonotis nepetifolia*, *Combretum molle* and *Coffea canephora*. Single preparations of these plants were orally administered as water extracts in variable dosages over varied time periods.

The antimalarial activities of *Z. chalybeum*, *M. foetida*, *A. indica* and *Melia azedarach* - whose active ingredient is gedunin, are known. Lacroix, Prado, Kamoga, Kasenene, Namukobe and Krief et al. (2011) itemized antiplasmodial plants used traditionally in Kiohima village, near the Kibale National Park in south-western Uganda (Table 7.7).

Again, the leaves of *V. amygdalina*, though potent against *Plasmodium* in Kiohima village, have strong cytotoxicity and therefore unsafe for antimalarial therapy. At an institution of Traditional Healers called Prometra-Uganda, *V. amygdalina*, *Bidens pilosa*, and *J. betonica* are common prescriptions for malaria (Adia, Anywar, Byamukama, Kamatenesi-Mugisha, Sekagya, Kakudidi, & Kiremire, 2014). Vernangulides A and B, two sesquiterpene lactones isolated from *V. amygdalina*, are responsible for the antiplasmodial activity (IC$_{50}$ = 2 µg/ml). Regrettably, the selectivity index of vernangulides A and B is very low (from 2 to 5.3); this may be the key reason *V. amygdalina* preparations are cytotoxic.

Polyacetylenidioc acid isolated from *Bidens pilosa* has potent activity against malaria parasites both *in vitro* and *in vivo*. Although *Markhamia lutea* has no antiplasmodial activity *in vitro*, it activates the host immune function which restrains *Plasmodium* parasites *in vivo*. It also has very low cytotoxicity, hence is a wonderful adjuvant remedy for malaria.

Other plants were: *Aloe dawei*, *Amaranthus hybridus*, *Rhus vulgaris*, *Combretum molle*, *Bridelia micrantha*, *Clerodendrum rotundifolium*, *O. grattisimum*, *Plectranthus caninus*, *Rosmarinus officinalis*, *Hibiscus surattensis*, *Cissampelos mucronata*, *Albizia grandibracteata*, *Ficus saussureana*, *Eucalyptus grandis*, *Syzygium cumini*, *Vangueria apiculata*, *Solanum nigrum* and *Zea mays* (Adia et al., 2014).

Namukobe, Kiremire, Byamukama, Kasenene, Akala, Kamau and Dumontet (2015) reported that extracts of the plant *Neoboutonia macrocalyx* are used as traditional medicine for malaria. They cite a study which showed the antiplasmodial activity of the stem extract. Another study isolated tigliane diterpenoids from the stem bark of the same plant. Cycloartane triterpenes were characterized from the leaves of *N. macrocalyx* and their antiplasmodial potential was demonstrated.

Namukobe et al. (2015) identified two *N. macrocalyx* diterpenoids, neoboutomacroin and montanin. Although these diterpenoids had good antiplasmodial activity (IC_{50} less than 10 μg/ml against D6 and W2 *P. falciparum* strains), both were were highly cytotoxic to MRC5 cells (IC_{50} less than10 μM).

Senegal

In the Dakar area, an ethnobotanical study documented seven plants used to treat malaria: *Cissampelos mucronata, Maytenus senegalensis, Terminalia macroptera, Bidens engleri, Ceratotheca sesamoides, Chrozophora senegalensis* and *Mitracarpus scaber* (Benoit-Vical, Soh, Salery, Harguem, Poupat, & Nongonierma, 2008). Crude extracts from the leaves and stems of *C. senegalensis* showed the best antiplasmodial activity, IC_{50} = 1.6 μg/ml, with no cytotoxicity. Life cycle observations illustrated that *C. senegalensis* extracts disrupted parasite DNA synthesis as well as the period of liberation and reinvasion of merozoites.

South Africa

Rood (2013) discoursed quite a few plant remedies used to prevent and treat malaria: bark extract of *Rhus undulata*, bark extract of *Rauvolfia caffra*, leaf infusion of *A. digitata* (baobab), bark decoction for *Warburgia salutaris*, beans and bark of *Croton megalobotrys* (large fever berry), root extract of *Securinega virosa*, and roots of *Pterocarpus angolensis* (wild teak). Other phyto-remedies are *Aloe ferox* leaf extract (prophylactic), roots of *Protasparagus capensis* (wild asparagus), fresh juice of the leaves of *Plantago cafra*, *Sorghum* species root extracts, root extract of *Securidaca longependunculata*, sap of the leaves of *Rumex acetosella*, root decoction of *Vangueria infausta* and root extract of *Gnidia cuneata*.

Twenty plants used to treat malaria by the Venda people were evaluated for their antiplasmodial efficacy and cytotoxicity (Bapela, Meyer, & Kaiser, 2014). Dichloromethane extracts of *Tabernaemontana elegans* (Apocynaceae) and *Vangueria infausta* subsp. *infausta* (Rubiaceae) displayed significant antiplasmodial activities, IC_{50} = 0.33 μg/ml and IC_{50} = 1.84 μg/ml, respectively. Selectivity indexes were 14 and 25, respectively. The non-polar root extracts of *Bridelia mollis* and *Cussonia spicata* demonstrated significant *in vitro* antiplasmodial activity (IC_{50} = 3 μg/ml) and selectivity indexes for malaria parasite strain NF54 were 17 and 15, respectively.

Rwanda

Muganga, Angenot, Tits, and Frédérich (2010) tested thirteen plants for antiplasmodial action: *Aristolochia elegans, Conyza aegyptiaca, Markhamia lutea, Microglossa pyrifolia, Mitragyna stipulosa, Fuerstia africana, Rumex abyssinicus, Rumex bequaertii, Solanecio mannii, Terminalia mollis, T. diversifolia, Trimeria grandifolia* and *Zanthoxylum chalybeum*. The results of the study showed that the majority of the plants had antiplasmodial activity. The highest activities were observed with dichloromethane leaf and flower extracts of *T. diversifolia*, leaf extract of *Microglossa pyrifolia* and root extract of *Rumex abyssinicus*, methanol leaf extract of *Fuerstia africana*, root bark extracts of *Zanthoxylum chalybeum* and methanol bark extract of *Terminalia mollis*. These extracts were active (IC$_{50}$ < 15 μg/ml) on both chloroquine-sensitive and resistant strains of *P. falciparum*; *Z. chalybeum, S. mannii* and *T. mollis* displayed the best selectivity indexes.

Muganga et al. (2010) quoted studies where *F. africana* was known to possess ferruginol, a compound with strong antimalarial activity (IC$_{50}$ = 1.95 μg/ml). But ferruginol is not a desirable antimalarial candidate because it is highly cytotoxic. Two antiplasmodial diterpenes, e-phytol and 6E-geranylgeraniol-19-oic acid, were identified from *M. pyrifolia* (IC$_{50}$ = 4.7μg/ml), a plant with high cytotoxicity. Other studies showed that mature stems of *T. diversifolia* contain an artemisinic acid analogue. This is likely to be the antiplasmodial principle. The aerial parts of *T. diversifolia* also contain tagitinin C, a lactone sesquitene with a very promising antiplasmodial activity. Unfortunately, tagitinin C is also cytotoxic.

Togo

Koudouvo, Karou, Kokou, Essien, Aklikokou and Glitho et al. (2011) listed plants used as antimalarial remedies in Togo. They identified 52 species belonging to 49 genera and 29 families. Some of the frequently cited plants were: *A. digitata, Alchornea cordifolia, A. boonei, A. indica, Borassus flabellifer, C. siamea, Clausena anisata, Dodonaea viscosa, Ficus exasperata, Holarrhena floribunda, Lippia multiflora, Mitragyna inermis, M. oleifera, N. latifolia, Nephrolepis biserrata, Ocimum canum, Pergularia daemia, Sansevieria liberica, T. indica, Tectona grandis* and *Zanthoxylum xanthoxyloides*.

Zambia

Fowler (2006) documented antimalarial plants in Zambia as reported by Vongo, Nair, Haapala, Palgrave and Storrs. Medico-botanical knowledge of some of these plants is given in Table 7.8.

Zimbabwe

Ngarivhume, Klooster, de Jong and Van der Westhuizen (2015) surveyed for plants used as antimalarial remedies in Chipinge District (Table 7.9). The authors refer to *Plumbago zeylanica* as an important medicinal plant in Africa and Asia. Other than being a remedy for malaria, *P. zeylanica* is also used to treat HIV/AIDS. Plumbagic acid glucosides, naphthoquinones and coumarins have been isolated from its roots. *Pavetta crassipes* contains flavonoids including a quercetin 3-O-rutinoside which has good antimicrobial activity. Its significant antimalarial activity was attributed to alkaloids.

India

P. falciparum and *P. vivax* are the two predominant malaria parasites in India. Nearly 22% of India's population is classified as being under high risk malaria transmission, 1 to 10 cases per 1000 population. Nagendrappa, Naik and Payyappallimana (2013) studied plants traditionally used for prevention of malaria in Cuttack, Gajapati and Koraput districts of Odisha state, eastern India. Their study revealed the use of 16 plant species belonging to 12 families for prevention of malaria. *Andrographis paniculata, A. indica, Nyctanthes arbor-tristis, Ocimum sanctum, Piper nigrum* and *Z. officinale* (ginger) were the most commonly reported plant extract decoctions for malaria prophylaxis.

In their assays of Indian plants, Singh et al. (2015) found high antiplasmodial activities ($IC_{50} \leq 5$ µg/ml) for leaf ethanol extracts of *Corymbia citriodora* (synonym *Eucalyptus citriodora*), *Calotropis procera* (contains cardenolides), *Annona squamosa* and bark ethanol extract of *Holarrhena pubescens*. Good antiplasmodial activity ($IC_{50} = 11\text{-}20$ µg/ml) was observed for leaf ethanol extract of *Bryophyllum pinnatum* and whole plant ethanol extract of *Catharanthus roseus*. *Annona squamosa* contains antiplasmodial alkaloids (Johns, Windust, Jurgens, & Mansor, 2011).

As explained by Singh et al. (2015), the active ingredients of *C. citriodora* are attributable to the anti-inflammatory agents eucalyptol and cineole. Antiplasmodial functions of *H. pubescens* (synonym *Holarrhena antidysenterica*), a traditional remedy for dysentery and diarrhoea, are probably founded in the abundance of alkaloids, the main one being conessine, with chemical similarity to quinine and quinidine.

Kaushik, Bagavan, Rahuman, Mohanakrishnan, Kamaraj and Elango et al. (2013) studied the antiplasmodial potentials of selected medicinal plants from Ghats, south India. Their results corroborate that antiplasmodial activities for *Cyperus rotundus* and *Z. officinale* were very good (IC$_{50}$ < 10 µg/ml). Good activities were displayed by *Ficus religiosa* and the curry tree *Murraya koenigii* (IC$_{50}$ = 10–15 µg/ml). *Ficus benghalensis* had moderate activity (IC$_{50}$ = 15–25 µg/ml).

Among the Sonitpur community of Tezpur in Assam, north-east India, antimalarial remedies were prepared from the following plants: *A. paniculata, Artemisia vulgaris, A. indica, Alstonia scholaris, Adhatoda vasica, Aegle marmelos, A. squamosa, Aristolochia indica, Centella asiatica, Caesalpinia volkensii, Coptis teeta, Cissampelos pareira, C. citratus* and *Clerodendrum infortunatum* (Namsa, Mandal, & Tangjang, 2011).

Namsa et al. (2011) also documented other plants: *Gymnopetalum cochinchinensis, Lantana camara, O. sanctum, Piper longum, Stephania hernandifolia, Vitex peduncularis, Withania somnifera* and *Zanthoxylum hamiltonianum*. The plants were also applied as mosquito repellents. *Artemisia vulgaris*, an antimalarial also used in Vietnam, is known to impede the growth of chloroquine-resistant *P. falciparum* strain FCR-3; EC$_{50}$ = 5.6 µg/ml for a methanol extract.

Malaysia

To make an inventory of plants traditionally used in the treatment of malaria, an inaugural community based ethnobotanical study in Peninsular Malaysia was conducted (Al-Adhroey, Nor, Al-Mekhlafi, & Mahmud, 2010). Nineteen species belonging to 17 families were identified. The plants were: *A. indica* (locally known as *Margosa*), *Brucea javanica* (infusion), *C. siamea, Cocos nucifera* (infusion), *Eurycoma longifolia, Labisia pumila, Languas galanga, Lansium domesticum* (infusion), *Morinda citrifolia, Nigella sativa* ((locally known as *Jintan hitam*, infusion), *Ocimum tenuiflorum, Phyllanthus niruri, Piper betle* (chewing), *Hibiscus rosa-sinensis* (infusion), *Tinospora crispa, Aeschynanthus* sp., *Alstonia angustiloba, Curcuma domestica* and *Elateriospermum tapos*.

The most widely used plants were *E. longifolia, L. pumila* and *T. crispa*. Most of the remedies were taken three times a day as decoctions prepared after boiling. *Piper betle* exhibits antiplasmodial action, antioxidant activity and is toxicologically safe to humans (Al-Adhroey, Nor, Al-Mekhlafi, Amran, & Mahmud, 2010).

Amazon Region

Giovannini (2015) provides results of the first ethnobotanical survey among the Achuar (Jivaro), indigenous people of Amazonian Ecuador and Peru. He documented the following plant remedies against malaria, known as *paludismo* in Spanish: *Bactris gasipaes* (decoction, taken orally and then vom ited), *Banisteriopsis caapi* (decoction is drunk and then vomited), *Cremastosperma cauliflorum* (decoction) and *Dieffenbachia* sp. (decoction is taken orally).

The Achuar people also use *Grias neuberthii* (scraped bark is mixed with water and boiled, decoction is drunk and vomited), *Guarea grandifolia* (powdered bark is mixed with water and taken orally, then vomited), and *Hamelia patens* (decoction is administered orally). Peeled and cooked roots of *Manihot esculenta* (cassava) are fermented to make chicha and juice from leaves of *Nicotiana tabacum* (tobacco) are added and drunk. A decoction of *Urera baccifera* is also drunk and vomited.

A cold suspension of dried powdered roots of the plant *Ampelozyziphus amazonicus*, locally called Indian beer or Saracura-mira, is used to prevent malaria in the Brazilian Amazon (Andrade-Neto et al., 2008). The preparation significantly reduces the number of schizonts in culture. It also inhibits the primary development of sporozoites in the host. Indian beer is rich in saponins and has low cytotoxicity to human cells.

The province of Loreto in the Peruvian Amazonia is classified by WHO as a malaria grade III zone because of its high frequency of chloroquine resistant strains. It is the epicentre of malaria in Peru. Ruiz, Ruiz, Maco, Cobos, and Gutierrez-Choquevilca (2011) detail pants used by native Amazonian groups from the Nanay River, Peru, for the treatment of malaria. Their antiplasmodial tests on strain FCR-3 confirm that *Abuta rufescens*, *Ayapana lanceolata*, *Capsiandra angustifolia*, *C. limon*, *C. paradisi*, *Minquartia guianensis*, *Potalia resinifera*, *Scoparia dulcis*, and *Physalis angulata* demonstrated good antiplasmodial activity ($IC_{50} < 10$ μg/ml).

Renaissance Europe

Nowadays, few people would ever think there was malaria in Europe. However, as Adams, Alther, Kessler, Kluge and Hamburger (2011) wrote, malaria was a part and parcel of Western civilization since antiquity and up into the 20th century. Until the Aare River was tamed between 1868 and 1891, the basin of central Switzerland (Mittelland) was badly hit by malaria (Bruce-Chwatt & De Zulueta, 1980). Malaria was present in the wetlands of the Isar River in Munich up to the 1940s.

Archangelsk in northern Russia, just 225 km from the Arctic Circle, suffered a malaria epidemic which killed 60,000 people in 1918. Up to the 1950s, Greece was considered the most malaria prone country outside Sub-Saharan Africa (Packard, 2009). With improvements in healthcare, changes in agricultural practices and living standards, the use of DDT and modern antiparasitics, the disease was only recently eradicated in Europe.

Adams et al. (2011) documented old herbal remedies for Malaria tertiana (*Plasmodium vivax*) or Malaria quartana (*Plasmodium malariae*) in 16th century and 17th century Europe. Three hundred and fourteen taxa were identified as herbals for this indication. But recent pharmacological data were only found for 5% of them.

The following plants were known to be among the remedies used to treat malaria in Europe during the 16th and 17th centuries (Adams et al., 2011): *Sambucus nigra*, *Viburnum opulus*, *Ferula assa-foetida*, *Peucedanum ostruthium*, *Asparagus officinalis*, *Achillea millefolium*, *Artemisia absinthium*, *Cichorium intybus*, *Eupatorium cannabinum*, *Humulus lupulus*, *Hypericum androsaemum*, *Mentha pulegium*, *Melia azedarach*, *Ficus sycomorus*, *Peganum harmala* and *Cinchona officinalis*.

A Closer Look at Malaria and Plants as Sources of New Antimalarials

Two main reasons for the high global burden of malaria include the increasing insecticide resistance of mosquito vectors and the escalating resistance of *Plasmodium falciparum* to antimalarial drugs. To address the growing challenge of parasite resistance to drugs, there is no denying that new antimalarial drug leads are urgently needed. As the question of malaria persistently badgers Africa, there has been no meaningful and concerted answer, sadly, among African countries - the hardest hit by malaria, to develop new antimalarial drugs.

Conspicuously, the lion's share of local and donor resources is still directed at roll-back malaria programmes which involve spraying the mosquito vector through indoor residual spraying of dangerous insecticides like DDT, manufactured and marketed by big western multinational companies. Much like tuberculosis, malaria is a low-profit disease whose medications have not really whetted the capitalist appetites of big pharmaceutical companies; reluctant to bring new innovative drugs to patients they consider too poor to buy their drugs.

Poor funding from African governments has left antimalarials research to the whims of donor charity. In the face of increasing HIV infections, malaria is also an orphaned disease, with little support from western donors who fear more about the risk of HIV transmission than they do for malaria. Global funding to malaria, including support for the development of new drugs, continues to dwindle.

It is acknowledged that malaria and HIV-1 cause bidirectional and synergistic interactions (Diou et al., 2009). For example, it has been demonstrated that malaria pigments can induce a severe impairment of phagocytic cells' functions. Dual infection of persons by malaria and HIV also complicates treatment success and adverse drug effects are especially common in regions where the two infections are superimposed. But there is still a paucity of data with regard to the mechanism(s) by which each pathogen impacts the other.

Despite the molecular mechanisms of *Plasmodium* inhibition, understanding the pathological mechanisms involved in *P. falciparum* and HIV-1 co-infection is of high importance because of possible therapeutic ramifications. Additional and more comprehensive basic studies are needed to fully understand the consequences of *P. falciparum*/HIV-1 interactions. This is vital for the discovery of promising drug combinations that can treat co-infected individuals.

Overall, malaria is still a complicated disease and it would seem that patients, too, have a complicated relationship with the use of plant-based antimalarial remedies. The complication is also reflected in the plethora of symptoms cited by persons that have suffered from malaria. Symptoms of malaria differ from patient to patient, depending on geographical and *Plasmodium* strain.

While nature provides a little protection against malaria to persons in endemic areas, for example through the sickle cell haemoglobin trait where the amino acid glutamate is replaced by valine, malaria is still a menace, infecting and killing millions of adults and children. Indeed, malaria is one of the reasons Sub-Saharan Africa is under-developed. Despite donor funding, mostly from the Global Fund and Bill/Melinda Gates Foundation, many countries in Africa are struggling to rollback malaria.

People in endemic areas still use plants as self-reliant remedies to treat malaria. Common food plants are used as antimalarials. Ethnobotany and Pharmacognosy provide a faster route to antimalarial drug leads; this principle has been reinforced by the discovery of artemisinin and quinine from *Artemisia* and *Cinchona* plant species, respectively. Hence, artemisinin-based combined therapy and quinine are currently the drug treatments of choice for malaria. However, treatment of malaria is threatened by the continuing development of resistance to available drugs.

Whilst the African continent is endowed with a high diversity of antimalarial plants, for example, plants in the family Annonaceae are often used to treat malaria in West Africa, there has been no political will, hitherto, to convert these plants into new drugs. Even in Kenya where numerous researches on antimalarial plants have been done, there were no clinical trials by 2011 for antimalarial drug candidates from plants. Data on *in vivo* antimalarial activities, posology (dosages), toxicities and mechanisms of action are also not readily available.

Although progress in most countries has been slow, several plant-derived formulations were taken to clinical trial and three plant-derived drugs (Manalaria®, Nsansiphos®, and Quinine Pharmakina®) have been licensed in the

DRC (Memvanga et al., 2015). This is a step in the right direction for a country that accounts for about 15% of the global mortality due to malaria.

Dike et al. (2012) reviewed various phytochemicals found in antimalarial plants: *A. occidentale* (tannins), *M. indica* (glycosides, saponims, steroids and tannins), *Alstonia congensis* (at least 15 alkaloids), *G. kola* (biflavonoids, xanthones and benzophenones) and *A. indica* which has about 135 different compounds including isoprenoids and its antiplasmodial derivative called gedunin. Other botanicals with putative antimalarial compounds were: *P. guajava* (flavonoids, carbohydrates and saponins), *C. citratus* (terpenoids, aldehydes), *M. lucida* (danacanthal), *N. latifolia* (flavonoids, saponnin, terpenoids and tannins), *M. charantia* (triterpenoids and balsaminols) and *Ficus exasperata* (tannins, saponins, flavonoids, steroids, anthraquinone glycosides and reducing sugars).

In the DRC, some structures of plant chemical compounds with high *in vitro* activity against various strains of *P. falciparum* (IC_{50} < 1 µg/ml) were elucidated: strychnogucine B, ancistrocongoline A, isochondodendrine, ancistrocongoline B, cocsoline, korupensamine, ancistroealaine B, ellagic acid, physalin B, ancistrolikokine D, cryptolepine, hydroxycryptolepine, neocryptolepine and yadanziolide (Memvanga et al., 2015). Eight iridoids were had antiplasmodial activity: Gaertneroside, acetylgaertneroside, methoxygaertneroside, epoxygaertneroside, dehydrogaertneroside, dehydromethoxygaertneroside, epoxymethoxygaertneroside and gaertneric acid. Given the enormous number of antimalarial plants, especially in Africa, more chacterization of active chemical compounds needs to be done.

Plants used in more than two African countries may be more effective in the management of malaria. A cross-check in the literature shows that certain African plant species are used in several countries (Chinsembu, 2015): *A. indica* (ten countries; Benin, Burkina Faso, Ghana, Guinea, Ethiopia, Kenya, Nigeria, Togo, Uganda and Zimbabwe), *N. latifolia* (nine countries; Benin, Cameroon, Gabon, Ghana, Guinea, Kenya, Nigeria, Senegal and Togo), *C. papaya*, *C. siamea*, *Ficus sur* (eight countries), *C. occidentalis*, *J. curcas*, *Maytenus* sp., *T. indica*, *V. amygdalina* (seven countries), *T. diversifolia* (six countries), *A. digitata*, *M. foetida* (five countries), *S. longepedunculata*, *Flueggea virosa*, *Ximenia americana* and *Z. chalybeum* (four countries).

Adebayo and Krettli (2011) discussed mechanisms of action for some of the plant active compounds: cryptolepine, an indole alkaloid isolated from *Sida acuta* and *Cryptolepis sanguinolenta* inhibits hemozoin polymerization in the parasite; gossypol, a disesquiterpene extracted from seeds of plants in the cotton genus *Gossypium*, inhibits *P. falciparum* lactate dehydrogenase (pfLDH), an essential enzyme for energy generation through glycolysis; gedunin isolated from *A. indica* and *M. azedarach* inhibits the parasite's HSP90 through alkylation; azadirachtin from *A. indica* interferes with the formation of mitotic spindles and the assembly of microtubules into typical axonemes in gametes, thus inhibiting the formation of mobile microgametes; and allicin works as a cysteine protease inhibitor that blocks the proteolytic processing of circumsporozoite protein by a parasite-derived cysteine protease, thereby preventing sporozoite invasion of host cells.

Conclusions and Recommendations

Chinsembu (2015) noted that the burden of malaria is decreasing. However, he lamented that parasite resistance to current antimalarial drugs and resistance to insecticides by vector mosquitoes threaten the prospects of malaria elimination in endemic areas. Corollary, there is a scientific departure to discover new antimalarial agents from nature. And, because the two antimalarial drugs quinine and artemisinin were discovered through improved understanding of the indigenous knowledge of plants, bioprospecting Sub-Saharan Africa's enormous plant biodiversity may be a source of new and better drugs to treat malaria. The antiplasmodial data, too, suggest an opportunity for inventing new antimalarial drugs from Sub-Saharan-African flora.

This chapter has mostly decribed antiplasmodial plants in Africa. In the African countries cited in this treatise, hundreds of plants are used as antimalarial treatments. The number of plant species is not exhaustive. Apart from plants, fungi and marine organisms are being studied for their antiplasmodial activities. Some potent active chemical compounds have been characterized from plants and other natural sources.

West African countries seem to have done more antimalarial plant research, mostly spearheaded by their collaborators in Europe, than countries in Southern Africa. West Africa, much like DRC, claims a lion's share of global malaria burden compared to Southern African countries. Only a small part of Limpopo Province has malaria, so the search for antimalarials from plants has no research priority in South Africa.

In Kenya, KEMRI has done excellent laboratory research on antimalarials from plants, but more needs to be done on clinical trials and commercialization of plant products. Like most African countries, Kenya also suffers from a lack of capacity in good manufacturing practices. Thus, most African countries continue to conduct ethnobotanical surveys without any meaningful attempts at identifying active chemical compounds, the prerequisite for new drug development.

It is urgent now for Sub-Saharan African countries affected by malaria to instigate a sustainable funding effort and agency to develop new antimalarial drugs from their own locally available antiplasmodial plants. Malaria is an island in the sea of African antimalarial plants. African governments should spare no effort and cent in tapping this natural pharmacy of antimalarial plants.

There is an urgent need for more research in the posology of plant remedies in general and antimalarial medications in particular. Extracts prepared strictly according to the practitioners' recipes should be screened for antiplasmodial activity and toxicity by in vitro and in vivo standard tests.

Plants used as herbal remedies for malaria, for example *Alstonia congensis*, are often distressed due to over-harvesting of leaves and barks, with barks often completely stripped off. Therefore, there is a compelling need for controlled harvesting of the most sought after species, as well as sustained cultivation of the same plants, in order to ensure continued growth and constant availability within malaria endemic communities.

Going by the biochemical mutations that have been selected to protect Africans from severe malaria and given the excellent African repertoire of antiplasmodial plants, nature's evolutionary tide against malaria is in Africa's favour. The continent should seize these evolutionary and natural odds against malaria.

Since plants contain a repertoire of chemical agents with multiple antiplasmodial valences, it would seem that nature is a powerful storehouse of antimalarial agents. Indeed, if there is a long-term remedy for malaria, it must lie in nature's potent antimalarial plants and other natural products. Even if some plants may be toxic, many of their chemical agents err on the side of antiplasmodial efficacy; they swing into action at the first signs of *Plasmodium*. Given the biochemical mutations that have been selected to protect Africans from severe malaria, and given the excellent African repertoire of antiplasmodial plants, nature's evolutionary tide against malaria is in Africa's favour. The continent should seize these evolutionary and natural odds against malaria. Most important, the antiplasmodial data suggest an opportunity for inventing new antimalarial drugs from Sub-Saharan-African flora, making malaria control and elimination a tractable challenge.

References

Abbah, J., Amos, S., Chindo, B., Ngazal, I., Vongtau, H.O., Adzu, B., ... & Gamaniel, K.S. (2010). Pharmacological evidence favouring the use of *Nauclea latifolia* in malaria ethnopharmacy: Effects against nociception, inflammation, and pyrexia in rats and mice. *Journal of Ethnopharmacology, 127*(1), 85-90.

Abdul-Ghani, R., Al-Mekhlafi, A.M., & Alabsi, M.S. (2012). Microbial control of malaria: Biological warfare against the parasite and its vector. *Acta Tropica, 121*(2), 71-84.

Abosi, A. O., Akala, H., Liyala, P., Majinda, R. R. T., Mbukwa, E., Midiwo, J. O., ... & Yenesew, A. (2006). *Vangueria infausta* root bark: *In vivo* and *in vitro* antiplasmodial activity. *British Journal of Biomedical Science, 63*(3), 129-133.

Abu-Raddad, L.J., Patnaik, P., & Kublin, J.G. (2006). Dual infection with HIV and malaria fuels the spread of both diseases in Sub-Saharan Africa. *Science, 314*(5805), 1603-1606.

Adams, M., Alther, W., Kessler, M., Kluge, M., & Hamburger, M. (2011). Malaria in the Renaissance: remedies from European herbals from the 16th and 17th century. *Journal of Ethnopharmacology, 133*(2), 278-288.

Adebayo, J.O., & Krettli, A.U. (2011). Potential antimalarials from Nigerian plants: a review. *Journal of Ethnopharmacology, 133*(2), 289-302.

Adia, M.M., Anywar, G., Byamukama, R., Kamatenesi-Mugisha, M., Sekagya, Y., Kakudidi, E. K., & Kiremire, B.T. (2014). Medicinal plants used in malaria treatment by Prometra herbalists in Uganda. *Journal of Ethnopharmacology, 155*(1), 580-588.

Aditya, N.P., Vathsala, P.G., Vieira, V., Murthy, R.S.R., & Souto, E.B. (2013). Advances in nanomedicines for malaria treatment. *Advances in Colloid and Interface Science, 201*, 1-17.

Affum, A.O., Shiloh, D.O., & Adomako, D. (2013). Monitoring of arsenic levels in some ready-to-use anti-malaria herbal products from drug sales outlets in the Madina area of Accra, Ghana. *Food and Chemical Toxicology, 56*, 131-135.

Agbaje, E.O., & Onabanjo, A.O. (1994). Toxicological study of the extracts of antimalarial medicinal plant *Enantia chlorantha. The Central African Journal of Medicine, 40*(3), 71-73.

Ajaiyeoba, E., Ashidi, J., Abiodun, O., Okpako, L., Ogbole, O., Akinboye, D., ... & Oduola, A. (2005). Antimalarial ethnobotany: *In vitro* antiplasmodial activity of seven plants identified in the Nigerian middle belt. *Pharmaceutical Biology, 42*(8), 588-591.

Ajaiyeoba, E., Ashidi, J., Abiodun, O., Okpako, L., Ogbole, O., Akinboye, D., ... & Oduola, A. (2005). Antimalarial ethnobotany: *In vitro* antiplasmodial activity of seven plants identified in the nigerian middle belt. *Pharmaceutical Biology, 42*(8), 588-591.

Akendengue, B. (1992). Medicinal plants used by the Fang traditional healers in Equatorial Guinea. *Journal of Ethnopharmacology, 37*(2), 165-173.

Al-Adhroey, A. H., Nor, Z. M., Al-Mekhlafi, H. M., & Mahmud, R. (2010). Ethnobotanical study on some Malaysian antimalarial plants: A community based survey. *Journal of Ethnopharmacology, 132*(1), 362-364.

Al-Adhroey, A.H., Nor, Z.M., Al-Mekhlafi, H.M., Amran, A.A., & Mahmud, R. (2010). Antimalarial activity of methanolic leaf extract of *Piper betle* L. *Molecules, 16*(1), 107-118.

Alemu, A., Shiferaw, Y., Addis, Z., Mathewos, B., & Birhan, W. (2013). Effect of malaria on HIV/AIDS transmission and progression. *Parasites and Vectors, 6*(18), 1756-3305.

Alker, A.P., Lim, P., Sem, R., Shah, N.K., Yi, P., Bouth, D.M., ... & Meshnick, S.R. (2007). pfmdr1 and in vivo resistance to artesunate-mefloquine in falciparum malaria on the Cambodian–Thai border. *The American Journal of Tropical Medicine and Hygiene, 76*(4), 641-647.

Andrade-Neto, V.F., Brandão, M.G.L., Nogueira, F., Rosário, V.E., & Krettli, A.U. (2008). *Ampelozyziphus amazonicus* Ducke (Rhamnaceae), a medicinal plant used to prevent malaria in the Amazon Region, hampers the development of *Plasmodium berghei* sporozoites. *International Journal for Parasitology, 38*(13), 1505-1511.

Asase, A., Akwetey, G.A., & Achel, D.G. (2010). Ethnopharmacological use of herbal remedies for the treatment of malaria in the Dangme West District of Ghana. *Journal of Ethnopharmacology, 129*(3), 367-376.

Asase, A., Hesse, D.N., & Simmonds, M.S. (2012). Uses of multiple plants prescriptions for treatment of malaria by some communities in southern Ghana. *Journal of Ethnopharmacology, 144*(2), 448-452.

Asres, K., Bucar, F., Knauder, E., Yardley, V., Kendrick, H., & Croft, S. L. (2001). *In vitro* antiprotozoal activity of extract and compounds from the stem bark of Combretum molle. *Phytotherapy Research, 15*(7), 613-617.

Atindehou, K.K., Schmid, C., Brun, R., Koné, M.W., & Traore, D. (2004). Antitrypanosomal and antiplasmodial activity of medicinal plants from Côte d'Ivoire. *Journal of Ethnopharmacology, 90*(2), 221-227.

Bapela, M.J., Meyer, J.M., & Kaiser, M. (2014). *In vitro* antiplasmodial screening of ethnopharmacologically selected South African plant species used for the treatment of malaria. *Journal of Ethnopharmacology, 156*, 370-373.

Bbosa, G.S., Kyegombe, D.B., Lubega, A., Musisi, N., Ogwal-Okeng, J., & Odyek, O. (2013). Anti-*Plasmodium falciparum* activity of *Aloe dawei* and *Justicia betonica*. *African Journal of Pharmacy and Pharmacology, 7*, 2258-2263.

Benoit-Vical, F., Soh, P.N., Salery, M., Harguem, L., Poupat, C., & Nongonierma, R. (2008). Evaluation of Senegalese plants used in malaria treatment: focus on *Chrozophora senegalensis*. *Journal of Ethnopharmacology, 116*(1), 43-48.

Bero, J., Ganfon, H., Jonville, M.C., Frédérich, M., Gbaguidi, F., DeMol, P., ... & Quetin-Leclercq, J. (2009). *In vitro* antiplasmodial activity of plants used in Benin in traditional medicine to treat malaria. *Journal of Ethnopharmacology*, *122*(3), 439-444.

Bhumiratana, A., Sorosjinda-Nunthawarasilp, P., Kaewwaen, W., Maneekan, P., & Pimnon, S. (2013). Malaria-associated rubber plantations in Thailand. *Travel Medicine and Infectious Disease*, *11*(1), 37-50.

Boniface, P.K., Verma, S., Shukla, A., Cheema, H.S., Srivastava, S.K., Khan, F., ... & Pal, A. (2015). Bioactivity-guided isolation of antiplasmodial constituents from *Conyza sumatrensis* (Retz.) EH Walker. *Parasitology International*, *64*(1), 118-123.

Borkow, G., & Bentwich, Z. (2004). Chronic immune activation associated with chronic helminthic and human immunodeficiency virus infections: role of hyporesponsiveness and anergy. *Clinical Microbiology Reviews*, *17*(4), 1012-1030.

Bourdy, G., Willcox, M.L., Ginsburg, H., Rasoanaivo, P., Graz, B., & Deharo, E. (2008). Ethnopharmacology and malaria: New hypothetical leads or old efficient antimalarials? *International Journal for Parasitology*, *38*(1), 33-41.

Boyom, F.F., Kemgne, E.M., Tepongning, R., Ngouana, V., Mbacham, W.F., Tsamo, E., ... & Rosenthal, P.J. (2009). Antiplasmodial activity of extracts from seven medicinal plants used in malaria treatment in Cameroon. *Journal of Ethnopharmacology*, *123*(3), 483-488.

Brahmbhatt, H., Kigozi, G., Wabwire-Mangen, F., Serwadda, D., Sewankambo, N., Lutalo, T., ... & Gray, R. (2003). The effects of placental malaria on mother-to-child HIV transmission in Rakai, Uganda. *AIDS*, *17*(17), 2539-2541.

Brentlinger, P.E., Behrens, C.B., & Micek, M.A. (2006). Challenges in the concurrent management of malaria and HIV in pregnancy in Sub-Saharan Africa. *The Lancet Infectious Diseases*, *6*(2), 100-111.

Bruce-Chwatt, L.J., & De Zulueta, J. (1980). *The rise and fall of malaria in Europe: A historico-epidemiological study*. Published for the Regional Office for Europe of the World Health Organization by Oxford University Press, Walton Street, Oxford OX2 6DP.

Cabrera, A., Neculai, D., & Kain, K.C. (2014). CD36 and malaria: friends or foes? A decade of data provides some answers. *Trends in Parasitology*, *30*(9), 436-444.

Carraz, M., Jossang, A., Franetich, J.F., Siau, A., Ciceron, L., Hannoun, L., ... & Mazier, D. (2006). A plant-derived morphinan as a novel lead compound active against malaria liver stages. *PLoS medicine*, *3*(12), e513.

Carrel, M., Patel, J., Taylor, S.M., Janko, M., Mwandagalirwa, M.K., Tshefu, A.K., ... & Emch, M. (2014). The geography of malaria genetics in the

Democratic Republic of Congo: A complex and fragmented landscape. *Social Science and Medicine*, 1-9.

Chen, X., Xie, S., Bhat, S., Kumar, N., Shapiro, T.A., & Liu, J.O. (2009). Fumagillin and fumarranol interact with *Plasmodium falciparum* methionine aminopeptidase 2 and inhibit malaria parasite growth in vitro and in vivo. *Chemistry and Biology*, *16*(2), 193-202.

Chen, Y., Yan, T., Gao, C., Cao, W., & Huang, R. (2014). Natural products from the genus *Tephrosia*. *Molecules*, *19*(2), 1432-1458.

Childs, L.M., Abuelezam, N.N., Dye, C., Gupta, S., Murray, M.B., Williams, B.G., & Buckee, C.O. (2015). Modelling challenges in context: Lessons from malaria, HIV and tuberculosis. *Epidemics*, *10*, 102-107.

Chinsembu, K.C. & Hedimbi, M. (2010). An ethnobotanical survey of plants used to manage HIV/AIDS opportunistic infections in Katima Mulilo, Caprivi region, Namibia. *Journal of Ethnobiology and Ethnomedicine*, 6:25.

Chinsembu, K.C. (2009). Model and experiences of initiating collaboration with traditional healers in validation of ethnomedicines for HIV/AIDS in Namibia. *Journal of Ethnobiology and Ethnomedicine*, 5:30.

Chinsembu, K.C. (2015). Plants as antimalarial agents in Sub-Saharan Africa. *Acta Tropica*, 152, 32-48.

Chinsembu, K.C., & Hedimbi, M. (2012). Ethnomedicinal study of plants used to manage HIV/AIDS-related disease conditions in the Ohangwena region, Namibia. *International Journal of Medicinal Plant Research, 1(1)*, 4-11.

Chinsembu, K.C., Hedimbi, M. & Mukaru, C.W. (2011). Putative medicinal properties of plants from the Kavango region, Namibia. *Journal of Medicinal Plants Research 5*(31), 6787-6797.

Chintu, C., Luo, C., Bhat, G., DuPont, H.L., Mwansa-Salamu, P., Kabika, M., & Zumla, A. (1995). Impact of the human immunodeficiency virus type-1 on common pediatric illnesses in Zambia. *Journal of Tropical Pediatrics*, *41*(6), 348-353.

Choomuenwai, V., Andrews, K.T., & Davis, R.A. (2012). Synthesis and antimalarial evaluation of a screening library based on a tetrahydroanthraquinone natural product scaffold. *Bioorganic and Medicinal Chemistry*, *20*(24), 7167-7174.

Choomuenwai, V., Schwartz, B. D., Beattie, K. D., Andrews, K.T., Khokhar, S., & Davis, R.A. (2013). The discovery, synthesis and antimalarial evaluation of natural product-based polyamine alkaloids. *Tetrahedron Letters*, *54*(38), 5188-5191.

Cocquyt, K., Cos, P., Herdewijn, P., Maes, L., Van den Steen, P.E., & Laekeman, G. (2011). *Ajuga remota* Benth.: From ethnopharmacology to phytomedical perspective in the treatment of malaria. *Phytomedicine*, *18*(14), 1229-1237.

Conway, D.J. (2015). Paths to a malaria vaccine illuminated by parasite genomics. *Trends in Genetics, 97(2)*, 97-107.

Cotter, C., Sturrock, H.J., Hsiang, M.S., Liu, J., Phillips, A.A., Hwang, J., ... & Feachem, R.G. (2013). The changing epidemiology of malaria elimination: new strategies for new challenges. *The Lancet, 382*(9895), 900-911.

Cuadros, D.F., Branscum, A.J., & Crowley, P.H. (2011a). HIV-malaria co-infection: effects of malaria on the prevalence of HIV in East Sub-Saharan Africa. *International Journal of Epidemiology, 40*, e931–9.

Cuadros, D.F., Branscum, A.J., Garcia-Ramos, G. (2011b). No evidence of association between HIV-1 and malaria in populations with low HIV-1 prevalence. *PLoS One, 6*, e23458.

Danno, K., Rerolle, F., de Sigalony, S., Colas, A., Terzan, L., & Bordet, M.F. (2014). China rubra for side-effects of quinine: A prospective, randomized study in pregnant women with malaria in Cotonou, Benin. *Homeopathy, 103*(3), 165-171.

De Morais Lima, G.R., de Sales, I.R.P., Caldas Filho, M.R.D., de Jesus, N.Z.T., de Sousa Falcão, H., Barbosa-Filho, J.M., ... & Batista, L.M. (2012). Bioactivities of the genus *Combretum* (Combretaceae): A review. *Molecules, 17*(8), 9142-9206.

De Ridder, S., Van der Kooy, F., & Verpoorte, R. (2008). *Artemisia annua* as a self-reliant treatment for malaria in developing countries. *Journal of Ethnopharmacology, 120*(3), 302-314.

Diarra, N., van't Klooster, C., Togola, A., Diallo, D., Willcox, M., & de Jong, J. (2015). Ethnobotanical study of plants used against malaria in Sélingué subdistrict, Mali. *Journal of Ethnopharmacology, 166*(2), 352-360.

Dike, I.P., Obembe, O.O., & Adebiyi, F.E. (2012). Ethnobotanical survey for potential antimalarial plants in south-western Nigeria. *Journal of Ethnopharmacology, 144*(3), 618-626.

Diou, J., Gauthier, S., Tardif, M.R., Fromentin, R., Lodge, R., Sullivan, D.J., & Tremblay, M.J. (2009). Ingestion of the malaria pigment hemozoin renders human macrophages less permissive to HIV-1 infection. *Virology, 395*(1), 56-66.

Djimdé, A.A., Fofana, B., Sagara, I., Sidibe, B., Toure, S., Dembele, D., ... & Doumbo, O.K. (2008). Efficacy, safety and selection of molecular markers of drug resistance by two ACTs in Mali. *The American Journal of Tropical Medicine and Hygiene, 78*(3), 455-461.

Dondorp, A.M., Nosten, F., Yi, P., Das, D., Phyo, A.P., Tarning, J., ... & White, N.J. (2009). Artemisinin resistance in *Plasmodium falciparum* malaria. *New England Journal of Medicine, 361*(5), 455-467.

Dondorp, A.M., Yeung, S., White, L., Nguon, C., Day, N.P., Socheat, D., & von Seidlein, L. (2010). Artemisinin resistance: current status and scenarios for containment. *Nature Reviews Microbiology, 8*(4), 272-280.

Duffy, R., Wade, C., & Chang, R. (2012). Discovery of anticancer drugs from antimalarial natural products: a MEDLINE literature review. *Drug Discovery Today*, *17*(17), 942-953.

Egharevba, O. H., Oladosu, P., Okhale, E. S., Ibrahim, I., Folashade, K. O., Okwute, K. S., & Okogun, I. J. (2010). Preliminary anti-tuberculosis screening of two Nigerian *Laggera* species (*Laggera pterodonta* and *Laggera aurita*). *Journal of Medicinal Plants Research*, *4*, 1235-1237.

Falade, M. O., Akinboye, D. O., Gbotosho, G. O., Ajaiyeoba, E. O., Happi, T. C., Abiodun, O. O., & Oduola, A. M. J. (2014). In vitro and In vivo antimalarial activity of *Ficus thonningii* Blume (Moraceae) and *Lophira alata* Banks (Ochnaceae), identified from the ethnomedicine of the Nigerian Middle Belt. *Journal of Parasitology Research*, Hindawi Publishing Corporation, Article ID 972853, 6 pages, Available at: http://dx.doi.org/10.1155/2014/972853. Accessed April 11, 2015.

Fowler, D.G. (2006). Traditional fever remedies: a list of Zambian plants. http://www. giftshealth. org/ritam/news/Traditional_Fever_remedies 1. pdf). Accessed April, 12, 2015.

Garcia-Alvarez, M.C., Moussa, I., Soh, P.N., Nongonierma, R., Abdoulaye, A., Nicolau-Travers, M.L., ... & Benoit-Vical, F. (2013). Both plants *Sebastiania chamaelea* from Niger and *Chrozophora senegalensis* from Senegal used in African traditional medicine in malaria treatment share a same active principle. *Journal of Ethnopharmacology*, *149*(3), 676-684.

Gathirwa, J.W., Rukunga, G.M., Njagi, E.N.M., Omar, S.A., Guantai, A.N., Muthaura, C.N., & Mwitari, P.G. (2007). *In vitro* antiplasmodial and in vivo antimalarial activity of some plants traditionally used for the treatment of malaria by the Meru community in Kenya. *Journal of Natural Medicine*, *61*, 261–268.

Gathirwa, J.W., Rukunga, G.M., Njagi, E.N.M., Omar, S.A., Mwitari, P.G., Guantai, A.N., ... & Ndiege, I.O. (2008). The *in vitro* antiplasmodial and in vivo antimalarial efficacy of combinations of some medicinal plants used traditionally for treatment of malaria by the Meru community in Kenya. *Journal of Ethnopharmacology*, *115*(2), 223-231.

Giovannini, P. (2015). Medicinal plants of the Achuar (Jivaro) of Amazonian Ecuador: Ethnobotanical survey and comparison with other Amazonian pharmacopoeias. *Journal of Ethnopharmacology*, *164*(1), 78-88.

Hadi, V., Hotard, M., Ling, T., Salinas, Y. G., Palacios, G., Connelly, M., & Rivas, F. (2013). Evaluation of Jatropha isabelli natural products and their synthetic analogs as potential antimalarial therapeutic agents. *European Journal of Medicinal Chemistry*, *65*, 376-380.

Hay, S.I., Okiro, E.A., Gething, P.W., Patil, A.P., Tatem, A.J., Guerra, C.A., & Snow, R.W. (2010). Estimating the global clinical burden of *Plasmodium falciparum* malaria in 2007. *PLoS Medicine*, 7, e1000290, doi:10.1371/journal.pmed.1000290.

Hermans, M., Akoègninou, A., & Van der Maesen, J. (2004). Medicinal plants used to treat malaria in southern Benin. *Economic Botany*, *58*(1), S239-S252.

Hiben, M.G., Sibhat, G.G., Fanta, B. S., Gebrezgi, H.D., & Tesema, S.B. (2015). Evaluation of *Senna (Cassia) singueana* leaf extract as an alternative or adjuvant therapy for malaria. *Journal of Traditional and Complementary Medicine*.

Hirt, H.M., Lindsey, K., & Balagizi, I. (2008). *AIDS and natural Medicine*. Anamed: Winnenden, Germany.

Holmgren, G., Hamrin, J., Svärd, J., Mårtensson, A., Gil, J.P., & Björkman, A. (2007). Selection of pfmdr1 mutations after amodiaquine monotherapy and amodiaquine plus artemisinin combination therapy in East Africa. *Infection, Genetics and Evolution*, *7*(5), 562-569.

Hsu, E. (2006). The history of qing hao in the Chinese materia medica. *Transactions of the Royal Society of Tropical Medicine and Hygiene*, *100*(6), 505-508.

Ilboudo, D. P., Basilico, N., Parapini, S., Corbett, Y., D'Alessandro, S., Dell'Agli, M., ... & Taramelli, D. (2013). Antiplasmodial and anti-inflammatory activities of *Canthium henriquesianum* (K. Schum), a plant used in traditional medicine in Burkina Faso. *Journal of Ethnopharmacology*, *148*(3), 763-769.

Ishola, I.O., Oreagba, I.A., Adeneye, A.A., Adirije, C., Oshikoya, K.A., & Ogunleye, O.O. (2014). Ethnopharmacological survey of herbal treatment of malaria in Lagos, Southwest Nigeria. *Journal of Herbal Medicine*, *4*(4), 224-234.

Iwalewa, E.O., Omisore, N.O., Adewunmi, C.O., Gbolade, A.A., Ademowo, O.G., Nneji, C., ... & Daniyan, O.M. (2008). Anti-protozoan activities of *Harungana madagascariensis* stem bark extract on trichomonads and malaria. *Journal of Ethnopharmacology*, *117*(3), 507-511.

Jain, K., Sood, S., & Gowthamarajan, K. (2013). Modulation of cerebral malaria by curcumin as an adjunctive therapy. *The Brazilian Journal of Infectious Diseases*, *17*(5), 579-591.

Jansen, F.H. (2006). The herbal tea approach for artemisinin as a therapy for malaria? *Transactions of the Royal Society of Tropical Medicine and Hygiene 100*, 285–286.

Jansen, O., Angenot, L., Tits, M., Nicolas, J.P., De Mol, P., Nikiéma, J.B., & Frédérich, M. (2010). Evaluation of 13 selected medicinal plants from Burkina Faso for their antiplasmodial properties. *Journal of Ethnopharmacology*, *130*(1), 143-150.

Jiofack, T., Ayissi, I., Fokunang, C., Guedje, N., & Kemeuze, V. (2009). Ethnobotany and phytomedicine of the upper Nyong valley forest in Cameroon. *African Journal of Pharmacy and Pharmacology*, *3*(4), 144-150.

Johns, T., Windust, A., Jurgens, T., & Mansor, S.M. (2011). Antimalarial alkaloids isolated from *Annona squamosa*. *Phytopharmacology*, 1, 49–53.

Kamatenesi-Mugisha, M., & Oryem-Origa, H. (2007). Medicinal plants used to induce labour during childbirth in western Uganda. *Journal of Ethnopharmacology, 109*(1), 1-9.

Kantamreddi, V. S., & Wright, C. W. (2008). Investigation of Indian Diospyros species for antiplasmodial properties. *Evidence-based Complementary and Alternative Medicine, 5*(2), 187-190.

Kaur, K., Jain, M., Kaur, T., & Jain, R. (2009). Antimalarials from nature. *Bioorganic and Medicinal Chemistry, 17*(9), 3229-3256.

Kaushik, N.K., Bagavan, A., Rahuman, A.A., Mohanakrishnan, D., Kamaraj, C., Elango, G., ... & Sahal, D. (2013). Antiplasmodial potential of selected medicinal plants from Eastern Ghats of South India. *Experimental Parasitology, 134*(1), 26-32.

Kigondu, E.V.M., Rukunga, G.M., Gathirwa, J.W., Irungu, B.N., Mwikwabe, N.M., Amalemba, G.M., ... & Kirira, P.G. (2011). Antiplasmodial and cytotoxicity activities of some selected plants used by the Maasai community, Kenya. *South African Journal of Botany, 77*(3), 725-729.

Kimbi, H.K., & Fagbenro-Beyioku, A.F. (1996). Efficacy of *Cymbopogon giganteus* and *Enantia chlorantha* against chloroquine resistant *Plasmodium yoelii nigeriensis. East African Medical Journal, 73*(10), 636-637.

Koudouvo, K., Karou, D.S., Kokou, K., Essien, K., Aklikokou, K., Glitho, I.A., ... & Gbeassor, M. (2011). An ethnobotanical study of antimalarial plants in Togo Maritime Region. *Journal of Ethnopharmacology, 134*(1), 183-190.

Kuete, V., Noumedem, J. A., & Nana, F. (2013). Chemistry and pharmacology of 4-hydroxylonchocarpin: A review. *Chinese Journal of Integrative Medicine, 19*(6), 475-480.

Kumar, V., Mahajan, A., & Chibale, K. (2009). Synthetic medicinal chemistry of selected antimalarial natural products. *Bioorganic and Medicinal Chemistry, 17*(6), 2236-2275.

Lacroix, D., Prado, S., Kamoga, D., Kasenene, J., Namukobe, J., Krief, S., ... & Brunois, F. (2011). Antiplasmodial and cytotoxic activities of medicinal plants traditionally used in the village of Kiohima, Uganda. *Journal of Ethnopharmacology, 133*(2), 850-855.

Lakshmanan, V., Rhee, K.Y., & Daily, J.P. (2011). Metabolomics and malaria biology. *Molecular and Biochemical Parasitology, 175*(2), 104-111.

Lekana-Douki, J.B., Bongui, J.B., Liabagui, S.L.O., Edou, S.E.Z., Zatra, R., Bisvigou, U., ... & Kombila, M. (2011). *In vitro* antiplasmodial activity and cytotoxicity of nine plants traditionally used in Gabon. *Journal of Ethnopharmacology, 133*(3), 1103-1108.

Liu, W., Li, Y., Learn, G.H., Rudicell, R.S., Robertson, J.D., Keele, B.F., ... & Hahn, B.H. (2010). Origin of the human malaria parasite *Plasmodium falciparum* in gorillas. *Nature, 467*(7314), 420-425.

Makler, M.T., & Hinrichs, D.J. (1993). Measurement of the lactate dehydrogenase activity of *Plasmodium falciparum* as an assessment of parasitemia. *The American Journal of Tropical Medicine and Hygiene, 48*(2), 205-210.

Makler, M.T., Ries, J.M., Williams, J.A., Bancroft, J.E., Piper, R.C., Gibbins, B.L., & Hinrichs, D.J. (1993). Parasite lactate dehydrogenase as an assay for *Plasmodium falciparum* drug sensitivity. *The American Journal of Tropical Medicine and Hygiene, 48*(6), 739-741.

Mallavadhani, U., Satyanarayana, K.V.S., & Mahapatra, A. (2004). Quantitative evaluation of anticancer marker levels of an Ayurvedic preparation, "Virala". *Pharmaceutical Biology, 42*(4-5), 338-341.

Manivasagan, P., Kang, K.H., Sivakumar, K., Li-Chan, E.C., Oh, H.M., & Kim, S.K. (2014). Marine actinobacteria: An important source of bioactive natural products. *Environmental Toxicology and Pharmacology, 38*(1), 172-188.

Maskey, R.P., Helmke, E., Kayser, O., Fiebig, H.H., Maier, A., Busche, A., & Laatsch, H. (2004). Anti-cancer and antibacterial trioxacarcins with high antimalaria activity from a marine streptomycete and their absolute stereochemistry. *The Journal of Antibiotics, 57*(12), 771-779.

Maude, R. J., Socheat, D., Nguon, C., Saroth, P., Dara, P., Li, G., ... & White, L. J. (2012). Optimising strategies for Plasmodium falciparum malaria elimination in Cambodia: Primaquine, mass drug administration and artemisinin resistance. *PLoS One, 7*(5), e37166.

Maude, R.J., Pontavornpinyo, W., Saralamba, S., Aguas, R., Yeung, S., Dondorp, A.M., ... & White, L.J. (2009). The last man standing is the most resistant: eliminating artemisinin-resistant malaria in Cambodia. *Malaria Journal, 8*(1), 31.

McCracken, S.T., Kaiser, M., Boshoff, H.I., Boyd, P.D., & Copp, B.R. (2012). Synthesis and antimalarial and antituberculosis activities of a series of natural and unnatural 4-methoxy-6-styryl-pyran-2-ones, dihydro analogues and photo-dimers. *Bioorganic and Medicinal Chemistry, 20*(4), 1482-1493.

Mekonnen, L.B. (2015). *In vivo* antimalarial activity of the crude root and fruit extracts of *Croton macrostachyus* (Euphorbiaceae) against *Plasmodium berghei* in mice. *Journal of Traditional and Complementary Medicine*.

Memvanga, P.B., Tona, G.L., Mesia, G.K., Lusakibanza, M.M., & Cimanga, R.K. (2015). Antimalarial activity of medicinal plants from the Democratic Republic of Congo: A review. *Journal of Ethnopharmacology*.

Mesfin, A., Giday, M., Animut, A., & Teklehaymanot, T. (2012). Ethnobotanical study of antimalarial plants in Shinile District, Somali Region, Ethiopia and *in vivo* evaluation of selected ones *against Plasmodium berghei. Journal of Ethnopharmacology, 139*(1), 221-227.

Mharakurwa, S., Thuma, P.E., Norris, D.E., Mulenga, M., Chalwe, V., Chipeta, J., ... & Mason, P.R. (2012). Malaria epidemiology and control in Southern Africa. *Acta Tropica, 121*(3), 202-206.

Mongalo, N.I., McGaw, L.J., Finnie, J.F., & van Staden, J. (2015). *Securidaca longepedunculata* Fresen (Polygalaceae): A review of its ethnomedicinal uses, phytochemistry, pharmacological properties and toxicology. *Journal of Ethnopharmacology, 165*, 215-226.

Motlhanka, D. M. T., & Nthoiwa, G. P. (2013). Ethnobotanical Survey of Medicinal Plants of Tswapong North, in Eastern Botswana: A Case of Plants from Mosweu and Seolwane Villages. *European Journal of Medicinal Plants, 3*(1), 10-24.

Muganga, R., Angenot, L., Tits, M., & Frederich, M. (2010). Antiplasmodial and cytotoxic activities of Rwandan medicinal plants used in the treatment of malaria. *Journal of Ethnopharmacology, 128*(1), 52-57.

Musila, M.F., Dossaji, S.F., Nguta, J.M., Lukhoba, C.W., & Munyao, J.M. (2013). *In vivo* antimalarial activity, toxicity and phytochemical screening of selected antimalarial plants. *Journal of Ethnopharmacology, 146*(2), 557-561.

Muthaura, C.N., Keriko, J.M., Derese, S., Yenesew, A., & Rukunga, G.M. (2011). Investigation of some medicinal plants traditionally used for treatment of malaria in Kenya as potential sources of antimalarial drugs. *Experimental Parasitology, 127*(3), 609-626.

Muthaura, C.N., Rukunga, G.M., Chhabra, S.C., Omar, S.A., Guantai, A.N., Gathirwa, J.W., ... & Njagi, E.N.M. (2007). Antimalarial activity of some plants traditionally used in treatment of malaria in Kwale district of Kenya. *Journal of Ethnopharmacology, 112*(3), 545-551.

Nagendrappa, P.B., Naik, M.P., & Payyappallimana, U. (2013). Ethnobotanical survey of malaria prophylactic remedies in Odisha, India. *Journal of Ethnopharmacology, 146*(3), 768-772.

Namsa, N.D., Mandal, M., & Tangjang, S. (2011). Antimalarial herbal remedies of northeast India, Assam: An ethnobotanical survey. *Journal of Ethnopharmacology, 133*(2), 565-572.

Namukobe, J., Kiremire, B.T., Byamukama, R., Kasenene, J.M., Akala, H.M., Kamau, E., & Dumontet, V. (2015). Antiplasmodial compounds from the stem bark of *Neoboutonia macrocalyx* Pax. *Journal of Ethnopharmacology, 162*(1), 317-322.

Nandakumar, D. N., Nagaraj, V. A., Vathsala, P. G., Rangarajan, P., & Padmanaban, G. (2006). Curcumin-artemisinin combination therapy for malaria. *Antimicrobial Agents and Chemotherapy, 50*(5), 1859-1860.

Ngarivhume, T., van't Klooster, C.I., de Jong, J.T., & Van der Westhuizen, J.H. (2015). Medicinal plants used by traditional healers for the treatment of malaria in the Chipinge district in Zimbabwe. *Journal of Ethnopharmacology, 159*(1), 224-237.

Nguta, J.M., & Mbaria, J.M. (2013). Brine shrimp toxicity and antimalarial activity of some plants traditionally used in treatment of malaria in Msambweni district of Kenya. *Journal of Ethnopharmacology, 148*(3), 988-992.

Njoroge, G.N., Bussmann, R.W., Gemmill, B., Newton, L.E., & Ngumi, V.W. (2004). Utilization of weed species as sources of traditional medicines in central Kenya. *Lyonia, 7*(2), 71-87.

Ogutu, A.I., Lilechi, D.B., Mutai, C., & Bii, C. (2012). Phytochemical analysis and antimicrobial activity of Phytolacca dodecandra, Cucumis aculeatus and Erythrina excelsa. *International Journal of Biological and Chemical Sciences, 6*(2), 692-704.

Ojewole, J. A., Mawoza, T., Chiwororo, W. D., & Owira, P. M. (2010). *Sclerocarya birrea* (A. Rich) Hochst. ['Marula'] (Anacardiaceae): A review of its phytochemistry, pharmacology and toxicology and its ethnomedicinal uses. *Phytotherapy Research, 24*(5), 633-639.

Okhale, S. E., Odiniya, E. O., & Kunle, O. F. (2010). Preliminary Phytochemical and Pharmacognostical Investigation of Pediatrics Antimalarial Laggera pterodonta (DC) Sch. Bip.: Asteraceae of Nigerian Origin. *Ethnobotanical Leaflets, 2010*(4), 9.

Oksman-Caldentey, K.M., & Inzé, D. (2004). Plant cell factories in the post-genomic era: new ways to produce designer secondary metabolites. *Trends in Plant Science, 9*(9), 433-440.

Olorunnisola, O.S., Adetutu, A., Balogun, E.A., & Afolayan, A.J. (2013). Ethnobotanical survey of medicinal plants used in the treatment of malarial in Ogbomoso, Southwest Nigeria. *Journal of Ethnopharmacology, 150*(1), 71-78.

Owuor, B.O., Ochanda, J.O., Kokwaro, J.O., Cheruiyot, A.C., Yeda, R.A., Okudo, C.A., & Akala, H.M. (2012). *In vitro* antiplasmodial activity of selected Luo and Kuria medicinal plants. *Journal of Ethnopharmacology, 144*(3), 779-781.

Packard, R.M. (2009). "Roll Back Malaria, Roll in Development"? Reassessing the Economic Burden of Malaria. *Population and Development Review, 35*(1), 53-87.

Prozesky, E. A., Meyer, J. J. M., & Louw, A. I. (2001). In vitro antiplasmodial activity and cytotoxicity of ethnobotanically selected South African plants. *Journal of Ethnopharmacology, 76*(3), 239-245.

Ramalhete, C., da Cruz, F.P., Mulhovo, S., Sousa, I.J., Fernandes, M.X., Prudêncio, M., & Ferreira, M.J.U. (2014). Dual-stage triterpenoids from an African medicinal plant targeting the malaria parasite. *Bioorganic and Medicinal Chemistry, 22*(15), 3887-3890.

Rood, B. (2013). *Nature's own pharmacy*. Pretoria, South Africa: Protea Book House.

RTS,S Clinical Trials Partnership (2015). Efficacy and safety of RTS,S/AS01 malaria vaccine with or without a booster dose in infants and children in Africa: final results of a phase 3, individually randomised, controlled trial. www.thelancet.com, http://dx.doi.org/10.1016/S0140-6736(15)60721-8. Accessed April 25, 2015.

Ruiz, L., Ruiz, L., Maco, M., Cobos, M., Gutierrez-Choquevilca, A.L., & Roumy, V. (2011). Plants used by native Amazonian groups from the Nanay River (Peru) for the treatment of malaria. *Journal of Ethnopharmacology, 133*(2), 917-921.

Rukunga, G.M., Gathirwa, J.W., Omar, S.A., Muregi, F.W., Muthaura, C.N., Kirira, P.G., ... & Kofi-Tsekpo, W.M. (2009). Antiplasmodial activity of the extracts of some Kenyan medicinal plants. *Journal of Ethnopharmacology, 121*(2), 282-285.

Santos-Magalhães, N.S., & Mosqueira, V.C.F. (2010). Nanotechnology applied to the treatment of malaria. *Advanced Drug Delivery Reviews, 62*(4), 560-575.

Seebaluck, R., Gurib-Fakim, A., & Mahomoodally, F. (2015). Medicinal plants from the genus *Acalypha* (Euphorbiaceae)–A review of their ethnopharmacology and phytochemistry. *Journal of Ethnopharmacology, 159*(1), 137-157.

Simoes-Pires, C., Hostettmann, K., Haouala, A., Cuendet, M., Falquet, J., Graz, B., & Christen, P. (2014). Reverse pharmacology for developing an anti-malarial phytomedicine. The example of *Argemone mexicana. International Journal for Parasitology: Drugs and Drug Resistance, 4*(3), 338-346.

Singh, N., Kaushik, N.K., Mohanakrishnan, D., Tiwari, S.K., & Sahal, D. (2015). Antiplasmodial activity of medicinal plants from Chhotanagpur plateau, Jharkhand, India. *Journal of Ethnopharmacology, 165*(1), 152-162.

Soonthornchareonnon, N., Ubonopas, L., Kaewsuwan, S., & Wuttiudom-ler, M. (2004). Lupinifolin, a bioactive flavanone from *Myriopteron extensum* (Wight) K. Schum. Stem. *Thai Journal of Phytopharmacy, 11*(2), 19-28.

Stangeland, T., Alele, P.E., Katuura, E., & Lye, K.A. (2011). Plants used to treat malaria in Nyakayojo sub-county, western Uganda. *Journal of Ethnopharmacology, 137*(1), 154-166.

Stanisic, D.I., Barry, A.E., & Good, M.F. (2013). Escaping the immune system: how the malaria parasite makes vaccine development a challenge. *Trends in Parasitology, 29*(12), 612-622.

Stolze, S.C., Deu, E., Kaschani, F., Li, N., Florea, B.I., Richau, K.H., ... & Kaiser, M. (2012). The antimalarial natural product symplostatin 4 is a nano-molar inhibitor of the food vacuole falcipains. *Chemistry and Biology, 19*(12), 1546-1555.

Tabuti, J.R. (2008). Herbal medicines used in the treatment of malaria in Budiope county, Uganda. *Journal of Ethnopharmacology, 116*(1), 33-42.

Tchouya, G.R.F., Souza, A., Tchouankeu, J.C., Yala, J.F., Boukandou, M., Foundikou, H., ... & Lebibi, J. (2015). Ethnopharmacological surveys and pharmacological studies of plants used in traditional medicine in the treatment of HIV/AIDS opportunistic diseases in Gabon. *Journal of Ethnopharmacology, 162*, 306-316.

Tegar, M., & Purnomo, H. (2013). Tea leaves extracted as anti-malaria based on molecular docking plants. *Procedia Environmental Sciences, 17*, 188-194.

Tepongning, R.N., Lucantoni, L., Nasuti, C.C., Dori, G.U., Yerbanga, S.R., Lupidi, G., ... & Habluetzel, A. (2011). Potential of a *Khaya ivorensis–Alstonia boonei* extract combination as antimalarial prophylactic remedy. *Journal of Ethnopharmacology, 137*(1), 743-751.

Titanji, V.P., Zofou, D., & Ngemenya, M.N. (2008). The antimalarial potential of medicinal plants used for the treatment of malaria in Cameroonian folk medicine. *African Journal of Traditional, Complementary and Alternative Medicines, 5*(3), 302.

Toyang, N.J., & Verpoorte, R. (2013). A review of the medicinal potentials of plants of the genus *Vernonia* (Asteraceae). *Journal of Ethnopharmacology, 146*(3), 681-723.

Tran, T.M., Samal, B., Kirkness, E., & Crompton, P.D. (2012). Systems immunology of human malaria. *Trends in Parasitology, 28*(6), 248-257.

Traoré, M.S., Baldé, M.A., Camara, A., Baldé, E.S., Diané, S., Diallo, M.S.T., ... & Baldé, A.M. (2015). The malaria co-infection challenge: An investigation into the antimicrobial activity of selected Guinean medicinal plants. *Journal of Ethnopharmacology.*

Traore, M.S., Baldé, M.A., Diallo, M.S.T., Baldé, E.S., Diané, S., Camara, A., ... & Baldé, A.M. (2013). Ethnobotanical survey on medicinal plants used by Guinean traditional healers in the treatment of malaria. *Journal of Ethnopharmacology, 150*(3), 1145-1153.

Tsabang, N., Fokou, P.V.T., Tchokouaha, L.R.Y., Noguem, B., Bakarnga-Via, I., Nguepi, M.S.D., ... & Boyom, F.F. (2012). Ethnopharmacological survey of Annonaceae medicinal plants used to treat malaria in four areas of Cameroon. *Journal of Ethnopharmacology, 139*(1), 171-180.

Valentin A., Mustofa M., Benoit-Vical F., Pelissier Y., Kone-Bamba D. and Mallie M., 2000. Antiplasmodial activity of plant extracts used in West African traditional medicine. *Journal of Ethnopharmacology, 73*(1), 145 -151.

Vamvaka, E., Twyman, R.M., Christou, P., & Capell, T. (2014). Can plant biotechnology help break the HIV–malaria link? *Biotechnology Advances, 32*(3), 575-582.

Van der Kooy, F., & Sullivan, S.E. (2013). The complexity of medicinal plants: The traditional *Artemisia annua* formulation, current status and future perspectives. *Journal of Ethnopharmacology, 150*(1), 1-13.

Van Eijk, A.M., Ayisi, J.G., Ter Kuile, F.O., Misore, A.O., Otieno, J.A., Rosen, D.H., ... & Nahlen, B.L. (2003). HIV increases the risk of malaria in women of all gravidities in Kisumu, Kenya. *AIDS, 17*(4), 595-603.

Van Zyl, R.L., & Viljoen, A.M. (2002). *In vitro* activity of Aloe extracts against *Plasmodium falciparum*. *South African Journal of Botany, 68*(1), 106-110.

Vargas, S., Ioset, K.N., Hay, A.E., Ioset, J.R., Wittlin, S., & Hostettmann, K. (2011). Screening medicinal plants for the detection of novel antimalarial products applying the inhibition of β-hematin formation. *Journal of Pharmaceutical and Biomedical Analysis, 56*(5), 880-886.

Vennerstrom, J.L., & Klayman, D.L. (1988). Protoberberine alkaloids as antimalarials. *Journal of Medicinal Chemistry, 31*(6), 1084-1087.

Wanyoike, G.N., Chhabra, S.C., Lang'at-Thoruwa, C.C., & Omar, S.A. (2004). Brine shrimp toxicity and antiplasmodial activity of five Kenyan medicinal plants. *Journal of Ethnopharmacology, 90*(1), 129-133.

Weathers, P.J., Jordan, N.J., Lasin, P., & Towler, M.J. (2014). Simulated digestion of dried leaves of Artemisia annua consumed as a treatment (pACT) for malaria. *Journal of Ethnopharmacology, 151*(2), 858-863.

White, N. J. (2008). *Plasmodium knowlesi*: The fifth human malaria parasite. *Clinical Infectious Diseases, 46*(2), 172-173.

White, N.J., Pukrittayakamee, S., Hien, T.T., Faiz M.A, Mokuolu, O.A., & Dondorp, A.M. (2014). Malaria. *The Lancet,* 383, 723–735.

Willcox, M.L., & Bodeker, G. (2004). Traditional herbal medicines for malaria. *British Medical Journal, 329*(7475), 1156-1159.

World Health Organization (2008a). *World Malaria Report 2008.* http://www.who.int/malaria/wmr2008/ malaria2008.pdf. Accessed on April 15, 2015.

World Health Organization (2008b). *Global malaria control and elimination.* http://apps.who.int/malaria/docs/elimination/MalariaControlElimination Meeting.pdf. Accessed April 14, 2015.

World Health Organization (2014). *World malaria report 2013.* Geneva, Switzerland: World Health Organization. Accessed April 14, 2015.

Wright, C.W. (2005). Traditional antimalarials and the development of novel antimalarial drugs. *Journal of Ethnopharmacology, 100*(1), 67-71.

Yetein, M.H., Houessou, L.G., Lougbégnon, T.O., Teka, O., & Tente, B. (2013). Ethnobotanical study of medicinal plants used for the treatment of malaria in plateau of Allada, Benin (West Africa). *Journal of Ethnopharmacology, 146*(1), 154-163

Table 7.1: Plant remedies for malaria in Cameroon

Annonaceae plant species	Methods of preparation	Posology and duration of treatment	Major symptoms and other diseases treated
Annickia chlorantha	Decoction of 500 g of stem bark removed by scraping with a machete in 3 l of water for 20 min	Take 250 ml decoction 3 times daily for 15 days	Aches, wounds, boils, vomiting yellow bitter, fever, chills, sore spleen in children†☼
Annona muricata	Decoction of a handful of leaves in 3 l of water for 20 min	Take 250 ml of decoction once a day for 7 days	Aches, back pains
Annona senegalensis	Decoction of 500 g of roots stem bark in 3 l of water for 20 min	Drink 250 ml of a decoction once a day for 15 days	Vomiting, muscle aches, tiredness, jaundice, fever, convulsions
Annona squamosa	Decoction of 150 g of leaves in 3 l of water for 20 min	Drink 250 ml of decoction 2 times daily for 10 days	Vomiting, muscle aches, tiredness, abscesses, fever, convulsions, digestive disorders and skin diseases
Anonidium mannii	Decoction of 500 g of stem bark from scraping with machete in 3 l of water, evaporating the decoction to 2/3	Drink 250 ml of decoction 3 times a day for 10 days	Fever ☼
Cleistopholis glauca	Decoction of 500 g of stem bark obtained from scraping with machete in 2 l of water for 24 h, or 100 g of leaves in 3 l of water for 20 min	Drink 250 ml of decoction once a day for 7 days	Fever, muscle ache
Cleistopholis patens	Decoction of 500 g of stem bark obtained from scraping with machete in 2 l of water for 24 h, or 100 g of leaves in 3 l of water for 20 mi	Drink 250 ml of decoction once a day for 7 days	Fever, muscle ache
Cleistopholis staudtii	Decoction of 500 g of stem bark obtained from scraping with machete in 2 l of water for 24 h, or 100 g of leaves in 3 l of water for 20 min	Drink 250 ml of decoction once a day for 7 days	Fever, muscle ache
Duguetia staudtii	Maceration of 500 g of stem bark in 3 l of water under sunlight for 6 h	Drink 250 ml every 12 h for 3 days	Vomiting, headache
Hexalobus crispiflorus	Decoction of 500 g of stem bark obtained from scraping with machete, or 100 g of	Drink 250 ml of decoction 3 times daily for 7 days	Convulsion, fever, muscle ache,

	leaves in 3 l of water for 20 min		
Isolona hexaloba	Infusion of 500 g of stem bark obtained from scraping with machete in 2 l of water for 24 h	Drink 250 ml of infusion once every 2 days during 2 consecutive weeks	Fever
Monodora brevipes	Decoction of one tea spoonful of stem bark and or the same amount of stem bark powder in 250 ml of water	Drink 250 ml of decoction twice a day for 10 days	Fever
Monodora myristica	Decoction of 1000 g of stem bark in 4 l of water for 20 min	Take a purge every 2 days	Joint pains, headache
Monodora tenuifolia	Decoction of 500 g of stem bark powder in 3 l of water for 20 min	Drink 250 ml of decoction 3 times a day for 7 days	Joint and muscle pain, headache
Polyalthia suaveolens	Decoction of 500 g of stem bark removed by scraping with a machete in 3 l of water for 20 min	Drink 250 ml of decoction 3 times daily for 15 days	Fever, jaundice, joint pains, headache †☼
Uvaria sp.	Decoction of 500 g of stem bark collected from scraping with machete in 3 l of water, evaporating the water to 1/2	Drink 250 ml of decoction 3 times a day	Fever, headache ☼.
Polyceratocarpus sp.	Decoction of 500 g of stem bark collected from scraping with machete in 3 l of water, evaporating the water to 1/2	Drink 250 ml of decoction 3 times a day	Fever, headache
Xylopia aethiopica	Decoction of one teaspoon of crushed dried stem bark in 1 l of water	Drink 250 ml 2 times daily for 7 days	Body aches, fever ☼
Xylopia hypolampra	Decoction of one teaspoon of crushed dried stem bark in 500 ml of water	Drink 250 ml of the resulting sauce 2 times daily for 15 days	Fever, chills
Xylopia parviflora	Decoction of 1000 g of stem bark in 3 l of water for 20 min	Drink 250 ml of decoction 3 times daily for 7 days	Body aches, headache, fever; †☼
Xylopia staudtii	Maceration of one teaspoon of crushed dried fruits in 500 ml water	Drink 250 ml of the mixture 2 times daily for 15 days	Fever, chills †

Adapted from Tsabang et al. (2012); †volatile extracts showing potency against Plasmodium falciparum in vitro; non-volatile extracts showing potency against Plasmodium falciparum in vitro

Table 7.2: Plant species used to treat malaria in Guinea

Plant species	Plant parts	Antiplasmodial activities in literature
Mangifera indica	Leaves	IC50 > µg/ml on strain FcB1
Pseudospondias microcarpa	Stem bark	IC50 = 26 µg/ml on strain FcM29
Vernonia colorata	Leaves	IC50 = 3 µg/ml on strain W2
Cassia siamea	Leaves	IC50 = 21 µg/ml on strain FcM29
Dialium guineense	Leaves	IC50 = 42.1 µg /ml on strain 3D7
Carica papaya	Leaves/root bark	IC50 = 15.19-18.09 µg /ml on strain FCK2
Cochlospermum planchonii	Root	IC50 = 80.11 µg/ml on strain 3D7
Cochlospermum tinctorium	Root	IC50 = 0.93 µg/ml on strain F32
Combretum micranthum	Leaves	IC50 = 0.7 -1.18 µg /ml on strain FCB1
Terminalia macroptera	Leaves/stem bark	IC50 = 1µg/ml on strain W2
Guiera senegalensis	Leaves	IC50 = 4.45–6.77 µg /ml on strain W2
Harungana madagascariensis	Leaves/stem bark	IC50 = 3.6 µg /ml on strain K1
Vismia guineensis	Leaves/stem bark	IC50 = 2 µg /ml on strain NF54
Azadirachta indica	Leaves	IC50 = 5.8-8.5 µg /ml on strain 3D7
Khaya senegalensis	Stem bark	IC50 = 47 µg /ml on strain 3D7
Trichilia emetica	Stem bark	IC50 = 3.61 µg /ml on strain K1
Dichrostachys cinerea	Leaves	IC50 > 5 µg /ml on strain K1
Ximenia americana	Leaves	IC50 = 0.8–6.25 µg /ml on strain FCB1
Gardenia ternifolia	Root bark	IC50 = 1.07 µg/ml on strain W2
Mitragyna inermis	Leaves	IC50 = 4.32 µg /ml on strain W2
Zanthoxylumzanthoxyloides	Stem bark	IC50 = 0.018 µg/ml on strain 3D7
Scoparia dulcis	Whole plant	IC50 = 6.6 µg /ml on strain FCR-3
Lantana camara	Leaves	IC50 = 5.7 µg/ml on strain W2

Adapted from Traore et al. (2013)

Table 7.3: Antiplasmodial activities and selectivity indices of plant extracts found in Kenya

Plant species/parts	Extraction solvent	Antiplasmodial activity IC$_{50}$ (µg/ml) and strains of *Plasmodium falciparum* used	Cytotoxicity	Selectivity index
Sericocomopsis hildebrandtii/ root bark	CHCl3	3.78 (D6)	>20 (KB)	>5.29
Artemisia afra/ leaves	MeOH	4.65 (W2)	594.85 (Vero E6)	149.46
Gutenbergia cordifolia/ leaves	CHCl3	4.40 (D6)	0.2 (KB)	0.045
Commiphora schimperi/ inner bark	CHCl3	4.63 (D6)	>20 (KB)	>4.32
Warburgia stuhlmannii/ stem bark	MeOH	1.81 (D6), 2.33 (W2)	233 (Vero E6)	128.7 (D6)
Warburgia ugandensis/ stem bark	CH2Cl2	2.2 (NF54), 1.4 (KI)	0.34 (L6)	0.24 (K1)
Boscia angustifolia/ root	Water	1.42 (D6), 4.77 (W2)	6720.0 (Vero E6)	4732.4 (D6)

Boscia salicifolia/ stem bark	MeOH	1.04 (D6) Water; 3.65 (D6)	304.92 (Vero E6)	293.19
Maytenus undata/ leaves	Water	0.95 (D6), 1.90 (W2)	3645.7 (Vero E6)	3837.6 (D6)
Maytenus putterlickioides/ root bark	MeOH	4.41 (D6)	112.4 (Vero E6)	25.5
Schkuhria pinnata/ whole plant	MeOH	1.30 (D6)	1 61.5 (Vero E6)	124.2
Vernonia lasiopus/ leaves	CHCl3	4.9 (NF54), 4.7 (KI)	>90 (L6)	>10.7
Cyperus robusta/ leaves	MeOH	3.41 (D6)	460.29 (Vero E6)	134.98
Flueggea virosa/ leaves	MeOH	2.28 (D6), 3.64 (W2)	682.6 (Vero E6)	299.3 (D6)
Acacia mellifera/ inner bark	CHCl3	4.48 (D6)	>20 (KB)	>4.46
Fuerstia africana/ whole plant	CHCl3	0.98 (D6), 2.40 (W2)	954.7 (Vero E6)	974.2 (D6)
Turraea robusta/ root bark	MeOH	2.09 (D6)	24.38 (Vero E6)	11.83
Ludwigia erecta/ whole plant	MeOH	4.10 (D6), Water; 0.93 (D6), 1.61 (W2)	3283.6 (Vero E6)	3530.7 (D6)
Rhamnus prinoides/ root bark	CHCl3	3.53 (D6)	>20 (KB)	>5.67
Clematis brachiata/ root bark	CHCl3	4.15 (D6)	>20 (KB)	>4.82
Balanites aegyptiaca/ root bark	CHCl3	3.49 (D6)	>20 (KB)	>5.73

Adapted from Muthaura et al. (2011); chloroquine-sensitive strains, D6, NF54, K39, K67, and M24; chloroquine-resistant strains, W2, KI, V1/S, ENT30, ENT36, and KIL9

Table 7.4: *In vivo* antimalarial activities of Kenyan plants that inhibit *Plasmodium berghei* in mice

Plant species/parts	Extraction solvent	Dose mg/kg/day (route)	*Plasmodium berghei* strain	% inhibition
Sclerocarya birrea/ stem bark	water	100 (ip)	ANKA	66.51
Lannea schweinfurthii/ stem bark	MeOH	100 (ip)	ANKA	91.37
Artemisia afra/ leaves	MeOH	100 (ip)	ANKA	77.45
Boscia angustifolia/ stem bark	MeOH	100 (ip)	ANKA	60.12
Vernonia lasiopus/ root bark	MeOH	500 (oral)	NK65	59.3
Flueggea virosa/ leaves	MeOH	100 (ip)	ANKA	70.91
Harungana madagascariensis/ leaves	water	100 (ip)	ANKA	88.04
Fuerstia africana/ whole plant	MeOH	100 (ip)	ANKA	61.85
Turraea robusta/ root bark	MeOH	100 (ip)	ANKA	78.2

Ludwigia erecta/ whole plant	MeOH	100 (ip)	ANKA	65.28
Rhamnus prinoides/ root bark	water	500 (oral)	NK65	51. 33
Clerodendrum eriophyllum/ root bark	MeOH	100 (ip)	ANKA	90.13
Clerodendrum eriophyllum/ root bark	Water	100 (ip)	ANKA	61.54
Rhus natalensis/ leaves	MeOH	100 (ip)	ANKA	56.24
Warburgia stuhlmannii/ stem bark	Water	100 (ip)	ANKA	84.95
Maytenus putterlickioides/ root bark	MeOH	100 (ip)	ANKA	78.66

Adapted from Muthaura et al. (2011); ip = intraperitoneal; ANKA, chloroquine- sensitive P. berghei strain; NK65, chloroquine-resistant P. berghei strain

Table 7.5: Plant species used as traditional medicines for Malaria in Namibia

Plant species used to treat malaria*	Known antimalarial or antiplasmodial activities cited in literature
Adansonia digitata	Ajaiyeoba, Ashidi, Abiodun, Okpako, Ogbole, and Akinboye et al. (2005); Fowler, (2006).
Albizia anthelmintica	Wanyoike, Chhabra, Lang'at-Thoruwa, and Omar (2004); Fowler, (2006).
Capparis tomentosa	Bapela et al. (2014); Fowler, (2006).
Clerodendrum ternatum	Motlhanka, and Nthoiwa, (2013); Fowler, (2006).
Combretum glutinosum	Asres, Bucar, Knauder, Yardley, Kendrick, and Croft, (2001); De Morais Lima, de Sales, Caldas Filho, de Jesus, de Sousa Falcão, and Barbosa-Filho et al. (2012).
Combretum lanceolatum	Fowler, (2006); De Morais Lima, de Sales, Caldas Filho, de Jesus, de Sousa Falcão, and Barbosa-Filho et al. (2012).
Combretum micranthum	Fowler, (2006); De Morais Lima, de Sales, Caldas Filho, de Jesus, de Sousa Falcão, and Barbosa-Filho et al. (2012).
Combretum psidioides	Prozesky, Meyer, and Louw, (2001); De Morais Lima, de Sales, Caldas Filho, de Jesus, de Sousa Falcão, and Barbosa-Filho et al. (2012).
Croton megalobotrys	Fowler, (2006).
Cucumis aculeatus	Njoroge, Bussmann, Gemmill, Newton, and Ngumi, (2004); Ogutu, Lilechi, Mutai, and Bii, (2012).
Dichapetalum cymosum	None
Diospyros sylvatica	Kantamreddi and Wright (2008).
Dichrostachys cinerea	Fowler, (2006).
Diospyros melanoxylon	Kantamreddi and Wright (2008).
Diospyros peregrina	Kantamreddi and Wright (2008).
Diospyros tomentosa	Kantamreddi and Wright (2008); Mallavadhani, Satyanarayana, and Mahapatra (2004).
Ficus exasperata	Hermans, Akoègninou, and van der Maesen (2004).
Ficus sur	Fowler, (2006).
Guibourtia tessmannii	Jiofack, Ayissi, Fokunang, Guedje, and Kemeuze (2009).
Laggera decurrens	Okhale, Odiniya, and Kunle (2010); Egharevba, Oladosu, Okhale, Ibrahim, Folashade, Okwute, and Okogun (2010).
Lophira alata	Falade, Akinboye, Gbotosho, Ajaiyeoba, Happi, Abiodun, and Oduola (2014); Ajaiyeoba, Ashidi, Abiodun, Okpako, Ogbole, and Akinboye et al.

	(2005).
Mundulea sericea	Kuete, Noumedem, and Nana (2013).
Schkuhria pinnata	Muthaura, Rukunga, Chhabra, Omar, Guantai and Gathirwa et al. (2007).
Sclerocarya birrea	Ojewole, Mawoza, Chiwororo, and Owira (2010).
Cassia occidentalis	Fowler, (2006).
Sesamum triphyllum	None
Tephrosia lupinifolia	Soonthornchareonnon, Ubonopas, Kaewsuwan, and Wuttiudomler (2004); Chen, Yan, Gao, Cao, and Huang (2014).
Terminalia sericea	Valentin, Mustofa, Benoit-Vical, Pelissier, Kone-Bamba and Mallie (2000).
Vangueria infausta	Abosi, Akala, Liyala, Majinda, Mbukwa, and Midiwo et al. (2006).
Vernonia amygdalina	Fowler (2006).
Xylopia sp.	Fowler (2006).
Xysmalobium undulatum	Fowler (2006).
Ziziphus mucronata	Fowler (2006).

*Some of the species are harvested in neighbouring countries

Table 7.6: Nigerian natural products with antiplasmodial activities and their cytotoxicity values

Plant species/isolated active compounds	IC50 (µg/ml) and strains used	Cytotoxicity IC50 (µg/ml) and cell-lines used	Selectivity index (cytotoxici-ty/activity)
Alchornea cordifolia	Ethanol: 2.30 (FcM29)	54.97 (Hela)	23.90
Anogeissus leiocarpa	Methanol: 2.60 (FcB1)	71.90 (L-6)	27.65
Azadirachta indica	Water: 4.17 (FcB1)	-	24.22
Casssia occidentalis	Petroleum ether: 1.50 (Nigerian strain)	-	-
Cocos nucifera (mestico variety)	Hexane: 10.6 (W2)	379.00 (Hep G2)	35.00
Ficus platypylla	Methanol: 13.77 (K1)	≥1500.00 (NBMH)	≥103.00
Nauclea latifolia	Water: 0.60 (FcB1)	400.00 (Human melanoma	666.67
Prosopis africana	Methanol: 14.97 (3D7)	≥1500.00(NBMH)	≥99.00
Terminalia avicennioides	Methanol: 12.28 (3D7)	≥1500.00(NBMH)	≥114.00
Tithonia diversifola	Ether: 0.75 (FCA)	-	-
Ellagic acid (*Alchornea cordifolia*)	0.080 (FcM29)	6.20 (Hela)	77.50
Gedunin (*Azadiracta indica*)	0.020 (W2)	2.30 (KB)	115.00
Tetrahydroharman (*Guiera senegalensis*)	1.30 (W2)	49.00 (THP1)	37.70
Guieranone A (*Guiera senegalensis*)	1.400 (W2)	90.000 (THP1)	64.28
Tagitinin C (*Tithonia diversifola*)	0.330 (FCA)	0.710 (HTC-116)	2.15

Adapted from Adebayo and Krettli (2011)

Table 7.7: Antiplasmodial and cytotoxic activities of selected Ugandan plants

Plant species	Plant parts	% inhibition of *Plasmodium falciparum* FcB1, 10µg/mL	Cytotoxic assay, % inhibition of KB cells, 10µg/mL
Vernonia amygdalina	Leaves	97.8±0.2	99.0±1.0
Erythrina abyssinica	Bark	83.6±16.0	89.0±2.0
Citropsis articulata	Roots bark	77.0±13.0	43.0±5.0
Funtumia latifolia	Leaves	68.1±9.0	57.0±2.0
Markhamia lutea	Leaves	70.8±11.0	4.0±5.0
Hoslundia opposita	Leaves	66.2±7.8	61.0±4.0
Parinari excelsa	Bark	66.5±9.9	54.0±1.0
Tagetes minuta	Leaves	61.0±1.8	nt
Taxotere® (cytotoxicity assay control)	--	--	93.0±0.3
Chloroquine (control)	--	98.1±0.3	--

Adapted from Lacroix et al. (2011); not tested

Table 7.8: Plant species used as remedies for malaria in Zambia

Plant species	Plant parts/ preparation/administration
Abrus fruticulosus; Abrus precatorius	Leaf decoction is used as a wash to treat fever; a leaf infusion is drunk like tea as a remedy for fevers (febrifuge)
Acacia nilotica; Acacia polyacantha	Fresh gum is used in a remedy for malaria; root decoction is drunk as a remedy for malaria
Adansonia digitata	Bark is used as a febrifuge and quinine-substitute; the powdered bark is made into a porridge and eaten as a remedy for malaria
Afzelia quanzensis	Infusion of the bark is drunk as a remedy for malaria; children weakened by malaria are bathed in a bark infusion
Albizia amara	Fruits are used as a remedy for malaria
Anisophyllea boehmii	Infusion of bark is given for malaria
Boscia angustifolia	Leaves are boiled and the extract used for vapour treatment
Brachystegia spiciformis	Infusion of chopped roots is used to wash the body in cases of light fever
Bridelia duvigneaudii	Leaves are used by the Bemba people for fever
Caesalpinia pulcherrima	Roots and flowers are used as a cure for fever
Capparis sepiaria	Shrub is used as a febrifuge
Carica papaya	Root infusion is drunk, and mixed with porridge
Cassia abbreviata	Leaf decoction is drunk, and the steam inhaled. A root infusion mixed with salt and drunk. Roots are soaked and boiled , and the vapour inhaled
Centella asiatica	Leaves are boiled and decoction is drunk
Cleome gynandra	Decoction of the roots is orally given to treat fevers
Combretum molle	Lenje people use a decoction of the leaves to bathe a feverish child
Corchorus olitorius	Leaf infusion is orally taken as a febrifuge
Crossopteryx febrifuga	Bark infusion is drank as a remedy for malaria
Croton gratissimus	Whole plant decoction is drank as a remedy for fevers
Dahlia variabilis	Tuber is used to produce a diaphoretic (induce sweating)
Desmodium gangeticum	Root decoction is drank as a febrifuge
Dicoma anomala	Decoction of roots is drunk

Diplorhynchus condylocarpon (D. mossambicensis)	Root infusion is used to bath body of the patient to treat fever; also drank
Elephantopus scaber L. sbsp. *plu-risetus*	Whole plant decoction is drank as a febrifuge
Euclea crispa	Whole plant is pounded and soaked, and the infusion drunk
Faidherbia albida	Decoction of the bark is taken as an emetic in fever treatment
Flueggea virosa	Infusion of the roots is mixed into beef broth as a remedy for malaria
Gardenia ternifolia	Fruit infusion is taken twice daily as a remedy for malaria
Helianthus annuus	Leaf infusion is drunk to treat malaria
Hibiscus micranthus	Whole plant decoction is used as a febrifuge
Jatropha curcas	Vapour of the leaves is used as a bath to treat fever
Lannea discolor	Infusion of the roots is orally taken to treat children's fevers
Ocimum americanum	Leaf vapour is used to steam body as a treatment for fever
Olax obtusifolia	Roots are boiled to make a steam bath
Parinari curatellifolia	Decoction of bark is orally taken as a remedy for malaria
Phyllanthus muellerianus	Leaf vapour is used to bathe the body in cases of fever
Pseudolachnostylis maprouneifolia	Roots are pounded and eaten in porridge; also pounded and applied to tattoos on painful joints
Pterocarpus angolensis	Decoction of the roots is used as a remedy for malaria
Ricinus communis (imonu, in Lunda)	Root infusion is drunk
Salix mucronata sbsp. *mucronata*	Root decoction is drank to treat malaria
Securidaca longepedunculata	Root decoction is drunk to treat fever
Sesbania sesban	Vapour from boiling leaves is inhaled
Steganotaenia araliacea	Root infusion is drank as a remedy for fever and to ease breathing; hot root decoction is used for vapour treatment
Syzygium cordatum	Roots are pounded and eaten in porridge
Tamarindus indica	Fruit pulp is used to make a refreshing drink to reduce fever
Ximenia caffra	Fresh leaves are chewed as a remedy for malaria
Xysmalobium undulatum	Root decoction is orally administered to treat malaria
Zanha africana	Roots are used to make snuff for sniffing; bark infusion is drunk or applied on tattoos on the forehead
Zanthoxylum chalybeum	Root bark infusion is orally taken to treat severe malaria
Ziziphus abyssinica	Infusion of the bark and roots is drunk

Adapted from Fowler (2006)

Table 7.9: Plants used in the treatment of malaria in Zimbabwe

Scientific name	Local name	Parts/preparation
Cassia abbreviata	Murumanyama	Root/bark; cold or hot infusion is drank
Strychnos potatorum	Mudyambira	Root; decoction taken orally
Crossopteryx febrifuga	Chikobengwa	Stem bark; cold infusion or take with porridge
Toddalia asiatica	Gato	Root; decoction taken orally
Ocimum angustifolium	Mufuranhema	Tuber; cold infusion is drank. May induce nausea
Erythrocephalum zambesianum	Muhloni	Root; cold infusion drank
Cissampelos mucronata	Chipombafodya	Tuber; hot infusion drank
Plumbago zeylanica	Mhisepise	Root; cold infusion drank
Momordica balsamina	Ngaka	Leaf; pumpkin leaves are cooked and eaten as vegetable relish
Euclea natalensis	Mushangura	Root; eaten with porridge; may cause diarrhoea
Momordica foetida	Muchukubaba	Leaf; leaves are cooked and eaten as vegetable relish

Adapted from Ngarivhume et al. (2015)

Last Word

On Sunday, 6th September 2015, as a pastor preached about the spectator syndrome, I kept thinking to myself that throughout the evolution of HIV and AIDS-related infections, plants have never in fact been spectators. In the world of plants, there is no 'bystander apathy'.

Plants and other natural products have always been involved. They always help victims of HIV and AIDS-related infections. They have always devoted and will always devote their chemical ingredients to the service of humankind; to nourish the nutrition and health of humans; and to heal humans from diseases such as HIV/AIDS.

Index

www.ingramcontent.com/pod-product-compliance
Lightning Source LLC
Chambersburg PA
CBHW062157270326
41930CB00009B/1567